REGENERATING ENGLAND: SCIENCE, MEDICINE AND CULTURE IN INTER-WAR BRITAIN

*Edited by Christopher Lawrence
and Anna-K. Mayer*

Amsterdam – Atlanta, GA 2000

First published in 2000
by Editions Rodopi B. V., Amsterdam – Atlanta, GA 2000.

Design and Typesetting by Alex Mayor, the Wellcome Trust.
Printed and bound in The Netherlands by Editions Rodopi B. V.,
Amsterdam – Atlanta, GA 2000.

British Library Cataloguing in Publication Data
A catalogue record for this book is available
from the British Library
ISBN: 90-420-0901-2 (Paper)
ISBN: 90-420-0911-X (Bound)

Regenerating England:
Science Medicine and Culture in Inter-war Britain –
Amsterdam – Atlanta, GA:
Rodopi. – ill.

(Clio Medica 60 / ISSN 0045-7183;
The Wellcome Institute Series in the History of Medicine)

Front cover:
Cover illustration, *Punch* October 23 1935.
Reproduced by kind permission.

Printed in The Netherlands

All titles in the Clio Medica series (from 1999 onwards) are available to
download from the CatchWord website: http://www.catchword.co.uk

Contents

Notes on Contributors

Michael Bartholomew was, until 1998, a Staff Tutor in the Yorkshire Region of the Open University. His original research interests were in Charles Darwin and Charles Lyell, but latterly he has moved backwards, with forays into eighteenth-century medicine, and forwards, with studies of Englishness in the 1920s and 30s.

Abigail Beach is a Research Fellow at the School of Health and Social Welfare at the Open University. She is currently working with Professor Celia Davies on a commissioned history of the United Kingdom Central Council for Nursing, Midwifery and Health Visiting, 1969-1998. She is co-editor (with Richard Weight) of *The Right to Belong. Citizenship and National Identity in Britain 1930-1960*, I. B. Tauris, 1998, and is preparing her doctoral study, 'Planning for Participation. The Labour Party and the Idea of Citizenship, 1931-1956' for publication.

Tim Boon is senior curator of public health at the Science Museum and has recently completed his doctoral thesis on 'Films and the Contestation of Public Health in Interwar Britain'. His publications include papers on smoke abatement and nutrition films and on the place of history in science museum curatorship. He is managing editor of the *Guide to the History of Technology in Europe* (1992, 1994, 1996). He worked on Health Matters (1994), the Science Museum's twentieth-century medicine gallery. He is currently deputy project director of the museum's new gallery on the history of technology since 1750. His continuing research work focuses on several aspects of the cultural history of public health.

Elizabeth Darling is a lecturer in architectural history at the School of Art and Design History, Kingston University. She is currently completing her Ph.D. on the housing consultant Elizabeth Denby. Her research interests include the social and material culture of twentieth-century social housing, gender issues in the production and consumption of the built environment and the cultural politics of the welfare state.

Lesley A. Hall is Senior Assistant Archivist, Contemporary Medical

i

Archives Centre, Wellcome Library for the History and Understanding of Medicine, and Honorary Lecturer in History of Medicine, University College London. Her publications include *Hidden Anxieties: Male Sexuality 1900-1950*, Polity Press, 1991, (with Roy Porter) *The Facts of Life: the Creation of Sexual Knowledge in Britain 1650-1950*, Yale University Press, 1995, and (as co-editor and contributor) *Sexual Cultures in Europe: National Histories and Themes in Sexuality*, Manchester University Press, 1999, as well as numerous articles and reviews. She is currently working on a biography of Stella Browne and an edited volume on venereal diseases in European social context (with Roger Davidson).

Rhodri Hayward is currently employed as a research associate in the new Wellcome Unit at the University of East Anglia. He studied at the universities of Lancaster and Edinburgh and previously worked as a research assistant to Roger Smith on his Wellcome Trust funded project 'The Brain and the Self: Popular Understanding of the Neurosciences in Twentieth-Century Britain'.

Christopher Lawrence qualified in medicine at the University of Birmingham in 1970. He is Professor of the History of Medicine at the University of London and at the Wellcome Institute for the History of Medicine. He has published numerous articles on the history of medicine from 1700 to the present day. He is the author of *Medicine in the Making of Modern Britain, 1700-1920*, London, 1994.

Anna Mayer is completing a Ph.D. on the emergence of professional history of science in Britain, 1916–59, at the University of Cambridge. In 1997–8, she ran the British Society for the History of Science Oral History Project: 'The History of Science in Britain, 1945-65'. She works for the Darwin Correspondence Project in the University Library, Cambridge. Her research interests are in the history of secondary and higher education, broadcasting and public perceptions of science.

Mathew Thomson is a Lecturer in the Department of History at the University of Warwick. His *The Problem of Mental Deficiency: Eugenics, Democracy and Social Policy in Britain, 1870-1959*, Oxford University Press, was published in 1998. He is now working on the the impact of psychological thought within British society during the first half of the twentieth century. He has published several essays deriving from this research.

Keith Vernon is a Senior Lecturer in Social History at the University of Central Lancashire. He has written on various aspects of state support for scientific research in the twentieth century, and is currently working on relationships between universities and the state in the late nineteenth and early twentieth century.

1

Regenerating England:
An Introduction

Christopher Lawrence and Anna-K. Mayer

In a radio broadcast of November 1932, H. G. Wells marvelled why there were so many professors and students of history working on the records of the past, when what the world needed were 'Professors of Foresight'.[1] In an ideal society, to his mind, it was the business of full-time professionals to predict the impact of innovations and discoveries. Such expert predictions would be reached, not by guessing blindly but by 'deduc[ing] the inevitable march of events arising out of already existing facts.'[2] In the absence of such incontrovertible expertise, however, the task of reading the signs of the time and of forecasting the fate of man fell upon the amateur – in this instance Wells himself. By offering advice in this latter capacity, Wells followed in the steps of a tradition that was being celebrated (and criticized) as peculiarly English, namely the tradition of the amateur-savant, whose wisdom distinguished him from his modern rival, the expert-professional. Wells's actual position (that of an amateur expecting that his advice be heeded) contradicts the content of his message (the call for an expert).[3] While it was contradictory, Wells's posture was, however, by no means untypical in inter-war Britain, that 'halfway house' (as Harold Perkin has called it) in which remnants of Victorianism co-existed with the harbingers of the future.[4]

Whether the best path of post-World War I regeneration would be found in the promises of science and technology, in continued and increased efficiency, in specialization and professionalization or whether the future of the nation depended on a rediscovery of older (and more authentic) English ways of doing things, on a defiant anti-modernism, was much debated in the inter-war years. Reconstruction rather than regeneration was the contemporary term for focusing on the future and, indeed, a Ministry of Reconstruction was set up in 1917. Reconstruction has a distinct modernizing and material ring about it however, and we have chosen the term 'regeneration' since as well as embracing vigorous renewal it also captures a sense, found in

1

the writings of many of the figures discussed in this volume, of the rebirth of a lost, more spiritual England.

A number of themes were prominent in the discourses on Britain's post-war regeneration, a regeneration that was, as we show below, usually discussed in terms of England. Such themes included Englishness itself, national character, citizenship, fitness, education, utopias, communities and so on. The chapters in the present volume address these themes, their relations to science and medicine and also to ideas of social and political 'health'. The reflections on the regeneration of England described here are part of what was mainly an amateur 'sociological' discourse. In contrast to the professional 'social thinkers', for example the circle around Sidney and Beatrice Webb, the present volume is mainly concerned with the social imagination of those whose professional expertise strictly speaking lay outside the social sciences. In Britain, there was a tendency to perceive social inquiry as a 'civic' rather than 'academic' pursuit.[5] Amateur reflections on the state of society (as opposed to formal academic analysis of society) were a traditional prerogative of the British intelligentsia and were explicitly counted among the many peculiarities of the British.[6] In the inter-war years, scientists and medical doctors, like their rivals and peers in the arts and, indeed, like members of other professions, continued to perceive it as part of their moral duty to publicize their social and moral insights. This amateur production of social thought, then, endured precisely during those decades that have also been read as constituting the road to the welfare state, in which society came to be managed by welfare professionals rather than the voluntary, amateur sector. How much the models for Britain after the Second World War owe to the social imagination of a pre-managerial era and to what extent they consciously depart from professional precepts is a question that emerges from this book. Although this and other questions of current pertinence arise, however, the chapters in this volume are focused more on the continuities and discontinuities of the inter-war world with the preceding culture and events.

Any study of cultural life in Britain in the years between the wars must take into account two things. First, the transformation in the economic, political and cultural life of the country at the turn of the century and, second, the impact on cultural perceptions of the First World War. 'The years between the 1860s and the First World War', writes Richard Shannon, 'transformed Britain more swiftly and more profoundly than any other comparable era.'[7] This was so both materially and culturally. By 1914, the Britain of the second industrial revolution was a thoroughly urbanized and suburbanized society. It was to a large extent secular, had a limited democracy and obligatory elementary education. Among many inventions, motor vehicles, tube trains, cinema, electric light, aeroplanes and the telephone testified eloquently to the transforming power of new technologies. Industry was becoming increasingly deskilled and scientifically managed. Modest welfare benefits for members of the working class had become legislative 'rights' as opposed to the stigmatizing concessions of the Poor Law. Most pertinent here is that these years had seen the fragmentation of the Victorian consciousness and the creation of distinctly modern sensibilities; many of these were obvious constituents of the works of those bent on regenerating England after 1918.[8] While this is so obviously the case, it is important to remember the importance of late Victorian assumptions and institutions – voluntarism, philanthropy etc. – in these years and through to the nineteen-forties. Jose Harris argues, 'late Victorian and Edwardian Britain resembled the Britain of the 1920s and 1930s and even of the 1940s and 1950s at least as much and in many ways far more than the Britain of the early and mid-Victorian years.'[9]

In separate essays, taken together, in their edited volume *Englishness: Politics and Culture 1880-1920*, Robert Colls and Philip Dodd make an important argument about national life in Britain at the time covered by their study. 'A capacious Liberalism,' writes Colls, 'remained the dominant force within the political culture [of Britain] between 1880 and 1920.' In the later part of this period the capacity of Liberalism was such that it was able to embrace 'a more visceral idea of the central State', presumably meaning, amongst other things, the endorsement of imperialism and more interventionist domestic policies, including, and particularly pertinent here, welfare reform.[10] Stefan Collini makes a similar judgement, observing that 'values and beliefs that had in the mid-nineteenth century been distinctively liberal had by the 1920s become assimilated as part of the received culture of the English educated classes.'[11]

For Colls and Dodd, a key element in maintaining the dominance of liberalism in these years was the refashioning of Englishness. It was through a new culture of Englishness, they argue, that different elements in society – notably the working class, women and non-English peoples – obtained new identities and legitimate spheres of activity.[12] Englishness was given a major role in the tradition that liberalism made for itself in the late nineteenth century and, indeed, many authors enrolled within the tradition had inextricably linked their political ideologies to conceptions of Englishness. In the seventeenth century, for example, the language of the freedom of the freeborn Englishman was common currency.[13] Well before the nineteenth century, authors ascribed to the English people various 'peculiarities' clustered around the ideas of freedom and liberty. This supposed fact was demonstrated by reference to a history in which the English increasingly institutionalized the defence of freedom and liberty in the nation's political structures; this Whig interpretation of the English past was articulated also in Victorian historiography.[14] For example in his *Short History of the English People* (1874), which (according to a 1927 Board of Education Report) made its influence truly felt in the 1920s, the liberal-radical J. R. Green conceptualized the history of the English 'as a forward march in which freedom broadened out from precedent to precedent'.[16] Not every Englishman or woman was, however, regarded as equally 'virtuous' and so, early authors in this tradition said, political management was entrusted to patricians. In the Whig conception of the body politic, public order was not imposed from above but had within it an active, voluntary element, denominated 'virtue'.[15]

In the nineteenth and early twentieth centuries, calls for wider participation of the public in the political sphere (many made by Liberals themselves) and the gradual extension of the franchise increasingly demanded modification of this account. For intellectuals, the acceptance (whether with reluctance or enthusiasm) of democracy created the problem of how to produce responsible or virtuous citizens. As the Victorian educated élite saw it, the issue was how to 'inculcate the moral qualities that would enable people to exercise ... [the powers of self-government] virtuously.'[17] The qualities that were required for such virtuous self-government included self-reliance, 'autonomy', 'self-realization', a mixture of initiative and obedience and what some Victorians called individualism.[18] Peter Mandler and Susan Pedersen have argued that Victorian intellectuals looked to three things to inculcate these and other qualities: the market economy, the education of the people and the bourgeois family. Many Victorian intellectuals also emphasized their own active role in the transition to democracy, seeing themselves as 'ideal agents of enlightenment and political acculturation, inducing successive sections of the population – suitably virtuous and instructed – into the liberal polity.'[19] This ethos endured in inter-war Britain and the British Broadcasting Corporation (BBC), with its mission to bring into every home all that was deemed best in every department of knowledge, endeavour and achievement, is a classic example.[20] Set up in the twenties, the Corporation was seen as a formidable engine for the transmission of values and broadcasting was soon regarded as a civilizing influence of the first order.[21]

Admission of the masses to the 'liberal polity' obviously provoked mixed responses. For many, wider enfranchisement promised less rather than more progress. For a number of nineteenth-century liberals democracy came too fast, outpacing civilization, leading to civic values 'being supplanted by caucus-driven municipal socialism or populist conservativism.'[22] Even for Victorian intellectuals who favoured democracy, such as John Stuart Mill, it was a key concern how democracy was to be reconciled with the cultural and aesthetic values equated with civilization. This concern turned on the question of *who* were the custodians and creators of culture. This issue persisted in the inter-war years when it remained a common assumption that innovation and progress were the work of enlightened minorities only.[23] John Reith, the first Director-General of the BBC, did not hesitate to define the task of the Corporation as 'to give the public what we think they need – and not what they want.'[24] Many inter-war intellectuals saw themselves as among the leaders and custodians of national moral life and despite a legacy of romanticizing the common (English) man, some had a marked distrust of the masses and the ways of ordinary people. In his inaugural lecture as the Regius Chair of Modern History, Oxford, in 1925, H. W. C. Davies typically argued:

> I can find no justification in history for the belief that what the masses think to-day society as a whole will infallibly believe to-morrow; that religions, philosophies, political ideas rise like exhalations from the cottage, the workshop, and the market-place. On the contrary, it would appear from what we know of the history of new ideas that, even if they do not fall like the rain from heaven, they make their first appearance somewhere near the summit of the social fabric and percolate downwards, not infrequently suffering adulteration or corruption in the process.[25]

A similar quote, no doubt, could be found dating from the late nineteenth century. Wells's plea, with which we began, is again apposite here, however, for the inter-war period saw contests being set up between older formations and newer ones for recognition as to who were the rightful bearers of culture and the nation's heritage. These new formations included professional groups in the sciences and the humanities and also new voluntary charitable bodies. If we consider the idea of culture in a general way we can take the case of health and medicine to illustrate this point: who, it was asked at this time, were the most appropriate custodians of and planners for the nation's health? There was no agreed answer in this period even though the medical profession, no doubt, considered itself the proper guardian of the health of the population. Yet, as Abigail Beach shows in her chapter on the experimental health centres at Peckham and Finsbury, there were tensions between the medical profession with its ideal of private health provision and the advocates of a public health service who envisaged national health to be the outcome of a collaboration between state salaried medical professionals and co-operating citizens. Moreover, in inter-war Britain voluntary organizations still pervaded the health domain and took considerable responsibility for the health of the people. For example, voluntary groups that were dedicated to the preservation of the English countryside advocated ideals of physical fitness for everyone through outdoor leisure activities; their propagandists developed what David Matless has called a 'normative ecology of pleasure', into which the English people were to be initiated under the eye of the expert educator.[26] Here again the moral and aesthetic preferences of the élites (operating through the voluntary sector) manifested themselves in prescriptive definitions both of what fitness was and of how the subject became fit for the national heritage.[27] Then, what did the people themselves want? As it turns out, they had their own ideas about the pleasures of outdoor leisure and, some said, they had considerably more right to knowledge and control of their bodies than others would grant them. The rise of the professional society brought with it new expert knowledge that was, however, not automatically accessible to those who had the right to vote. As Lesley Hall shows in her chapter, this was a central issue in Stella Browne's campaign for women to gain access to knowledge which would give them greater control of their sexual and reproductive activities.

In the early twentieth century, the issue of the compatibility of democracy with liberal ideals of civilization was played out in, among other things, debates about the rights and duties of citizenship. These issues seemed all the more pressing in the light of two questions. First, was the growth of state-supported welfare services sapping the virtues of self-reliance and weakening the charitable impulses of the better off? This question was answered optimistically by C. S. Loch, secretary of the Charity Organization Society, who, after the passing of the National Insurance Act of 1911, noted that the 'fear of moral injury which the state may cause is decreasing.'[28] While it was perhaps decreasing, many public statements of inter-war intellectuals testify to the fact that this fear did not disappear entirely. Also, as

Mandler and Pedersen insist, among the liberal intelligentsia it remained an expectation that the enabling state would whither away once the virtuous had bettered themselves.[29] The second question was a version of an earlier one but was given a new urgency largely as a political consequence of the war: had the admission of nearly all adult males to electoral politics in 1918 and almost every woman in 1928 come too fast?

As noted, central to the question of the reconciliation of democracy and responsibility was the issue of how individuals (notably those in the working classes and women) were to be made responsible (docile even) members of their own groups and at the same time citizens actively participating in the life of the community. It is here, Colls and Dodd argue, that the creation of Englishness in new cultural terms was central to the stabilization of British life. It was in the later part of the nineteenth century, Dodd writes, that a large number of now typically English 'educational and, more generally, cultural traditions and institutions were forged.'[30] The establishment located Englishness in projects such as: publications, for instance, the *New English Dictionary* (1884-1928) and the *Dictionary of National Biography* (1885-1900); academic disciplines, such as History and English Literature, which professionalized in this period; institutions, for example, the National Portrait Gallery and the National Theatre; traditions, in music, language and literature, in which a vision of the English landscape was associated with the South, and so on.[31] At this time too 'darkest England' was explored and a new literary genre 'Into unknown England' was created. In response to this 'discovery', charitable enterprises multiplied in the attempt to rescue those who dwelt in this world. However, in the course of these latter endeavours it also became clear to middle class observers that 'the working class was not simply without culture or morality, but in fact possessed a "culture" of its own.'[32]

The creative strongholds of the new Englishness were the male dominated (and masculinity promoting) public schools and the ancient universities. What is important here is that the new institutions of state education, professional groups, voluntary organizations and societies and the media, became the vehicles by which the population in general, and the working class especially, were 'invited' to adopt a new cultural identity. This, to a great extent, is what they did.[33] The working class male, for example, was largely agreeable to participating in a national culture in which he was portrayed as the forthright, heroic, physical labourer, unsuited to and contemptuous of theoretical matters. Englishness, it is important to note, was not imposed – not least since such a view would imply some concerted conspiracy – rather it was negotiated, 'active consent' on the part of the subordinated was required. Dodd rightly points out that 'an Englishness that centred exclusively on ... [national] institutions could hardly hope to mobilize the people in its defence.'[34] Notions of Englishness were replicated in the concrete local circumstances of people's lives, in their clubs, societies, co-operatives, village halls, churches, etc.[35] Thus it was that a 'little London factory hand' could tell the journalist H. V. Morton in the First World War that the England he was fighting for was the England of Epping Forest.[36] Likewise, an élitist London architect, the anti-modernist Sir Reginald Blomfield, could declare that 'as an Englishman and proud of this country', 'I am for the hill on which I was born.'[37] In nationalism, the 'base metal of the local and the temporary' (as Collini has put it) was somehow 'transmuted into the precious ore of the universal and timeless.'[38]

Rather than just an ideology, the emerging ideal of 'Englishness' became embodied in what we call 'cultural tradition'. As Patrick Wright has recently argued for the more recent but related case of the 'Heritage Culture', this distinction between mere ideology and a real cultural tradition is important.[39] Englishness was not merely administered but grew into a set of practices that were shared on national, local or regional levels. As Dodd argues, 'a great deal of the power of the dominant version of Englishness during the last years of the nineteenth century and the early years of the twentieth century lay in its ability to represent both itself to others and those others to themselves.'[40] For this reason Englishness, it needs be recognized, embraced, or at least defined, the Scots, the Welsh and the Irish. It is notable too that the state that was constituted by these various groups was frequently and increasingly analogized in this period to a biological organism. Such analogies offered ways of resolving the tensions between a community perceived horizontally – the English nation – and a social order, clearly hierarchical and unequal.[41] The biological analogy demonstrated to the satisfaction of many how different social groups had different responsibilities and functions in ensuring the smooth operation of the whole.

The second factor central to any understanding of the cultural life of the inter-war years is of course the Great War itself. Historians are divided over whether or not the war had a cataclysmic effect on European attitudes, notably to progress, and whether it produced a disillusionment that shaped the whole of inter-war discourse.[42] Thankfully there is no need to take sides on that issue here. What does matter, however, are the ways in which the thinkers and authors addressed here *said* that disillusionment (or, indeed, a rejuvenated faith in scientific progress) informed their values and projects. Also of importance is how the Great War changed perceptions of pre-war England. Englishness was frequently defined in contrast to "Prussianism" and Germanic models of modernism, as many in this volume indicate (see, e.g. the chapters by Anna-K. Mayer, Mathew Thomson and Keith Vernon). One of the reactions to the war was heightened nostalgia. As Richard Harman observed a world war later, 'in an age of destruction there is a reawakened interest in the things that "endure".'[43] The war undoubtedly was vital to intensifying the 'back to nature urge' that had become so prominent with the pre-war 'disintegration of the Victorian synthesis', manifesting itself in movements for social, moral and aesthetic reform such as the Garden City Movement.[44] During the war and after there was a strong sense that England had once been a rural Arcady: 'Gardeners camouflaged as soldiers' was how one RSM described his men.[45] After the war, as before, this sensibility was drawn to an ideal England perceived as comprising small communities in rural shires. The cottage and the village dominated in ideology and architecture: suburbs were built on village layouts, their 'arteries dubbed Gardens, Drive, Rise or Way in preference to Street or Road ... Along with the village layout went a villagey style for the façades and decoration of the suburban home; half-timbering, gables, tiles and diamond-paned "leaded" windows outdoors; oak beams, panelling, chunky tables and chairs and even big Tudor overmantels indoors.'[46] Along with the material village came an inter-war admiration of supposedly rural virtues: simplicity, privacy and domesticity.[47] For many in the middle class, Stanley Baldwin embodied the modest, domestic, rural Englander.[48] As Raphael Samuel observed:

> The historians of the period – Eileen Power and Sir Lewis Namier provide interestingly contrasted examples – enter into an altogether more affectionate relationship with their subjects, celebrating them no longer for their heroism but for their ordinariness. In history, as in the rhetoric of Baldwin and MacDonald, England appears as a land of villages. The more aspiring (Evelyn Waugh's Mr Samgrass in *Brideshead Revisited* is a well-chosen figure) began to haunt the muniment rooms of the country house; the more democratic (one might speculate) took part in such symptomatic historical initiatives of the period as the Place-Names Society (founded by Frank Stenton and Professor Mawer in 1923). In economic history ... the Arcadian

9

note, if less premeditated than in the rhetoric of Baldwin and MacDonald, is unmistakeable. ... Eleonora Carus-Wilson discovered the remote origins of capitalism in the fulling mills of the thirteenth-century estate, Eileen Power picturesquely associated it with the Woolsack and Perpendicular churches; Clapham and Ashton set the industrial revolution not in dark Satanic mills but in the rural setting of the Pennines.[49]

In connection with the ideal of village society the biological analogy continued to appear, for in rural life observers found 'a model of society – an organic and natural society of ranks, and of inequality in an economic and social sense, but one based on trust, obligation and even love.'[50]

In one way or another the following chapters in spite of their diversity deal with three related questions that permeate inter-war writings, lectures, broadcasts, films, exhibitions, etc., in other words, public intellectual culture in all its manifestations. What will (or does) a better world (England) look like, how is it to be made and who is to make it? The answers to these questions were to a great extent shaped by using broad assumptions framed before the war, many of which were outlined above. But conditions in the twenties and thirties were not quite as they were before the war and details of the answers to questions of regeneration were not simple repetitions of pre-war formulas. To begin with, the freeborn Englishman and woman seemed to be exercising a great deal more of their freedom than heretofore. Further and related, the huge growth of the news and entertainment industry, including cinema, radio and mass circulation newspapers, raised all sorts of issues about who was to determine the nation's culture.[51] It is not by accident that, in the wake of the war, English Literature became the focus of a new guardianship of national values: following the report of the Newbolt Committee, *The Teaching of English in England* (1921), English was systematically installed in British secondary and higher education. The mission of English was not merely aesthetic and intellectual, but also explicitly social, moral and political.[52] As George Sampson, one of the members of the Newbolt Committee, put it in his best-selling *English for the English* (1923), English aimed at 'making everyone forget that classes existed'; that is, it aimed at a unification of the English people not through material equality, but through what Sampson called 'immaterial communism'.[53] This was the new programme of national regeneration and moral rearmament, directed at a new, emerging England.

Alongside the two older images of an aristocratic, romantic, rustic

England and of a capitalist, industrial, depressed England, J. B. Priestley in 1933 identified a third face of the nation: a functional England characterized by mass society and mass production.[54] Responses to this modernist England were far from universally favourable. In a broadcast debate of 1934, for example, Blomfield (whom we cited earlier) deplored modernism as alien to true England, not least of all politically: it had 'spread like a plague to this country … whether it is communism or not, modernismus is a vicious movement which threatens the literature and art which is our last refuge from a world that is becoming more and more mechanised every day.'[55] His *Modernismus* (1934) grew out of the sensibility that 'the cataclysm of the war has thrown everything into the melting pot.'[56] David Dean has remarked that the book was plainly written 'out of moral duty, a sense that a Gadarene society must be called back from the cliff edge to the broad pastures of Edwardian empire.'[57] Such fears of a modernist, mechanised, materially more equal England were fuelled by the collapse of liberal democracies around the world. The rise of Fascism and communism further challenged any residual Victorian assumptions about the inevitability of progress.

The rural myth was a potent antidote to the faces of modernism and was peddled extensively in the inter-war years by the journalist H. V. Morton, the subject of Michael Bartholomew's chapter. For Morton the way forward was backward, to the simple, cap-doffing, religion-observing England he had found, he said, in his travels. What is important is not that this world never existed but that millions of people wanted to read about it and, presumably, were ready to lay down their lives for it in the long-expected next war, in the same way that many had died for it in the previous one.[58] What is striking, given the sheer volume of Morton's sales, is not that the myth appealed to a middle class facing a relative decline in the servant population but that it probably appealed to that population itself.[59]

After the war, as we indicated earlier, the propertied and privileged continued to feel they had the responsibility to mould national life. Particularly pertinent to the papers collected here were the challenges that the voluntary sector and increasingly professionals made to this view and how they felt or claimed they had, more than any other group, the highest responsibility for the efficient running of society. In his book on the rise of professional society, Perkin argues that this move was part of the transition from Old to New Liberalism; in other words, the political arrival of the opinion that the rights of persons and the welfare of the community came before the rights of property.[60] The professional voice (rather than that of a landed or industrial interest) was increasingly loud in its claim that it represented the values which constituted civilization as a whole and Englishness in particular. Chris Lawrence's chapter deals with an élite circle of doctors who in many ways spanned both groups. Like many of their Victorian middle class forebears, the doctors in this group identified with the leisured classes and 'developed the morality of professional service into their equivalent of *noblesse oblige*'.[61] These 'patricians' found much work for the rural myth to do, for they used it to picture a society in which the doctor took his place as gentleman and individual, safe from the predations of specialization and division of labour in medicine.[62]

Other public moralists of the period likewise found much to admire in the rural myth. As Mayer indicates in her chapter, traditionalists from the liberal-humanistic side of the intelligentsia tended to focus on science and technology as the moral and political enemy of an ideal England and they demanded that a stop be put to the process of scientization, specialization and mechanization of human societies. This movement was supported by Christian intellectuals and members of the churches, but it also included secular intellectuals, most prominently F. R. and Q. D. Leavis and the circle around the journal *Scrutiny*.[63] The notion that English culture was to be found in the past was a general one and symptomatic of it was a sentimental chorus of calls to stop the clocks, cries for a holiday from science and demands even for a return to the Middle Ages. Such entreaties grew out of a more general perception that Victorian *laissez-faire* and the second industrialization must be viewed as a social and aesthetic disaster. Yet, while this catastrophic interpretation of industrialization was widespread, sentimental pastoralism by no means exhausted the spectrum of responses. Indeed, the imitation of the ways of the ancestors was much ridiculed. Priestley noted with irony that 'nothing is said about killing off nine-tenths of our present population, which would have to be the first step [to return to Old England].'[64] Targeting those who mourned the passage of time, the marxist scientist J. D. Bernal mockingly exclaimed: 'how much safer it would be to be back in the ordered security of the pre-industrial eighteenth century, so prettily described in Voltaire's *Candide*.'[65] The film maker Paul Rotha, as Tim Boon shows in his chapter, hoped for 'an orderly march of progress' rather than a regress and the architect Arthur Eden, in Boon's judgement, rather than unduly romanticizing the English village, looked to it being adapted into a 'machine for living in'.[66] While the catastrophic interpretation of industrialization was indeed widely shared, a significant portion of the British intelligentsia agreed with Arnold Toynbee when, in his monumental *A Study of History* (1934-61), he identified in 'archaism' a pernicious tendency to admire the ways of the ancestors over those of contemporary personalities: archaism was a 'lapse from the dynamic movement of civilization'; it was 'invariably catastrophic'.[67]

One of the lessons some drew from the nineteenth century was the idea that the disorder generated by rampant *laissez-faire* required order and planning. Thus arcadian nostalgia and the promotion of scientific modernizing could coexist. Rotha like Priestley looked back to an idyllic, rural, pre-industrial England and like Priestley too he saw the Industrial Revolution as a blight on life and landscape. Unlike Priestley, however, he did not look pessimistically at the post-war world: Rotha saw in modernity the potential for liberating the poor and regenerating the landscape. In his film *The Face of Britain* (originally entitled *The Face of England* until his attention was drawn to Scotland), Rotha closed with a vision of electrical power bringing a clean, fresh start. There were also other varieties of combining the arcadian vision with scientific modernizing, as Rhodri Hayward shows in his chapter on Morley Roberts, a journalist and novelist, and Arthur Keith, one of the anatomists who in 1912 had vouched for the authenticity of Piltdown man.[68] Roberts and Keith both used the analogy between social and somatic pathology to redescribe the human body and human society as a whole, identifying a natural aristocracy of intellectuals as the *telos* of evolution. While, as Hayward argues, Roberts' idea of 'biopolitics' ultimately harboured an anarchist ideology, Keith's programme of national regeneration took the form of an atavistic eugenics: he insisted that the ideal Englishman possessed a darker side, 'a vicious evolutionary inheritance which persisted beneath the thin veneer of civilisation.'[69] Keith's radical modernizing through racial purification under the supervision of a scientific élite carried the seeds of a rival programme of Englishness, a programme that, as Hayward and Mayer both show, was conceived in a deliberate contrast to the Christian or liberal-humanistic vision which had identified Englishness with the civilized values of freedom, tolerance and fair play. In contrast to the bulk of their contemporaries, Roberts and Keith viewed war as an activity that was not only part of man's nature but also guaranteed the progress of the nation.

It should be noted that the war did not enter British national life exclusively in the role of the destroyer and devourer or, as for Keith, as 'nature's pruning hook'.[70] It had other cultural effects. For instance,

13

it was used to make a case for national education. As one commentator remarked in 1916, there already was 'a very great amount of literally first-class ability in this country going to waste for lack of opportunity'.[71] The Great War turned educational reform into a public concern and fostered debates about 'fellowship' and the development of 'personality' (but not an excessive kind of individualism) as active ingredients of civic life. Concerns about educating the nation's future élites appeared in debates on the form of the best educational institutions for developing young people's skills and talents. Keith Vernon's chapter addresses these questions by examining the inter-war debates over the provision of a suitable environment for students at red brick universities. By and large halls of residence were seen as the answer to the need to nurture the broader social skills of the nation's future experts and intellectuals. It should be noted that, once again, the rural vision permeated these projects: ideals of small scale, village-like communities informed the ideas of planners.

As before the war, one sector of society that had a major role in the smooth running of modern life was that consisting of the voluntary organizations. Particularly important and relevant here were those organizations that were concerned with 'social hygiene'.[72] Such was its breadth, social hygiene scarcely admits of definition. At one level it was a comprehensive attention to individual well-being, bringing science and medicine to bear on issues such as reproduction, child care, mental health and physical fitness. On another it was an ideology for disciplining and civilizing the poor. Central to its programme were national efficiency and the physical condition of the working class. Eugenic issues underlay many of the activities carried out in its name. Although social hygiene was a concern of government, voluntary organizations such as the People's League of Health (founded in 1917) played a major part in its promotion. The members of these organizations carried out a range of activities: education, research, debating, publicizing, planning, lobbying, home visiting etc. Membership included the landed gentry and professionals, notably doctors, lawyers and churchmen. During the inter-war years many of these bodies became increasingly conservative politically.

Women were very significant members of such organizations. Pat Thane has observed that the women's movement from the late Victorian period to the thirties

> should be seen, more than it has been, as part of the broad ferment of discussion about how viable democracy was to be achieved and

14

practised in an advanced industrial society; how the growing body of individuals who were acquiring or demanding rights of full citizenship could actively participate in the decision-making of an increasingly powerful and centralized state; and how power and centralization could be controlled.[73]

These themes – voluntarism and the women's movement – are brought together in Elizabeth Darling's chapter describing the professional career of a woman in a world dominated by men and voluntary organizations. Elizabeth Denby was a kind of social worker involved in planning inter-war housing schemes. Although describing a person who might be considered a thoroughly modern woman, Darling's chapter also harks back to those of Bartholomew, Lawrence and Mayer with its reminder of the grip the small, village-like community ideal had on the most forward-looking professionals. The notion of an 'urban village' grew out of a cultural heritage (or a tradition of 'Englishness') stipulating that village life was the embodiment of all those personal and civic values that secured individual and collective happiness. Kensal House, the 'urban village' Denby developed in collaboration with the modernist architect Maxwell Fry, exemplified the contemporary hope that architecture (informed by sound social thinking) would solve the social problems of the modern world by transporting traditional values into the modern era. Before redevelopment could begin, Denby insisted, the structure of each town needed to be examined and 'the new areas [related] to the best traditions of the past'.[74] Darling's chapter, like Vernon's, investigates the important question of the physical environment and the shaping of citizens and sheds light on debates about the appropriate environment for shaping particular *sorts* of citizens. This is also an important consideration for understanding the ideas behind the purpose-built health centres of inter-war London described in Beach's chapter. In these institutions, virtuous citizenship was to be fostered through the cultivation of positive health, a fact that reminds us once more of the national efficiency and eugenic concerns of these years. Again the village hall-like image of these institutions seems inescapable.

Important though positive health was, practically everyone agreed it was pointless to extend the promotion of it to everyone. There would always be some members of the population unfit to work, bear arms, reproduce and vote. Mathew Thomson's chapter explores this question through the inter-war definition and management of 'defectives'. The category of the 'defective' is a key to understanding the assumptions about citizens' rights in these years, for in the definition of 'defective' (or non-citizen), citizenship itself was being constructed. Again, the centrality of the idea of 'citizenship' within post-World War I reconstruction exemplifies contemporary concerns with moral regeneration as much as with material reconstruction.

The final two papers in the volume address many of the themes outlined here but introduce a new dimension. Not all those who had schemes for regenerating England in the inter-war years thought in national terms only. Like Wells, some had a much more global perspective on the country's future. Hayward's chapter, as indicated, analyses the biological sociology of the journalist Morley Roberts. Roberts is interesting in that his circle included some of the patrician doctors discussed by Lawrence, yet he did not seem to share their English liberal ideology. Rather, he espoused an idiosyncratic anarchism based on evolutionary biology. Stella Browne, the subject of Lesley Hall's chapter, likewise rejected the authoritarian attitude of established élites (in her case medical doctors) and thought in global rather than national terms. Browne developed a cosmopolitan radicalism early in her life from which she never seems to have deviated. A militant feminist she campaigned consistently and persistently for the right of all women to control their bodies. Apparently not the slightest shadow of rural sentimentalism clouded her public pronouncements. In an English cathedral town that most likely would have provoked idyllic rapture in H. V. Morton, what most took Browne's eye were the squalid insanitary streets. Browne is important in this book in that many of her pronouncements challenged assumptions that a majority of the characters described here took for granted.

As the present volume shows, the amateur production of social thought endured in the inter-war years. This is true not only of the most obvious suspects – political figures, dons and the literati, certain prominent individuals from the voluntary sector, the clergy even – but also of private individuals and the members of a variety of less likely professions involved in concerns such as housing, health, education, civil rights and other areas of public life. No doubt national regeneration depended on the government, the experts it co-opted and the few great inter-war thinkers whose names tend to inevitably crop up in the historiography of the British intelligentsia and who are so often credited with the achievement of having shaped 'their age'. In the present volume, however, we have tapped into a world that was not exclusively populated by the Eliots, the Leavises, the Frys, the

Woolfs, the Temples, the Stopeses, the Tawneys, the Keyneses and so on. We have looked at people who have not become canonical figures of the inter-war intelligentsia and whose activities and pronouncements have interested historians of that era fairly little. Also, we have recruited our agents and voices more from science and medicine rather than from the humanistic side of the two-culture-divide; a side which historians have somehow favoured as a source for representative statements of the intelligentsia. Moreover, we have largely focused on people who were trying to solve concrete problems, rather than those who became famous for their theoretical acumen. This collection, we hope, opens up a slightly different vista on inter-war Britain, by looking at how the then current issues permeated social and political perceptions and actions one level down from what is considered the intellectual aristocracy. Many features of these perceptions and actions seem sufficiently familiar to suggest that they are merely derivative. At the same time, there is no denying the innovativeness of many of the individuals discussed in the chapters below. This goes for Morton's self-fashioning as the priest of bucolic travel fiction, for Elizabeth Denby and her centrality to the architectonic and social experiment that was Kensal House, for the reinvented Englishness of Arthur Keith or Morley Roberts, for Lawrence's élite physicians and their holist approach to clinical medicine, for the prophets of reconstruction described by Mayer, for Stella Browne's appropriation of the ideal of individual liberty to create a discourse on women's fundamental right to control their bodies, for Rotha's vision of an electrified landscape of Britain, for the planners of red brick campuses in the inter-war period and so on.

Combining materials from their cultural context, many of these people produced distinctive inter-war models of regeneration. These models were part of their self-fashioning: the construction of models of regeneration was part of the process by which they acquired their social identities and in many instances their professional ones. The activity of recycling familiar materials and of creating platforms for their personal expertise proved many of the apparently intellectually second-rate to be innovative. Intellectual historians have not always seriously questioned H. W. C. Davies' model of innovation that we quoted earlier, according to which great ideas are born near the summit of the social fabric and then 'percolate downwards, not infrequently suffering adulteration or corruption in the process.' We need a historiography of British cultural life that is an addition to the existing appreciation of intellectual aristocracy on the one hand and the celebration of the authenticity of working class culture on the other. Looking at some of the individuals in this volume puts a different spin on the historiography of the British intelligentsia in the twentieth century; a historiography which has tended focus on the intellectual élites and the processes by which they gain and loose moral and cultural authority. The following chapters show that the groups that 'made' inter-war Britain included other and more people than just so many canonical figures from the donnish dominion. This is not to denigrate the high cultural and intellectual achievement of the latter, but to point to a broad context of concrete reality in which variations of regeneration were produced and replicated. This concrete reality is the backdrop before which the highest cultural and intellectual achievement stands out; it is, however, also the realm in which regeneration was practised.

Notes

1   H. G. Wells, 'Wanted – Professors of Foresight!', in *The Listener*, 23 November 1932, pp. 729–30.
2   *The Listener*, 23 November 1932, 736 (leader).
3   Fifteen years later Ernest Barker still celebrated amateurism along with gentlemanliness, voluntarism, eccentricity and youthfulness among the enduring characteristics of the English. Ernest Barker, 'An Attempt at Perspective', in *The Character of England*, Ernest Barker (ed.), Westport, 1947, pp. 550–75 at 565f.
4   Harold Perkin, *The Rise of Professional Society. England since 1880*, London, 1989, 218.
5   The views of Patrick Geddes and his followers, for example, exercised an influence far into the inter-war period. According to them, a healthy community and ultimately a regenerated Britain were to be constituted locally through volunteers and not through academic professionals. Martin Bulmer, *Essays on the History of British Sociological Research*, Cambridge, 1985, pp. 10–11.
6   On the 'peculiarities of the British' and for a new look at the alleged failure of the British to produce a body of sociology comparable to other Western country in the first half of the twentieth century, see e.g. Jose Harris, 'Platonism, Positivism and Progressivism: Aspects of British Sociological Thought in the Early Twentieth Century', in *Citizenship and Community: Liberals, Radicals and Collective Identities in the British Isles, 1865-1931*, Eugenio F. Biagini (ed.), Cambridge, 1996, pp. 343–60.
7   Richard Shannon, *The Crisis of Imperialism, 1865-1915*, London, 1974, 11.
8   For a number of individuals who were born in the Victorian era and

who subsequently 'made' inter-war Britain, see *After the Victorians. Private Conscience and Public Duty in Modern Britain. Essays in Memory of John Clive*, Susan Pedersen and Peter Mandler (eds), London and New York, 1994.

9 Jose Harris, *Private Lives, Public Spirit: a Social History of Britain 1870-1914*, Oxford, 1993, 252.

10 Robert Colls, 'Englishness and the Political Culture', in *Englishness: Politics and Culture 1880-1920*, Robert Colls and Philip Dodd (eds), London, New York and Sydney, 1986, pp. 29–61 at 29–30.

11 Stefan Collini, *Public Moralists: Political Thought and Intellectual Life in Britain 1850-1930*, Oxford, 1993, 338.

12 *Englishness*, Colls and Dodd (eds).

13 See e.g. Christopher Hill, *The Century of Revolution 1603-1714*, London and Edinburgh, 1961.

14 See J. W. Burrow, *A Liberal Descent: Victorian Historians and the English Past*, Cambridge, 1981.

15 In this context, it may be worth noting that Charles Townshend, in his recent study of the English way of preserving social peace, describes the tradition of 'humanist republicanism' as a practice that takes virtue to be the active component of public order. In this tradition, order 'arises out of the co-operative interaction of self-disciplined individuals'. The people do not merely constitute an administrative problem, but are relied on for their 'consensual capacity – ranging from "sense of community" or "civic responsibility" through to full-blown "national consciousness"'. Order is constituted locally, by co-operation, and it is fundamentally dependent on the right man being in the right place. It seems plausible that the rising system of state secondary education was to guarantee that s/he existed and that s/he was in the right place. See Townshend, *Making the Peace. Public Order and Public Security in Modern Britain*, Oxford, 1993.

16 On Green, see Raphael Samuel, 'Epical History', in *idem, Island Stories: Unravelling Britain. Theatres of Memory*, vol. 2, Alison Light (ed.), with Sally Alexander and Gareth Stedman Jones, London and New York, 1998, pp. 3–20 at 16.

17 Peter Mandler and Susan Pedersen, 'The British Intelligentsia after the Victorians', in *After the Victorians*, Pedersen and Mandler (eds), pp. 1–28 at 4.

18 See John Plamenatz, 'Liberalism', *Dictionary of the History of Ideas*, 5 vols, New York, 1973, vol. 3, pp. 36–61 at 50.

19 Mandler and Pedersen, 'British Intelligensia', 5.

20 For the founding of the BBC, see Asa Briggs, *The History of*

Broadcasting in the United Kingdom, vol. 1: *The Birth of Broadcasting*, Oxford and New York, 1995.

21 Asa Briggs, *The History of Broadcasting in the United Kingdom*, vol. 2: *The Golden Age of the Wireless*, Oxford and New York, 1995, pp. 172–210; D. L. LeMahieu, *A Culture for Democracy: Mass Communication and the Cultivated Mind in Britain between the Wars*, Oxford, 1988; Kate Whitehead, *The Third Programme: A Literary History*, Oxford, 1989, 10.

22 Mandler and Pedersen, 'British Intelligensia', 6.

23 See for example Collini on Henry Maine in *Public Moralists*, 274.

24 Whitehead, *The Third Programme*, 8.

25 H. W. C. Davis, 'The Study of History', given 4 November 1925, repr. in *Henry William Carless Davis, 1874-1928. A Memoir by J. R. H. Weaver and a Selection of his Historical Papers*, J. R. H. Weaver and Austin Lane Poole (eds), London, 1933, pp. 65–80 at 78.

26 David Matless, 'Moral Geographies of English Landscape', in *Landscape Research*, 22 (1997): 141–55 at 152.

27 David Matless, 'Moral Geographies'; *idem*, '"The Art of Right Living". Landscape and Citizenship, 1918-39', in *Mapping the Subject*, S. Pile and N. Thrift (eds), London and New York, 1995, pp. 93–122.

28 Cited in Collini, *Public Moralists*, 117.

29 Mandler and Pedersen, 'British Intelligentsia', pp. 7–8; L. T. Hobhouse, *Liberalism*, London, 1911.

30 Philip Dodd, 'Englishness and the National Culture', in *Englishness*, Colls and Dodd (eds), pp. 1–28 at 1. This 'Englishness' was of course built on earlier cultures of nationhood, see Linda Colley, *Britons: Forging the Nation, 1707-1837*, New Haven and London, 1992, but see also Peter Mandler, *The Fall and Rise of the Stately Home*, New Haven and London, 1997, who argues that Colley stresses the aristocracy at the expense of the plebeian and middle class makers of nineteenth-century national culture. More significant here, Mandler (pp. 114, 132) also argues that a sense of Englishness was created in the mid-Victorian period and that in the late Victorian and Edwardian eras the nation that was appealed to was Britain. However, strangely, in this very important book he does not at any point address Colls and Dodd, *Englishness*, which is now virtually the *locus classicus* of the argument that Englishness in many senses was created at this time.

31 Dodd, 'Englishness'; also Collini, *Public Moralists*, ch. 9: 'The Whig Interpretation of English Literature: Literary History and National Identity', pp. 342–73; Alun Howkins, 'The Discovery of Rural

England', in *Englishness*, Colls and Dodd (eds), pp. 62–88. On the privileging of the South see also Mandler, *Fall and Rise*, pp. 143–4, and Townshend, *Making the Peace*, 20.

32 Gareth Stedman Jones, 'Working Class Culture and Working Class Politics in London, 1870-1900: Notes on the Remaking of a Working Class', in *Languages of Class: Studies in English Working Class History 1832-1982*, Cambridge, 1983, pp. 179–238 at 183.

33 Dodd, 'Englishness', 22.

34 *Ibid.*, 7.

35 On working class communal life between the wars see Perkin, *Professional Society*, pp. 283–4.

36 See Bartholomew's chapter in this volume.

37 Blomfield in the broadcast debates: 'Is Modern Architecture on the Right Track?', *The Listener*, 26 July 1933, pp. 123–32 at 124; 'For or against Modern Architecture', *The Listener*, 28 November 1934, pp. 885–8 at 886.

38 Collini, *Public Moralists*, 361.

39 Patrick Wright, *On Living in an Old Country: the National Past in Contemporary Britain*, London, 1985, pp. 79–80.

40 Dodd, 'Englishness', 2.

41 On horizontal communities and hierarchical societies see Benedict Anderson, *Imagined Communities: Reflections on the Origin and Spread of Nationalism*, London, 1983.

42 See Daniel Pick, *War Machine: the Rationalisation of Slaughter in the Modern Age*, New Haven, 1993; Harris, *Private Lives, Public Spirit.*

43 *Countryside Mood*, Richard Harman (ed.), London, 1943, 5. Cited after Patrick Wright, *On Living in an Old Country*, 85.

44 Shannon, *Imperialism*, pp. 282, 284. For the Garden City Movement, see Standish Meacham, *Regaining Paradise. Englishness and the Early Garden City Movement*, Yale, 1999.

45 Cited in Paul Fussell, *The Great War and Modern Memory*, London, 1975, 234.

46 Mandler, *Fall and Rise*, pp. 229–30.

47 On domesticity see Alison Light, *Forever England: Femininity, Literature and Conservatism Between the Wars*, London, 1991.

48 See Dennis Smith, 'Englishness and the Liberal Inheritance after 1886' in *Englishness*, Colls and Dodd (eds), pp. 254–82; Mandler, *Fall and Rise*, 241.

49 Raphael Samuel, 'Empire Stories: the Imperial and the Domestic', in *idem, Island Stories*, pp. 74–97 at 82.

50 Alun Howkins, 'The Discovery of Rural England', 80. On organic or holistic thinking in biology and medicine in these years see the essays

in *Greater than the Parts: Holism in Biomedicine 1920-1950*,
Christopher Lawrence and George Weisz (eds), New York, 1998.

51 LeMahieu, *A Culture for Democracy.*

52 *The Teaching of English in England* (Report of the Newbolt
Committee), HMSO, 1921. On the cultural and political mission of
the Newbolt Committee and its report, see Chris Baldick, *The Social
Mission of English Criticism, 1848-1932*, Oxford, 1987; Stephen Ball,
Alex Kenny, David Gardiner, 'Literacy, Politics and the Teaching of
English', in *Bringing English to Order: the History and Politics of a
School Subject*, I. Goodson and P. Medway (eds), Falmer, 1990, pp.
47–86 at 52.

53 George Sampson, *English for the English*, Cambridge, 1923,
introduction.

54 J. B. Priestley, *English Journey: Being a Rambling but Truthful Account
of what one Man saw and heard and felt and thought during a Journey
through England during the Autumn of the Year 1933*, London, 1934;
see also Perkin, *Professional Society*, 268.

55 Blomfield, 'For or against Modern Architecture', 885.

56 Reginald Blomfield, *Modernismus*, London, 1934, 52.

57 David Dean, *The Thirties: Recalling the English Architectural Scene*,
London, 1983, 37.

58 It has been suggested that popular support for the war in Britain was
motivated by the desire 'to preserve a world' and 'to preserve and
restore'. See e.g. Modris Eksteins, *Rites of Spring: the Great War and
the Birth of the Modern Age*, New York, 1989.

59 On the relative decline of the servant population see Perkin,
Professional Society, 283; A. J. P. Taylor, *English History 1914-1945*,
Harmondsworth, 1970, 383.

60 Perkin, *Professional Society*, 140.

61 Shannon, *Imperialism*, 216.

62 On the profound changes in the organization of medicine in these
years see Steve Sturdy and Roger Cooter, 'Science, Scientific
Management, and the Transformation of Medicine in Britain
*c.*1870-1950', *History of Science*, 36 (1998): 421–66.

63 Francis Mulhern, *The Moment of Scrutiny*, London, 1979; Ian
Mackillop, *F. R. Leavis: A Life in Criticism*, London, 1995.

64 Priestley, *English Journey*, 372.

65 J. D. Bernal, 'Can We Control the Future?', *The Listener*,
Supplement of 21 December 1932, 894.

66 For the expression 'machine for living in', see Le Corbusier, *Towards
a New Architecture*, tr. Frederick Etchells, London, 1927.

67 Arnold Toynbee, *A Study of History*, vol. 6, *The Disintegration of*

Civilization (continued), Oxford, 1939, pp. 49–96.

68 For the Piltdown affair, see Jonathan Sawday, '"New Men, Strange Faces, Other Minds": Arthur Keith, Race and the Piltdown Affair (1912-53)' in *Race, Science and Medicine, c.1700-1960*, W. Ernst and B. Harris (eds), London, 1999, pp. 259–88.

69 See Hayward's chapter.

70 Quoted in Pick, *War Machine*, 13. See also Hayward's chapter.

71 *Times Educational Supplement*, 7 September 1916, 113. In evidence of his statement William Temple, the future archbishop, cited a report by Albert Mansbridge, the founder of the Worker's Educational Association. A. Mansbridge, *University Tutorial Classes. A Study of the Development of Higher Education among Working Men and Women*, London, 1913.

72 See Greta Jones, *Social Hygiene in Twentieth Century Britain*, London, 1986. Pauline Mazumdar, *Eugenics, Human Genetics and Human Failings: the Eugenics Society, its Source and its Critics in Britain*, London and New York, 1991.

73 Pat Thane, 'Women, Liberalism and Citizenship, 1918-1930', in *Citizenship and Communiy*, Biagini (ed.), pp. 66–92 at 66.

74 Denby, quoted after Lionel Esher, *A Broken Wave: The Rebuilding of England 1940-1980*, London, 1981, 29.

2

H. V. Morton's English Utopia

Michael Bartholomew

Morton, Utopia and the First World War

H. V. Morton (1892–1979) produced one of the inter-war years'
most characteristic and popular visions of utopia. He presented this
utopia in his enormously successful *In Search of England* (1927) and
developed it in subsequent books.[1] His utopian vision is of a rural,
agricultural, tranquil, hierarchical and socially cohesive England, and
it is set against a competing vision of an urban, threatening, ugly,
industrial and commercial England. 'Utopian' may seem too grand a
term to describe the contents of books which declare themselves to
be straightforward records of actual journeys around England, of the
sort that anybody might make. But although the journeys recorded
in the books are plainly based on the actual topography of England
and although places are described in great detail, the essential
England remains tantalisingly just out of reach. Its emblem is the
frontispiece of *In Search of England*, captioned by Morton simply 'A
Lane in England' (see Figure 1).

The precise whereabouts of the essential England are not fully
disclosed or elaborated in the books, but the reader is given the
assurance that in quiet corners of the shires, an untroubled, essential
England is going peacefully about its ways. It is this just-out-of-
reachness and the yearning associated with it, that makes Morton's
England a utopia. He was, of course, hardly original in promoting
such an Arcadian vision; it figures, implicitly or explicitly, in much
inter-war thought and art. Indeed, in one form or another, it is a
cultural universal. But Morton's particular – and highly profitable –
version of it found a huge, receptive audience during the twenties
and thirties, and by supplying this market he left a substantial mark
on the wider culture of the period.

The vision of England that Morton presented was especially
seductive to the generation who served in, or lived through the Great

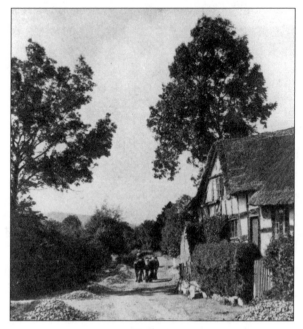

Figure 1
Frontispiece to *In Search of England* (1927)

War. The bugles that Wilfred Owen made faintly to call for the slaughtered in his 'Anthem for Doomed Youth' sounded not from the industrial towns that were likely to have been the youths' homes, but from 'sad shires'. Industrial, modern England could not, it seems, supply images deemed to be worth fighting for. A remark that Paul Fussell makes about Edmund Blunden's writing can apply more generally. In *The Great War and Modern Memory*, Fussell writes that attention was constantly addressed by Blunden to 'pre-industrial England, the only repository of criteria for measuring fully the otherwise unspeakable grossness of the war.'[2] In his later book, *Abroad*, Fussell suggests that a great deal of travel writing was released by the ending of the war: writers who had for years been cramped and desolated left England and went South for the sun.[3] Other writers, with whom Fussell is less concerned, stayed at home, willing themselves deep into an English landscape untouched by slaughter and destruction. Their books found a ready market. Any second-hand bookshop yields dozens of titles. A typical trawl fetched up Major General J. E. B. Seeley's *Forever England* (1932), A. Bonnet Laird's *This Way Arcady* (1926), W. S. Shears's *This England: a Book of the*

Shires and Counties (1936), the Batsford anthology *The Legacy of England* (1935) – with a contribution from Edmund Blunden on 'The Landscape' – and C. Henry Warren's *England is a Village* (1940).

Morton fits this specification of the devotee and purveyor of the Arcadian vision of England well. He started work as a newspaper reporter in Birmingham and joined the army in 1915, a year after the Great War had broken out. When peace returned he resumed his life as a journalist, now in London, working successively on the *Evening Standard,* the *Daily Express* and the *Daily Herald.* In 1925 he published between hard covers the first collection of his newspaper travel pieces. The success of this book turned him into a prolific travel writer. He published over 30 titles, starting with books about London, then England, Wales, Scotland and Ireland and moving on to books about Italy, Spain, the Middle East and South Africa. He has been picked up by recent scholars in studies both of the construction of what has become known as 'Englishness' and of between-the-wars writers, but he has not been marked out for special attention.[4] My aim in this chapter is to put him a bit more firmly on the map.

Although Morton is in many ways the archetypal presenter of an enduring and popular Arcadian vision of England, from time to time he breaks the conventions of this genre and presents a clashing vision of a troubled, depressed England, a vision which is closer to and, in my view, sometimes more penetrating than, those of canonised writers like George Orwell or J. B. Priestley, whose observations, made as they travelled round the country during the thirties, are supposed to have been particularly insightful. There is rather more to Morton than the half-invention, half-discovery of England that his books embodied. First, although he was, for most of the time, mesmerising himself and his readers into what Orwell called 'the deep, deep sleep of England', there are moments of self-awareness in his writing.[5] In places, he begins to identify what is now routinely known as 'the heritage industry' – the cultural and commercial forces that persuade us that we can take day trips to the past; a past signified by items whose original significance, however earnestly we may seek it, is effaced by the glamour that inescapably accompanies the designation 'heritage'.[6] For example, Morton connects the medieval Canterbury pilgrims who made their way to the shrine of Thomas Becket with those modern-day pilgrims who trek to see 'the spot where Nelson fell, Shakespeare's cradle, the bed that Queen Elizabeth slept in and Jane Austen's pen-wiper.' Who is to say, he reflects, that the modern objects of pilgrimage are more absurd than the medieval? Both are the product of 'a longing to make contact with something outside normal experience', a longing that is compulsive, but illusory and rarely satisfied.[7]

Second, although Morton's strong inclination is generally to seek out the picturesque, the rural, the archaic and places associated with the pageantry of history, he was by no means blind to aspects of England that could not easily be accommodated to this version of the nation's character. Traditionally, cities have tended to be characterised as sites of, on one hand, alien industry and commerce, and, on the other, squalor and poverty. Morton did not avoid industrial towns and, as I show below, when he wrote about them he often ran against the grain of the Merrie England mode by presenting them as places that, despite the disgrace of their slums, were exhilarating. And his accounts of the slums are at least as penetrating as later ones written by Orwell and Priestley.

Third, the sheer popularity of his writings commands attention. By 1943 there were 29 editions of *In Search of England* and twelve of the companion volume *The Call of England* in circulation. All of his books went through edition after edition (as the shelves of any second-hand bookshop will testify). Translations were common. Precise figures of the numbers of his books in circulation are hard to come by. The records of his publisher, Methuen, give no quantities, but one commentator asserts that over a million copies of *In Search of England* were sold in Britain alone.[8] It is likely, then, that Morton was among the most widely read inter-war writers, and therefore, was one of the more influential shapers of the English peoples' image of themselves and their country. Furthermore, he started publishing in the mid-twenties, and went on issuing books on England right up to the middle of the Second World War. He therefore registers a number of modifications to the myth and demonstrates how it was put to use when war broke out again.

Last, Morton repays attention because he was, in most respects, an absolutely standard practitioner in a genre which was pervasive between the wars. Critical interest obviously tends to follow the extraordinary and the innovatory but it can be revealing to pay close attention to the commonplace, in order to inspect the formulae that governed the production and reception of so many books. This is not to say that Morton was merely a mass-producer of banalities about cottages and hedgerows: he was a painstaking researcher and an engaging writer. Eyemouth, he writes, 'stands facing the sea like someone warding off a blow'; Birmingham is 'the city whose buttons hold up the trousers of the world'; Robert Burns was a poet 'whose songs have curled up like an old dog on the hearthstone'.[9]

Morton's best known book and the one upon which his status as a Merrie England ruralist is founded is *In Search of England*. His first five books, however, were little collections of vignettes of London life. Morton presents himself in these books as a self-deprecating, vaguely patrician and modestly intrepid narrator who roves round the city, by day and by night, bringing back accounts of the people: cabmen, river policemen, office cleaners, Billingsgate porters, Kensington Gardens nannies, chorus girls, down-and-outs, Harley Street doctors and dozens of others. He also describes places and events: Petticoat Lane street market, the Royal Mint, a night club, a boxing match, a city church, a Bloomsbury boarding house and so on.[10]

Morton does not attempt to combine all the observations in his London books into a single, integrated vision, projected from a clear moral viewpoint; he is content to leave them as an assortment of vignettes of a variegated, cosmopolitan city. His London is neither united by a particular set of characteristics, nor riven by social conflict, even though he is at pains to point out the dismal wages on which many of the people he writes about have to scrape along. Above all, for a writer who was later to become such a staunch promoter of a rural vision of England, the early books on London are a positive celebration of the variety and vitality of city life. No stereotypical version of England has emerged, and we are, by definition, save for one passage, a long way from the green shires.

The exception is the passage on the grave of the Unknown Warrior in Westminster Abbey. The Unknown Warrior, Morton writes, 'lies not only at the heart of London, but also at the heart of England.' Morton had served during the war with the Warwickshire Yeomanry, although he left no record of what he did, beyond his training on Salisbury Plain as a cavalry officer. In his later travel books, he always comments, often in great and passionate detail, on the war memorials erected in the town and villages he passes through. It is therefore perhaps not surprising that in the London books, despite their general lack of symbolic, unifying images, Morton should have given especial significance to the grave of the Unknown Warrior. In identifying the 'heart of England' as this grave in Westminster Abbey, he is seemingly cutting himself off from the symbolic potential of the green shires but he goes on to draw them in. The Unknown Soldier sleeps in 'the silence of a mighty church, a silence as deep and lovely as though he were lying in some green country graveyard steeped in peace, above him a twilight in which the stored centuries seem to whisper happily of good things done for England'.[11] Symbolically, then, the soldier is lying simultaneously in London and in a country graveyard and he is calling forth echoes of *Henry V.*

In Search of England

The green shires themselves came into view when, a year or so after the publication of his books on London, Morton published *In Search of England*. Fussell, in his book on travel writing between the wars, has drawn attention to the way in which travel books are shaped. They are not, he persuasively argues, artless chronicles of one incident after another but careful constructions, with characters and plots that have beginnings, climaxes and resolutions. The customary division between the supposedly truthful travel book and the frankly fictional novel is hard to sustain.[12] It is instructive, therefore, to see *In Search of England* as a shaped narrative, rather than an artless travel diary. The time frame of the journey, for example, runs from April – echoes here of *The Canterbury Tales* – through to harvest time, although the events recorded can hardly have actually taken five or six months. Morton's books are written in the first person, but the narrator is not necessarily identical with Morton himself: the narrator is a *persona*, a literary device. The distance between Morton and his narrator is often very small, and when he started writing books he is unlikely to have been aware that he was constructing a *persona*, but later in life, when he reflected on his enterprise, he recognised that the H. V. Morton who spoke through the books was not always the person he felt himself to be.

In Search of England opens with a short introduction in which Morton speaks directly, in a tone rather different from the self-deprecating, whimsical, emotional, patrician tones of the narrator of the book itself. The point of the formal, direct introduction is to tell readers that they must not interpret the book that follows as no more than a diary of a light-hearted jaunt through the highways and byways. Morton wants his project to be taken seriously; he says that he is addressing a momentous question. 'Never before', he writes, 'have so many people been searching for England.' His identification of the cause of this search is unremarkable: people are alienated from the lives and homes assigned to them in an urban and industrial society and, despite their living nominally in a country called England, they feel an urge to go in search of a place that will be recognised and felt as the *real* England. Morton does not develop this distinction between the real and what must be, in some sense, the unreal, bogus, inauthentic England in which people are compelled to pass their lives. We are now thoroughly habituated to this supposed distinction between the real and the inauthentic. Holiday firms routinely stake their whole claim on their ability to transport their customers to the real Provence or the real Tuscany, in implied contrast to some other version of these places. It is not at all an obvious distinction, but Morton and writers like him do not need to stop and reflect on it, so sure are they that their readers will unquestioningly recognise it.

Continuing his own introduction, Morton says that the search for the real England has lately been made easier, for cheap road transport now penetrates every part of the country, facilitating the instinctive search for the rural 'common racial heritage'. What will the searchers find, though? Is the rural heartland in good shape? It is not; 'behind the beauty of the English country is an economic and social cancer.' Old estates are being taxed out of existence and broken up, cheap imported food is undermining farmers' livelihoods. What is the solution? It is idle to think that the 'intellectual solitude in which the rustic evolved his shrewd wisdom' can be sustained: the radio, roads and newspapers are irreversibly bringing villages into a wider culture. But the nation as a whole will flourish only when attention is paid to the rebuilding of secure, prosperous and traditional agricultural communities, supporting 'a contented and flourishing peasantry', to which the town-bred searchers can go for spiritual and physical refreshment.[13]

Morton's is hardly a profound analysis. The twenties and thirties were full of such jeremiads which, in turn, have a lineage that stretches back through the Edwardian and Victorian social critics to the earliest commentators on the social effects of the Industrial Revolution. What makes Morton interesting is the unreflecting way in which he can trundle out this routine analysis of the ills of England shortly after having produced books about the vivid lives of Londoners. Cramped and hard as some of these London lives were, Morton had not presented them as inauthentic. Collectively and even in the absence of any overt, personal statements, Morton's London books testify to an exciting, authentic urban culture. Yet the Arcadian myth, with its stock formulations of the degenerate city contrasting with the wise and profound countryside, is waiting to sweep him (and dozens of writers like him) off in search of the eternal verities. No doubt the buoyancy of the market for the myth had a lot to do with it: *In Search of England* went through three editions *a year* in its first four years. No journalist – which is what Morton was – is likely to ignore a market like that. At a less commercial level and as I have suggested, it may be that the extraordinary market during the twenties for books like Morton's was driven partly by a compulsion among readers to locate a realm of the enduring and beautiful in the face of the dislocation, brutality and meaningless of the Great War.[14]

Following Morton's own introduction, the opening of chapter one of *In Search of England* is very much in the mode of the officer in the trenches dreaming of the English shires. In fact the incident recorded actually occurred after the war, when Morton was on a newspaper assignment. The narrator opens with a recollection of a moment in Palestine in 1923 when, ill and fearful of dying, he was stirred by a picture of England that arose in his mind:

> ... a village street at dusk with a smell of wood smoke lying in the still air and, here and there, little red blinds shining in the dusk under the thatch. I remembered how the church bells ring at home, and how, at that time of year, the sun leaves a dull red bar low down in the west, and against it the elms grow blacker minute by minute. Then the bats start to flicker like little bits of burnt paper and you hear the slow jingle of a team coming home from the fields.

The narrator goes on to record his recollection that there and then, he vowed to himself that if he survived, he would 'go home in search of England, and the little thatched cottages of England.' He hoped to 'lean over English bridges and lie on English grass, watching an English sky.' He says too that his vision is widely shared. 'A little London factory hand' whom he had met during the war had said 'when pressed, and after great mental difficulty' that the England he was fighting for was the England of Epping Forest, not the England of the streets in which he actually lived.[15]

In Search of England is nominally a record of a motor journey that Morton undertook when he had returned safely back to England. Morton later disarmingly confessed that on the journey he had 'deliberately shirked realities' by making 'wide and inconvenient circles to avoid modern towns and cities.' He had devoted himself 'entirely to ancient towns and cathedral cities, to green fields and pretty things.'[16] The journey opens with the narrator heading south and west from London.[17] His first, supposedly chance encounter is in Berkshire, where he meets 'the last bowl-turner in England' who plies his craft on a primeval lathe in a tumble-down hut lost in a maze of muddy lanes. As the reader expects, the bowl-turner, in suitably rustic terms, rejects the cash nexus: '"Money?" he said with a slow faun-like smile, "Money's only storing up trouble, I think. I like making bowls better than I like making money".'[18] And so it goes, as the narrator drives in a great loop down to Land's End, up to Carlisle, across to Newcastle and down the East side of the country, through Lincolnshire, over to Warwickshire and back to London. The citizens of village, market town and cathedral city step obligingly and generally deferentially forward, as if straight from Central Casting, to utter, in formulaic dialect, gems of traditional legend, custom and wisdom. Between these encounters, Morton keeps the momentum up by sketching in, very effectively, colourful romantic historical background and by having his narrator pause to reflect sonorously on the spirit of the places he visits: 'At night, especially under this witching moon, the streets of Shrewsbury take you back to Old England. Butcher Row at night is perfect.'[19]

This is not the whole story. Powerful and seductive as the myths of Arcady and Merrie England are, Morton is not entirely swept away by them. For example, at a tiny village in Cornwall, the narrator is put up for the night by an old farming couple. He elaborately builds up a picture of a Cornish Eden. But the culmination of this taste of paradise is his being invited up the lane to hear a neighbour's new battery radio that, after much tuning, beams in an evening of dance-band music from the Savoy. The proud owner of the radio tells the narrator how closely it had kept them in touch with news of the General Strike ('"we liked that Mr Baldwin, for he wor as plain as if he wor in this room."'). Morton's artful juxtaposition of the metropolitan sophistication of the Savoy, the placid timelessness of rural Cornwall and the world of urgent political action is left to do its own work. No doubt the reader is supposed to sigh over the intrusion into Eden of vulgar modernity and the brutal world of politics but Morton does not step out of the narrative and deliver a personal castigation. He leaves it at the elegaic but noncommittal level of 'the new picture of rural England; old heads bent over the wireless set in the light of a paraffin lamp.'[20]

The narrator is more direct when he reaches Wigan, a town that later, in Orwell's account, achieved symbolic status. The narrator says that, feeling conscious of having avoided the industrial regions, he turned down a road to Wigan as a sort of penance. He is agreeably surprised, partly because he finds the town less ugly than he had imagined, but chiefly because it was remarkably easy to get out of it, into pleasant neighbouring fields. He does his rather condescending best with the town, and – high praise from Morton – notes that 'it has one of the few good war memorials I have seen in England.'[21]

The plot of *In Search of England* starts to build toward its climax when the narrator reaches Warwickshire, birthplace of Shakespeare and the region in which Morton spent his youth. He is recaptivated by Stratford. Shakespeare and England bond there. The narrator gives a fanciful account of glimpsing Titania, Peaseblossom and the

rude mechanicals from *A Midsummer Night's Dream* in a nearby
wood and declares the view of the river from the churchyard to be
'one of the supremely English views'. But here, when the most potent
elements of Englishness are in play, an ironic, deflating note is
sounded. As a youth, he recalls, he had worshipped Frank Benson,
the actor-manager who had been responsible for the annual
Shakespeare festivals at Stratford from 1886 to 1919. Morton recalls
having heard Benson proclaim that

> only through Stratford, the common meeting-place of the English-
> speaking world, could we heal the pains of Industrialism and make
> England happy again. We were to make the whole world happy,
> apparently, by teaching it to morris-dance and sing folk-songs and to
> go to the Memorial Theatre. With the splendid faith of Youth we
> pilgrims believed that England could be made 'merrie' again by
> hand-looms and young women in Liberty gowns who played the
> harpsichord. Then, I seem to remember, shortly after that war was
> declared. However ...[22]

The culminating point of the book is the narrator's account of
another casual, though actually highly improbable, encounter, this
time with the vicar of an unnamed hamlet, seemingly near Warwick.
The incident is immaculately stage-managed. The narrator
encounters the vicar in the churchyard and, among the ancient
graves, hears him ruminate on the continuity of village life. The vicar
invites him to stay overnight. They drink old port from Georgian
glasses. Their talk is of the ancient, naturally hierarchical tradition of
the place, and the mournful prospect of the break-up of the local
estate when death duties are demanded. In the morning, the vicar
conducts the harvest festival service in the church, before a
contented, ruddy-faced congregation. And finally, in a passage which
would have qualified for three stars on the *Cold Comfort Farm* purple
passage scale:

> I took up a handful of earth and felt it crumble and run through my
> fingers, thinking that as long as one English field lies against another
> there is something left in the world for a man to love. "Well," smiled
> the vicar, as he walked towards me between the yew trees, "that, I am
> afraid, is all we have." "You have England," I said.[23]

The England for which the narrator has been searching has been
found. Its unsurprising identifying features are: remoteness from
industrial cities and all traces of modernity, the palpable presence of
ancient, benign landowning and church authority, a contented

population of agricultural workers and a tinge of Shakespeare. Open politics has no place in England, although a vaguely specified, but nonetheless fundamental sense of the rightness of the old order – the almost comically old, eighteenth century, or even Tudor social order – is built into its very foundations. This is very much the England Chris Lawrence describes in his chapter as being conjured up by the inter-war physicians as the idyllic scene of Edward Jenner's country practice.

I noted earlier that *In Search of England* is 'nominally' a record of a motor trip around the country. But it is not a guide book. It would be impossible for the reader faithfully to trace the narrator's route. Indeed, in some passages – the passages recording the Berkshire bowl-turner and the Warwickshire harvest festival, for example – he is extremely evasive about precise location. What, then, is the purpose of the book and how do we account for its extraordinary popularity? The 'search' motif is important. We have to imagine a reader who is not so much looking for a guide book or gazetteer for a journey he or she is planning, but who wants reassurance that there is, somewhere out there, an essential England. Morton's book convinces the reader that such an England has successfully been sought and found, even though the locations of its quintessential sites are not disclosed. The reassuring knowledge that England is there and that Morton has found it and described it for us, is maybe all the reader needs. Morton works simultaneously in the realms of topography and the imagination.

A year later, in 1928, four editions of *In Search of England* were comfortably in the bag. Morton had evidently succeeded in constructing an authorial *persona* that was attractive to a large readership. He had struck gold and he worked the rich seam for fifteen years. The money that his writing brought in enabled him eventually to set himself up in a handsome medieval farmhouse in Hampshire. He never lived the life of the yeoman. Even if he did enjoy the rural view from his study window, he probably preferred the view from a cab window as it bowled down Piccadilly, taking him to dinner at the Ritz.[24] The gap that opened between the suave Harry Morton and the genial narrator of the books re-emphasizes Fussell's point about the constructedness, artfulness and fictionality of the seemingly transparent 'travel' book.

Later Books on England

Morton quickly followed up the success of *In Search of England* with a companion volume, *The Call of England* (1928). Setting aside

Morton's commercial imperative, the purpose of the new book was to make redress to the North of England, a region he had neglected on his first tour. In his new book he wanted to introduce those Home Counties readers, who, like him, tended instinctively to turn south and west whenever they sought the real England, to great tracts of what he had delightedly discovered to be equally English country, north of the Trent. He also wanted to do justice to the Northern industrial cities. In practice, the two objectives work against each other and, predictably enough, the rural North gets far more attention than the industrial North. It is the Yorkshire moors and ruined abbeys, the Northumberland coast, the cathedral cities of Durham and York and the ancient small market towns like Clitheroe, Beverley and Ripon that call forth his most effusive praise: 'you feel in little places such as Ripon that you touch the sturdy roots of England firmly locked in a distant and important past.'[25]

Morton's narrator does go to the big industrial centres. The interesting thing, though, is that somewhat inconsistently, he does not fly to the opposite extreme and picture them as affronts to the essential England. Instead, he responds rather affirmatively to their confident style and enormous vitality. Manchester and Liverpool win him over completely. He does mention the expected black puddings, clogs and shawls but his imagination is really caught by the glamour of the Manchester Cotton Exchange, the raffish pubs, Liverpool Pier Head and the Great Dock Road, 'a magnificent epic of commerce'. Even Sheffield, which, as a steel town, was overwhelmingly smoky and grimy, impressed him: 'The hard ugliness is queerly grand.'[26] He was not entirely blind, however, to the sorts of miseries that were, a decade later, to dominate the imaginations of travellers from the south like Orwell. The description, for instance, of the desperate world of the Liverpool casual dockworker is forthright and stark. Overall, his response to the industrial cities – including, later, Birmingham where Morton grew up – is positive, very much in the way that his earlier response to London had been positive. Indeed, for all the clogs and shawls and rolling moors aspects of the North, he will allow no absolute disjunction between South and North. He points out that desperate casual dock work is as much a feature of London as of Liverpool life. He later wrote a piece about casual workers in the London docks who were recruited for the dangerous and filthy job of scraping out the sludge from oil-fired ships' fuel pumps.[27]

In *The Call of England*, then, Morton attempted to integrate North and South, industry and country, into a more comprehensive vision of England. The North-South integration is a success, but he was unable successfully to incorporate industry into the essential England. At the book's close, as at the close of his first England book, the narrator is magnetically drawn to Stratford-upon-Avon in the Warwickshire heartland. He finds a seat, close to Shakespeare's tomb, and reviews his journey. The highlights that he recalls are not the industrial cities but the ancient northern cathedrals and the moorland abbeys. The essential features of England were not, it seems, under serious threat of redefinition.

These two books on England encouraged Morton to devise searches for the rest of the British Isles. *In Search of Scotland* (1929), *In Search of Ireland* (1930) and *In Search of Wales* (1932) quickly followed and were highly successful. These books lie outside the scope of this chapter but it is important to note that they are substantial works, not just dashed-off afterthoughts. Scotland was soon, like England, given a companion volume, *In Scotland Again* (1933). Morton emphatically did not regard Ireland, Scotland and Wales as insignificant, vaguely comic or romantic appendages to England. The books are informed by a vivid sense of the autonomous histories of the four countries (especially of Highland, Jacobite Scotland) but, like those on England, the texts are regulated by prior notions of the essences of the countries he is visiting. In the book on Wales, for example, there is a painstaking, detailed and entirely sympathetic account of the life and work of Glamorgan coal miners. The narrator goes down a mine (which reminds him of being in the trenches), gets to know the miners and their wives and makes as plain as he can what family life is like when short time working and layoffs are always just round the corner and where the basic wage of just over two pounds a week is pitiful. Morton offers no political commentary, beyond tersely observing: 'It is, of course, all wrong.'[28] The important point, in this study of Morton and Englishness, is that he was far readier to see the Glamorgan miners as the embodiment of something essential to the entity called Wales than he was to see their English equivalents as embodying anything essentially English. A stereotype is being struck here: to the English, the real Wales *includes* coal miners, just as it includes Snowdon.

This brings us to the books Morton wrote about England during the thirties and forties, the decades that saw Orwell and Priestley taking their own, more celebrated, though in my view often less searching, journeys to the industrial areas. Morton's descriptions of life in the slums are as acute as Orwell's, even though they are set within a comparatively weakly formulated political perspective. Morton's most trenchant publication started life as a series of pieces for the *Daily Herald*. In these pieces the gap between Morton and his narrator narrows, for they were not written with the conventions of the travel book in mind. The series was reprinted in 1933 by the Labour Party, with a forward by George Lansbury, as a little twopenny pamphlet called *What I Saw in the Slums*, with photographs by James Jarché. In his introduction, Morton declares that he is not a member of any political party but that he wished urgently to present 'a perfectly frank account of a short journey through the slums of six great industrial cities of England.' Close-up descriptions of squalid housing are interleaved with grim public health statistics. Political analysis, however, is not entirely absent. Slums, he says, cannot be cleared away by the unregulated private enterprise that produced them in the first place. Civic intervention is necessary. Sheffield's Labour council is singled out for praise.

The relationship Morton assumes with the poor and wretched people he meets is, as in his other books, patrician; he evidently feels no awkwardness in intruding into their lives and homes. Indeed, he points out that he was positively welcomed when he made clear that he was there to expose the wickedness of slum landlords, about whom he is unreservedly contemptuous: 'In a perfect state of society they would be stripped to the waist and whipped squealing through their own kennels.' He presents the people who live in the slums as engaged in a desperately unequal battle to preserve decency and respectability, symbolised by the women's Sisyphean practice of forever whitening their front doorsteps. The women particularly impress him: 'What a ghastly life they lead in mean streets. Always washing. Always cooking minute quantities of food. Always cleaning something that cannot be cleaned. Always enriching the earth. Always worried about something. This waste of energy is awful.'[29] In this short pamphlet, Morton offers no reflections on the relationship between the slums that have so outraged him and the essential, utopian England that is the quest of his other books. Implicitly, though, he presents the slums as a particularly grim legacy of the aberrant industrial revolution that has blighted an essentially green and pleasant land.

Morton and the Second World War

Morton continued to publish throughout the Second World War. He evidently felt a real threat of defeat and it wrung from him even more intense evocations of the England that stood in jeopardy. In the summer of 1939, certain that war was close, he set off on yet another tour of England, to capture what he thought might be a final vision of it. He published his findings as *I Saw Two Englands*, the two being England at peace and England at war. His tour, worked up into the now familiar format of the genially-narrated journey, took him first to Kent, where he progressed from stately home to stately home (Penshurst, Knole, Hever, Chevening), and then in a clockwise loop, ending at Peterborough, where he watched gas masks being issued and realised that war was only weeks away.

A dozen years had passed since his first tour of England and he registers the difference by remarking on the mock Tudor houses that were springing up along the new bypasses. The fashion for the Tudor, he writes,

> may be deplorable or amusing, and it is easy to make fun of it, but it seems to express a longing for something good and, above all, something English. In a better world, our rulers and our educationalists would seek out the meaning of it, and if they found, as I think they might, that it expresses a turning away from a pitilessly mechanised age which is even now thinking of tearing itself to bits, they would see what could be done to deepen that instinct, to develop it and save it from the speculator.[30]

The narrator himself does not press forward with a response to his own challenge.

The second half of the book is the record of a tour in October 1939, plainly undertaken with a good deal of official help in the form of petrol coupons and passes to government installations, to inspect and report on the war effort. His conclusion is that England is fundamentally as 'sound as a bell' but is waiting for a leader.[31] The book ends with a highly-wrought postscript, written in the dark days of 1940. It ranges once again over the question of the identity of the essential England. The postscript describes two nights in the life of a rural Home Guard unit (during this period, Morton was living in his farmhouse in Hampshire and was commanding the local Home Guard unit). On the first night, the narrator leads his men, some of them veterans of the trenches of the First War and all intimately familiar from youth with every hedge and tree in the locality, in a sweep across the moonlit harvest stubble fields in search of reported German parachutists. 'The combined local knowledge of farmer, poacher, and sportsman had been pooled for a moment in order to hunt the invader from our corner of England.' On the second night, the narrator stands watch on the tower of his village church and uses the quiet night to muse on what the war was doing to England. The slums, the industrial towns, the mock-Tudor bypass houses do not invade his musings. The threat posed by Hitler has pushed all the troubling aspects of England aside and has revealed the underlying, enduring England:

> ... it comes to me that one of the most remarkable things about this war is the quiet way England has ceased to be a country or even a county for many of us, and has become a parish. All over our land, villages once proclaimed dead and done for have awakened to arms. ... my parish has become England ... [The danger of war] has accomplished for the villages of England what musical young men from Oxford, with bells at their knees, and earnest women in Liberty silk gowns hoped to do a decade ago; it has made England almost "merrie" again.[32]

Two years later, and still fearful of defeat, Morton published his one and only novel, *I James Blunt.* It was commissioned by the Minister for Information, Brendan Bracken, and Morton surrendered his royalties for the war effort. The novel, just 56 pages long and printed on cheap wartime paper, bound in flimsy covers, takes the form of a diary by a James Blunt, a 61 year old resident of a southern English market town who records his experiences of life following the successful invasion of Britain by the Germans. A swastika flies over the town hall. Jews and trade unionists have been rounded up. Blunt's grandchildren have been corrupted by Nazi propaganda at the village school. In the bar of his local pub, the sporting prints have been taken down from the wall and replaced by pictures of Hitler. The novel ends with the writer of the diary breaking off half way through an entry as a sinister knock comes on the door in the dead of night. The novel has no literary pretensions but it went through three editions within a month of publication, making Morton wonder if he had maybe been too self-sacrificing in surrendering his royalties. The book was, as it was designed to be, a piece of propaganda intended to chill the complacent. Its significance for this study of Morton's sense of the essential England is that, unsurprisingly, when he wished to symbolise the beleaguered nation, he unhesitatingly reached for 'a peaceful English country town', where 'everything blends beautifully, as English things do', near Farnham, in Surrey.[33]

The final text to be surveyed is a little book Morton published in 1943, *Atlantic Meeting.* Morton was evidently well-connected, for he was asked, at short notice and under conditions of strict secrecy, to be one of only two journalists accompanying Winston Churchill on his voyage across the Atlantic in August 1941, to confer with

Franklin Delano Roosevelt and, as Morton saw it, to persuade America to join the war. Morton observes Churchill at close quarters during the voyage and ventures a conclusion about what he considers to be his unique qualities of leadership. They derive, Morton says, from his being deeply rooted in a pre-industrial, pre-class, 'old, warm, emotional England'. He notes that Churchill was not afraid to weep openly during affecting scenes in the commercial feature films that were shown in the destroyer's wardroom and which Churchill relished. According to Morton, Churchill calls forth a response from the whole English People – the Scots, Irish and Welsh vanish in this account – because he is not identified with sectional, class, regional or industrial interests; he rises above all the jarring elements of a potentially riven country and speaks from, and on behalf of, the essential England that subsumes them all:

> I have sometimes studied the effect of Churchill's voice and words upon an ordinary gathering of men in a public house. Why, I have wondered, should they have been so firmly held, so silent until the last word? And I have wondered if it may not be that he speaks with the voice of an older England, that we recognise the voice, not of an industrialist, but of one who speaks to us as if from the deck of the Golden Hind.

Churchill's voice is also classless. He has no public school accent. Like the Elizabethans, he speaks, says Morton, not as an Etonian but as an Englishman.[34]

Conclusion

Morton made a highly successful career out of writing books whose chief object was to serve the insatiable market for the myth that over that horizon, round that bend in the lane, across that field, lies an authentic England, untouched by the Industrial Revolution, by suburbia, by the anxieties of modern life. The myth was extraordinarily appealing to Morton's generation. People clung to it during the incomprehensible slaughter of the Great War. They pursued it on foot, on bicycles and in cheap motorcars down the open roads of the twenties and thirties and clung to it once again in 1939 when fears of a German invasion revived. The myth generated a sub-genre of books on England and within that sub-genre, Morton was the most successful author. In many passages of his hugely popular books he is absolutely archetypal, but he was not entirely consumed by the myths he served. He forced himself to become acquainted with features of English life that were distinctly un-merrie and he described them vividly. But he never fully integrated his vision of England: the focus of his most popular books always, in the end, narrows to the parish, the rural, the utopian. The most poignant speeches given to the narrator tend to be descriptions of an England that can never actually be visited or lived in. In Housman's phrase, it is a 'land of lost content'.

By the end of the war, the gap between Morton and the *persona* he had created for the narrator of his books had widened to a gulf. Contemplating, from his now servantless Surrey home, the forthcoming years of austerity, he chose not to put his weight behind the national task of post-war reconstruction. Instead, he sold up and bought land near Cape Town where he built himself a fine house. Back in the twenties and thirties, when he had been conjuring up his utopian vision of England, he no doubt believed what he was writing, or at least believed it at the moment he was actually writing. But by 1948 he had neither the desire nor the need to go on searching. The dream of the English shires gave way to the view from his terrace of Table Mountain.

Acknowledgements

A somewhat different version of this paper appeared in *The Representation and Reality of War: Essays in Honour of D. G. Wright*, K. Dockray and K. Laybourn (eds), Stroud, 1999.

Notes

1 H. V. Morton, *In Search of England*, London, 1927.

2 P. Fussell, *The Great War and Modern Memory*, Oxford, 1975, 268. See especially Chapter 7, 'Arcadian Resources'.

3 P. Fussell, *Abroad: British Literary Travelling Between the Wars*, Oxford, 1980. See also D. Matless, *Landscape and Englishness*, London, 1998.

4 On 'Englishness' and for passing references to Morton, see *Englishness: Politics and Culture, 1880-1920*, R. Colls and P. Dodd (eds), London, 1986; M. J. Wiener, *English Culture and the Decline of the Industrial Spirit, 1850-1980*, Cambridge, 1981, repr. Penguin, 1985; P. Wright, *On living in an Old Country*, London, 1985; V. Cunningham, *British Writers of the Thirties*, Oxford, 1988; *Writing Englishness*, J. Giles and T. Middleton (eds), London, 1995; A. Calder, *The Myth of the Blitz*, London, 1991. Chapter 9.

5 G. Orwell, *Homage to Catalonia*, 1938, repr. Penguin, 1989, p187.

6 Wright, *Living in an Old Country*; R. Hewison, *The Heritage Industry*, London, 1987; *The Museum Time Machine*, R. Lumley (ed.), London, 1988.

7 H. V. Morton, *I Saw Two Englands*, 2nd edn, London, 1942, pp. 82–3.

8 K. Fields, 'The Travel Books of H. V. Morton', *Book and Magazine Collector*, 58 (January 1989): 50–56. No source is given for the figures.

9 Did the Burns phrase originate with Morton, or is he quoting? *In Search of Scotland*, 17th edn, London, 1932, 268.

10 H. V. Morton, *The Heart of London*, London, 1925; *A London Year*, London, 1926; *London*, London, 1926; *The Spell of London*, London, 1926; *The Nights of London*, London, 1926. Save for *A London Year*, these books were reprinted together as *H. V. Morton's London*, London, 1940.

11 H. V. Morton, *The Spell of London*, 10th edn, London, 1932, 15. Compare his comments on the Cenotaph, 'that mass of national emotion frozen in stone', *H. V. Morton's London*, 13th edn, London, 1945, 19. On war memorials and their significance in general, see S. Hynes, *A War Imagined: the First World War and English Culture*, London, 1990, esp. p. 270 *et seq*.

12 Fussell, *Abroad*, 174.

13 Morton, *In Search of England*, 12th edn, London, 1930, pp. vii–xi.

14 The suggestion is made, for example, by Hynes, *War Imagined*.

15 Morton, *In Search of England*, pp. 1–3.

16 H. V. Morton, *The Call of England*, 6th edn, London, 1930, vii.
17 Alan Howkins has argued that the essential England that was
    constructed in the early decades of the twentieth century, was
    located in *southern* England. Non-southern features could be
    incorporated only if they conformed with the southern pattern of
    field, hedgerow, lane and thatch. Moors and mountains are not
    English. See A. Howkins, 'The Discovery of Rural England', in
    Englishness, Colls and Dodd (eds), pp. 62–88. Morton initially fits in
    well with this model. He heads south and west, rather than north
    and east. But he is not finally trapped by the model, for he
    rhapsodises over Yorkshire, Northumberland, Northampton, and
    (particularly) Warwickshire – where he was brought up.
18 Morton, *In Search of England*, 10.
19 *Ibid.*, 180.
20 *Ibid.*, pp. 78–85. Morton works exactly the same trick of a dance
    band coming over the airwaves into the remote countryside in his
    account of a night spent in a remote bothy in the Cairngorms. See
    In Scotland Again, 10th edn, London, 1944, pp. 304–6.
21 Morton, *In Search of England*, pp. 187–90.
22 *Ibid.*, pp. 255–60. Morton himself trails off with the suspension
    points at the end of the quoted paragraph.
23 *Ibid.*, 280. Stella Gibbons's *Cold Comfort Farm*, London, 1932
    satirised earthy, ruralist books. She alerted readers to purple passages
    in her book by signifying them with one, two, or three stars, on the
    Baedeker principle.
24 This emerges from the diary (now in private hands) that Morton
    kept from 1939–1945.
25 Morton, *Call of England*, 6th edn, 1930, 64.
26 *Ibid.*, pp. 150, 172.
27 H. V. Morton, *Our Fellow Men*, 2nd edn, London, 1936, pp. 66–9.
28 H. V. Morton, *In Search of Wales*, 8th edn, London, 1936, pp.
    246–67.
29 H. V. Morton, *What I Saw in the Slums*, London, 1933, pp. 9, 29.
30 H. V. Morton, *I Saw Two Englands*, London, 1942, 65.
31 *Ibid.*, 282.
32 *Ibid.*, 288. This passage is virtually identical to one quoted earlier
    (fn. 22).
33 H. V. Morton, *I James Blunt*, London, 1942, 8.
34 H. V. Morton, *Atlantic meeting*, London, 1943 pp. 80–1. In fact
    Churchill went to Harrow School, not Eton.

3

Edward Jenner's Jockey Boots and the Great Tradition in English Medicine 1918–1939

Christopher Lawrence

The responses of élite groups to the cultural changes, economic upheavals and political crises of inter-war Britain have recently come under scholarly historical scrutiny.[1] Many intellectuals who had been brought up in the bright sun of Victorian liberalism and took a relatively optimistic view of the future retreated in the twenties and more particularly the thirties to more pessimistic positions. In many cases such pessimism was coupled with condemnations of mass production and mass culture. These denunciations were often associated with an appeal for the creation of, or a return to, an organic society. In this period too many scientists turned to organic models of nature.[2] Élite doctors, who I have elsewhere dubbed 'patrician', summoned up organic ideals of the body, emphasized the importance of the healing power of nature and warned of the dangers of the unrestricted proliferation of laboratory science. The latter was seen by some of them as an embodiment of the division of labour, the destroyer of an individualism that, clinicians held, was the bedrock of sound medical practice.[3]

No simple model encompasses the variety of views about modernity held by these doctors but a number of themes repeatedly appeared in their writings including: gardening, England, humanism, the priesthood, individualism and citizenship. One of the motifs that underlay these themes was the perceived peculiarity of the English mind. It was stressed by many medical authors that the English mind was of an empirical bent, a fact that made English medicine a particularly suitable heir to Hippocrates. There was, it was said, an English empirical tradition, notably exemplified by William Harvey, Thomas Sydenham, John Hunter, Edward Jenner, Richard Bright and Joseph Lister that gave English medicine its natural historical turn and its down-to-earth, commonsensical quality. This quality was contrasted with the theoretical tendency of continental medicine that, in some way, was part of a frame of mind that gave rise to dangerous things such as Fascism and communism. Admittedly John Hunter was a Scotsman, but what was being created in this genealogy was an *English* medicine, in the same way that the *Dictionary of National Biography* was a series of volumes about English culture, notwithstanding its Celtic component.[4] One did not have to be English to contribute to English literature, merely write it.

In describing a 'great tradition' that these doctors venerated and saw themselves as heirs to, I am of course alluding to F. R. Leavis and his 'great tradition' in English literature. Constructing traditions was an important constituent of the making of English cultural identity, not that ancestors had to be English.[5] Two members of Leavis's tradition were not native born, Henry James and Joseph Conrad, but they were easily accommodated. James 'belonged by birth and upbringing to that refined civilization of old European America' his 'congenial soil and climate were in Europe.' *Portrait of a Lady*, wrote Leavis, describes the English country-house with 'idealizing charm' (and, of course, James lived in Sussex from 1896 until his death in 1916). As for Conrad his 'themes and interests demanded the concreteness and action ... of English.'[6] There are many similarities between the Leavisites and the doctors. Both stressed the importance of concreteness and both expressed distaste for abstractions, features, Mannheim noted, of conservative ideologies.[7] Leavis's nostalgia for an organic society and his denunciations of 'standardization' and 'the machine' are well known.[8] The apparent difference between Leavis and the doctors was that Leavis and the Scrutineers (Leavis's journal was *Scrutiny*) were to some extent engaged in *overthrowing* a gentleman-scholar tradition. Mulhern in his illuminating *Moment of Scrutiny* argues that 'neither birth nor occupational status fitted its members for the role of scholar-gentlemen. They were, for the most part, petit or lower bourgeois in origin.' Similar things could be said of the origins of some of the doctors. Thomas, Lord Horder was a draper's son. In addition medicine had never been fully accepted as a gentleman's profession. None the less, neither background nor professional status stopped the doctors adopting the role of gentlemen. I argue it is more accurate to see the Scrutineers engaged in overthrowing the *critical apparatus* employed in a scholar-gentleman tradition but by no means its gentlemanly elitism. Mulhern offers no evidence that the Scrutineers did not adopt the social forms of their predecessors. The reverse seems rather the case. Leavis relished his Huguenot-ducal ancestry.[9]

To the point here, is that both groups constituted élites that found in the past a Golden Age in which there was an organic

England. For the Leavisites it was associated with the metaphysical poets, particularly John Donne. Clinicians too found the Elizabethan era Golden. Sir Walter Langdon Brown, consulting physician at St. Bartholomew's hospital specifically compared the passing of Elizabethan high civilization into Jacobean 'disillusionment' with the periods before and after the First World War.[10] The patricians, however, also found in the late eighteenth-century doctor, Edward Jenner, the icon of a lost or ideal world. Jenner, they insisted, was the lone country practitioner, who had saved civilization from a dreadful disease, small pox, through simple natural historical inquiry. As such Jenner could be made to embody many of the things they valued.

The ways in which the empiricism of English medicine, past and present, were stressed in the inter-war years scarcely does justice to the long intellectual history underlying this view. It would no doubt be possible to trace the celebration of empiricism in English medicine and its coupling with an ideology of sturdy individualism to at least the seventeenth century. Nor would this be an exercise in tracing an idea without substance. The substantive empiricism of English medicine is part of the history of English empiricism generally. There are ways in which overt system building *is* more characteristic of the Continent and Scotland than it is of England. Thus the combined celebration of English empiricism and the peculiarities of the English mind has a long history in many spheres.[11] For example, contemporary with the doctors considered here, many English historians were expressing their approval of empiricism in their discipline and, some of them at least, were condemning continental theory.[12] As Collini records 'in characteristic and unselfconscious hunting metaphor' Ernest Barker noted at mid century 'the Engish mind has baulked and stumbled at the fence of philosophy.'[13] The relativity of empiricism, however, is nowhere more nicely illustrated than in judgement of a nineteenth-century American doctor who seemed to speak for many of his compatriots when he condemned English doctors for being 'wonderful metaphysicians.'[14] Rather than trace here the long domestic history of the praise of empiricism in English medicine, I look at it first as a living tradition in one of the teachers admired by some, and possibly all, of the men who are the subject of this study.

One of the most esteemed of the late Victorian clinicians who revered empiricism in general and its appearance in the English mind in particular was the Bart's hospital consultant, Samuel Gee, physician to the Prince of Wales. For Gee, experience was the essence of the practical art of medicine. Experience was to be gained on the ward and then supplemented by hours in the post-mortem room; for it was morbid anatomy that gave meaning to much bedside examination. The vast majority of clinical signs were explicable by morbid anatomy, a discipline regarded by men such as Gee as a branch of natural history, as was the description of diseases at the bedside. Tommy (as he was known) Horder, perhaps Gee's most devoted disciple, was to write in 1939 in the manner Gee might have written fifty years earlier: 'The doctor is a naturalist, having the human animal as his subject ... observation is vital, so vital that the earlier the habit is cultivated the better.'[15] Natural history was regarded by English doctors as one of the highest forms of scientific investigation. John Pickstone has persuasively connected such views to the courtly culture with which this sort of medical practice had long been associated.[16]

In his book on auscultation and percussion of the chest of 1893, Gee's clinical precepts were legitimated by an appeal to tradition and in particular to Hippocrates.[17] Gee cast his clinical observations as aphorisms in imitation of the Greek physician. In Gee's account English (not British) doctors were deemed the most appropriate heirs of Hippocrates. This view can also be found Gee's address 'Sects in Medicine'. Even though, at the turn of the nineteenth and twentieth century many were claiming the new sciences were transforming medicine, Gee held that the unchanging 'constitution of the human understanding' ensured 'that the sects are essentially the same in our time as they were in the early days of medicine.' Gee dealt first with the dogmatist who practised medicine 'reasoned from his theory of disease', although no dogmatists, he said, had been in evidence since the days of Albrecht von Haller in the eighteenth century.[18] In 1924, echoing Gee's essay, Horder called morbid anatomy a 'fundamental institution' in medicine, one which exercised 'salutary control ... over the natural tendency of the human mind to dogmatize.'[19] Unlike dogmatists, however, methodists still flourished. Methodists were practitioners who endeavoured 'to make the data of pathology and therapeutics as few as possible in number, and as universal as possible in extent.' Homeopaths were the most obvious modern example. But '[t]he English mind', Gee observed, 'is averse from methodism' adding 'Van Helmont and Stahl, Brown [a Scotsman] and Broussais, were not English.' Next were the physiological pharmaceutists, a sect 'at least as old as the days of Thomas Willis' who proceeded as follows: 'Ascertain the manner in which the healthy body is affected by a drug ... and you have a principle to guide you to the use of the drug in disease.' Too rapid an application to clinical medicine of physiological knowledge gained by vivisection was the potential danger in this approach. For, said Gee, 'physiological experiment has hitherto contributed very little to practical therapeutics.'[20] In 1950, the physiologist, Sir Henry Dale recalled Gee teaching him that: 'When you enter my wards your first duty is to forget all your physiology. Physiology is an experimental science – and a very good thing no doubt in its proper place. Medicine is not a science, but an empirical art.'[21] Gee, wrote J. Wickham Legg, who knew him well, 'went so far as to doubt the value of experiment in the natural sciences.'[22] The sect to which Gee proclaimed allegiance was the empiric. The empirical physician practised on the basis of personal experience. Empiricism, he explained, begins by compiling 'a history of diseases' so that the individual's complaint can be compared with a 'standard of reference.'[23] This was diagnosis, the cornerstone of medicine. The untheorized nature of empiricism underlay its aphoristic style of transmitting knowledge, as in some of the Hippocratic texts. Horder, indeed, collected his teacher's aphorisms for publication and brandished empiricism when needed. [24] In 1924 he referred to 'all of us who are empiricists in the proper sense of that word.'[25]

As already noted I have designated the sort of medicine practised by Gee and his contemporaries and pupils 'patrician', meaning that such doctors evidenced a commitment to a professional self-styling shaped in part by the values of a royal, aristocratic and generally wealthy clientele. The doctors were committed to clinical individualism and there is a sense in which they adopted the very old role of physician as counselor.[26] Their various shared values, commitments and interests can be understood in a number of ways. Élite doctors from the 1890s to the 1930s practised privately among the wealthy and the aristocracy and many had the valued duty of charitable practice at prominent voluntary hospitals. They were themselves wealthy and lived in a style not unlike that of the plutocrats they treated. They enjoyed aristocratic leisure activities, such as dining well, gardening and motoring (Horder had a vast estate in Sussex and a Rolls Royce). The order in which they moved and of which they approved was patronage-based. It depended on face-to-face encounters to maintain and promote social relations and attract clientele. It was a social order institutionalized at the great London voluntary hospitals, in Harley Street houses, at the Royal College of Physicians, the Royal College of Surgeons and the ancient universities. At the end of the nineteenth century, Gee and his like were the so-called 'Great' of the London Hospitals.[27] They cultivated the role of gentlemen, moral advisors and custodians of culture (in many senses, including the aesthetic) and valued clinical experience as the highest medical good.[28] To men such as these, many of whom had royal appointments, the figure of the queen or king represented all that they approved of and regal metaphors frequently appeared in their writings. Once the patient has entered the consulting room, he, 'like the person of the king, is sacred', wrote Horder in his maturity.[29]

Among the many things that distinguished the inter-war generation from its predecessor was the intensity of its anxiety about the decline of the clinician which was, I suggest, a focused anxiety about the decline of civilisation. In the inter-war years, Eric Hobsbawm has noted that 'survivors from the nineteenth century were perhaps most shocked by the collapse of values and institutions of the liberal civilization their century had taken for granted.'[30] Langdon Brown, also a pupil of Gee, observed to the Abernethian Society at Bart's in 1931 that John Maynard Keynes (Brown's nephew), speaking of those brought up around the 1870s, had said, 'they regarded the then existing state of affairs as normal, certain, and permanent, except in the direction of further improvement, and any deviation from it as aberrant, scandalous, and avoidable.' 'Few would deny', Brown added, 'that the War brought disillusionment.'[31] In the writings of most of the men considered here (nearly all brought up in the 1870s and 1880s) the familiar antimodernist targets, for instance mass production, urban growth and the death of rural England, are apparent. Their pronouncements on these matters sometimes displayed the physician's traditional disdain for trade. Francis Crookshank, a Wimpole Street doctor, wrote that in the world of '"big business" ... intelligence unaccompanied by brutality is at a discount.'[32] Langdon Brown complained in 1936 that 'the division of labour in a large factory has reached such a pitch that in many occupations craftsmanship is dead and the workman has become a robot.'[33] In the same year Horder lamented that 'the large town [far from] being essential for the development of genius, as some hold ... tends to stultify initiative and resource, which are the very root of genius.' Because 'we cannot face the company of our own souls', he wrote, 'we crowd into huge cities.'[34] Brown considered that '[i]t is one of the drawbacks of these vast new suburbs, mere dormitories, which radiate out like huge tentacles from London, destroying the countryside as they grow, that they offer so few opportunities for communal life and a social background.'[35] Mass consumption and entertainment (notably cinema going, an object of particular contempt for the Leavisites) the patricians found equally enervating.

'We don't read any more', lamented Horder,

though we decorate our rooms with the classics, and in the most expensive bindings. The best authors have given way to the best sellers. And even these pall on us, and we substitute the yellow newspaper and the nearly-as-yellow illustrated magazine. For sport, we watch the professionals play our games for us. For amusement, we crowd into "the pictures".[36]

Crookshank linked 'jazz-bands' to people of the 'coarsely sensual kind' and noted of the 'kinema' it was the 'greatest enemy of the epoch to intellectual culture', specifically associating the lower stages of evolution with 'the shiftiness of the monkey, the film star and the imbecile.'[37] Such public sentiments, A. J. P. Taylor suggests, were coupled with private ones about the character and availability of domestic servants. He noted:

> The number of private domestic servants did not increase even during the Depression. Only about 5 per cent of private households had a resident domestic between the wars. The cynical observer will not forget this fact when he reads lamentations from the comfortable classes about the decline of civilization. The lamentations only meant that professional men were having to help with the washing-up.[38]

Science, which all these men venerated in many ways, could also be seen as contributory to the post war malaise. 'Science', said Langdon Brown, 'on the one hand offers material comfort, on the other intellectual abstractions. This leads to a mechanized world without moral direction.'[39] I have explored elsewhere how these general worries appeared in the language of bedside medicine, how general clinicians expressed concern that the organization of laboratory science was usurping clinical skill to the detriment of good medical care. I have noted that their response to these worries was to stress clinical individualism, the organic nature of health, the non-reducibility of disease to laboratory categories and the body's natural healing powers.[40] Here I examine how, to counter cultural change in general and to defend clinical individualism and, relatedly, what was perceived to be the most open, organic and democratic society in the world, that of England, the empirical tradition in English medicine was summoned up. This tradition was deemed to begin with Hippocrates [sic] and the patricians discussed below saw themselves as inheriting it. Thus Sir George Newman, Chief Medical Officer of Health, but a staunch defender of the individual clinician, after noting how, in the twentieth century, specialism dominated medicine and that a 'profound change' separated past and present doctors, added, '*[b]ut the practitioner remains*' the 'heir of two centuries.'[41] More pointedly, Horder observed, 'after just two hundred years, the Tradition comes down to *us*.'[42]

When the patricians summoned tradition, some drew superficially on history but most had considerable historical learning. I deal with their writings thematically, aggregating work from the twenties and thirties although I am aware that a chronological treatment might bring out subtle changes of sentiment over the two decades. The former approach, however, emphasizes the consistency with which certain themes were reiterated. To the great tradition in English medicine, the English mind was reckoned fundamental. Sir D'Arcy Power, consulting surgeon at Bart's, found the virility and particularity of English medicine to lie in the quality of the 'English mind [that] has always preferred facts to theories and it is not surprising therefore that English physicians have been very careful to verify their diagnoses by constant visits to the post-mortem room.'[43] As the Oxford physician Alexander Gibson, observed in a discussion of a work of John Locke's on medicine:

> It has somewhere been said that the British doctor excels in practice rather than in science; it is true that most of our great figures in Medicine, Sydenham, Hunter, Radcliffe, Jenner, Bright, have been great practitioners, but a few of them only have been men of science. They were, however, the outstanding figures of a common type and have shown a sanity and breadth of outlook, a directness in method, and a skill in action which have made a lasting name for their art.[44]

Tommy Horder expressed a similar sentiment explicitly linking these mental qualities to the survival of civilization:

> For the doctor there can be no left or right. For him there is only expert knowledge and a rooted adherence to truth and horse-sense. That formidable British mixture is our equipment in what is perhaps the most lethal fight that we, as individuals and as a nation, have ever had to face: the fight for stability of mind and body in the interest not only of national existence but of the existence of civilization.[45]

More subtly, Gibson noted: 'Gardeners and ploughmen, rather than the profound philosophers, are the makers of fair gardens and fruitful fields.'[46] No doubt his readers knew that the English made the fairest gardens as well as producing the flowers of medicine. '[T]he ranks of the famous physicians' said John Ryle in an essay on 'The Physician as Naturalist' of 1931, 'are chiefly filled with men belonging to the observational school.'[47] If Hippocrates and William Osler count as honorary Englishmen, aside from Laennec and Trousseau, eight of the ten physicians named as examples of this school were English. Not a single German (or Scot) was mentioned. It is notable that what gave the English mind its peculiar qualities was scarcely ever addressed in this literature. Certainly only on the rarest occasions was racial essence invoked, as when Sir St Clair Thomson noted that Lister was a "'true-born Englishman.'" None of the nations which make up our United Kingdom can claim he had any "'Celtic fringe'".[48]

The development of the quintessential English medicine made by this mind was chronicled by a number of these authors especially D'Arcy Power. In 1930, Power's *Medicine in the British Isles* appeared. In the preface, dated 1930 from London, England, he noted how the powerful corporations of London, Edinburgh and Dublin had exercised considerable influence on the development of medicine and '[t]he history of medicine, therefore, in *this country* is mainly a history of its corporate bodies.' Although Power gave a generous and learned account of medicine in all parts of he British Isles, recurrently England seemed to stand for the area as a whole. For example, in the chapter 'Some Masters of British Medicine', William Harvey was accounted 'one of the greatest masters in English medicine.' Yet when attempting to adjudicate between the greatness of the Hunter brothers he could not decide who was 'the greater master in medicine.'[49] The point is that Power did not recognize a Scottish medicine any more than T. S. Eliot recognized a Scottish literature.[50] The Celts were simply to rejoice in a national culture (English literature or medicine) to which they had contributed. Similarly, elsewhere, describing specialism, Power observed, '[d]ermatology in England began with Dr. Robert Willan' but no mention was made of dermatology elsewhere.[51]

Bizarre though may seem, the English tradition in medicine began with Hippocrates, not least because Sydenham, 'the English Hippocrates' of the seventeenth century, was deemed to have thoroughly comprehended the ancient physician's mind and method. This had been possible because of Sydenham's own down-to-earth, open, non-speculative, independent, empirical mind. Ryle noted Hippocrates 'was literally the founder of the observational method' and that Sydenham had 'faithfully followed the Hippocratic system.'[52] Gibson could scarcely have made a clearer statement of the importance of the tradition and his own place within it, for he published John Locke's manuscript fragment 'De Arte Medica' with 'an attempt to expand' Locke's thoughts. In a small volume, handsomely produced by the Clarendon Press, Gibson attested to the continuity of twentieth-century English medical practice with that of Locke and Sydenham and in turn with Hippocrates. Gibson's expansion of Locke was a discourse on the medical art and the impossibility of its reduction to a science. Science could only supplement art, 'the principles of … [which] are unchanged, and … the method of attack against disease is the same now as in the days of Hippocrates.' Carefully tutored experience taught the art and, as Sydenham said, 'our art is not to be better learned than by its exercise and use.' Gibson's text created continuity in the history of the medical art between antiquity and the seventeenth century by ascribing identity to the knowledge and practices of Sydenham and Hippocrates. For instance, the statement that Sydenham gave the advice that sometimes it was good practice not to intervene medically was followed by the observation that: 'Hippocrates also knew well that the body tends to overcome disease.'[53]

Sir George Newman's *Interpreters of Nature* appeared in 1927. Chapter two (written in 1924) was devoted to 'Thomas Sydenham, Reformer of *English* Medicine'. Entirely appropriately, such a reformer was born in a manor-house standing in the idyllic English countryside. Writing in a mode which, as Michael Bartholomew shows in his chapter on H. V. Morton, was of immense popular appeal in these years, Newman began: 'In the soft and pleasant country which lies to the west of Dorchester, and which has been made familiar to us in the Wessex novels of Thomas Hardy, there stands a grey old manor-house with gables, porch, and mullioned windows.' Newman described how Sydenham studied at Oxford and learned much from Bacon but '[a]bove all … he walked alone.' Newman linked Sydenham's approach to his Puritan independence through rural metaphor: 'Ploughing his lonely furrow, discarding tradition', said Newman, Sydenham 'bends himself to his great task.' His 'straightforwardness' allowed him to see 'that to follow the principles of Hippocrates meant reality and thoroughness.' He pursued 'the scientific method of observation and induction.' Thus Newman constructed Sydenham as the true disciple of Hippocrates *because of* Sydenham's Englishness. Sydenham, said Newman, was 'the embodiment of the two immortal ideas of Hippocrates – love of craft and love of man.' His 'apprehension of the scope and function of the medical practitioner … gave to English Medicine an enduring foundation.' There was a sense too in which national identities were conflated for 'Sydenham was a Coan', that is spiritually from Cos, Hippocrates' birthplace, and thus home of the sect considered, at this time, to have produced the observational books of the Hippocratic corpus as opposed to the Cnidians who supposedly supplied the classificatory works.[54] Although this was a judgement about medical traditions it was presumably not hard for an Englishman to consider there was a special kinship between his country and Greece.

If Hippocrates was the spiritual father of the English tradition and Sydenham its earthly one, it was the clinicians of the eighteenth century who, for Newman, became 'the successors of Thomas Sydenham as he himself followed Hippocrates.'[55] Usually invoked next in the tradition was John Hunter (and occasionally William), but Hunter was a Scot and a surgeon and not primarily a clinician and seems to have presented minor difficulties for the tradition makers, much as Charles Dickens did for Leavis. Perhaps of all the doctors admitted to the tradition it was Hunter's pupil Edward Jenner who was most clearly shaped into the sort of doctor the patricians admired. He was, all agreed, a country gentleman who rode to hounds and wrote poetry for recreation. He lived, a family man with his servants, in an organic, rural, patriarchal community where he dutifully did his rounds, serving his patients who in turn felt and showed gratitude. Finally he was an inquisitive, acute observer, a great natural historian; a pure empirical mind unfettered by theory. He stood for the England and the medicine that was being lost. Of course Jenner was not made that way between the wars, a Romantic Jenner had already been crafted in the nineteenth century, but this Jenner was ready made for inter-war nostalgia. What could be added to the myth was that his achievements had been possible without sophisticated science and technology.

In Power's edited *British Masters of Medicine* of 1936, Sir Buckston Browne recorded that Jenner 'came of sound English clerical stock.'[56] After noting that he was born in Berkeley, Gloucestershire, F. Dawtrey Drewitt observed that it was 'an ideal spot for one destined to be a devoted lover of the English countryside' since it was a 'little old town, standing on a gentle eminence, with its feudal castle, [that] overlooked the rich pasture lands of the Vale of Berkeley and the river Severn.'[57] In 1935, Sir William Hale-White, consulting physician to Guy's Hospital, set the scene of Jenner's life, conjuring up a past England through one which was still present:

> Half-way between Bristol and Gloucester, a country lane turns west from the main road. After going about two miles along it you reach Berkeley, once a town, now a characteristic English village, peaceful, unspoiled by motor traffic and still just as it was two centuries ago. Adjacent to the east end of the village is Berkeley Castle, the seat of the Earls of Berkeley ...[58]

It is not clear by what form of transport Hale-White reached Berkeley. Newman, invoking English town and village names, related that '[a]fter schooldays at Wotton-under Edge and Cirencester' came Jenner's apprenticeship. 'The boy', said Buckston Browne, 'was devoted to natural history from his childhood.'[59] 'Before he was nine', recorded Drewitt, 'he had made a collection of dormice nests.'[60] In his manhood, stated Newman, he 'lived the happy and busy life of a country practitioner.'[61] He was, Browne told his readers, 'a modest unassuming country doctor.'[62] Newman cited Edward Gardner, Jenner's friend, on his appearance, 'everything about him showed the man intent and serious and well prepared to meet the duties of his calling … He was dressed in a blue coat and yellow buttons, buckskins, well-polished jockey boots and handsome silver spurs; and he carried a smart whip with a silver handle.'[63] He escaped, said Drewitt (who also noticed the well-polished boots), from 'the smokey air of London.' He thus did not have to learn 'that indifference to neighbours … which comes to all who have to struggle everyday in a crowd.'[64] He practised medicine, said Hale-White, 'thoroughly happy, riding through the beautiful country' and 'led the happy life of the perfect country doctor.'[65] Buckston Browne, after repeating Gardner's description of the jockey boots, noted that Jenner was 'a clean-shaven, good-looking man.'[66] Horder simply referred to this 'blue-eyed, handsome, easy, almost debonair Saxon, this West Country doctor, spending his days, booted and spurred, in riding to hounds, and his evenings in writing light verse.'[67] Browne, weaving his text with references to Jane Austen and George Eliot (the other two authors in Leavis's tradition), noticed in a portrait of Jenner his 'clear blue eyes' and 'well-formed right hand.' He told his readers that Jenner 'loved his flute and violin' and that Jenner's friends thought, 'had he cared, he might have become a distinguished poet.' In addition to all this, he had 'insatiable curiosity.'[68] He 'delighted', recounted Hale-White, 'in landscape gardening.'[69] Jenner's skills as a naturalist were stressed by all the biographers as being the basis of his work on smallpox. It was his 'enquiring mind' that enabled him to describe 'cow-pox as he saw it in Nature', said Newman.[70] Browne noted that Jenner had 'nothing to assist him save his simple surgery and the farmsteads around him.'[71] This latter observation signals one of the many reasons why Jenner was important to these men: without laboratory science or complex technology, a clinician-naturalist had, they said, discovered a means of preventing one of the scourges of humankind. Another reason why Jenner figured so highly in the great tradition was his embodiment of what, for the patricians, was a great English virtue. Drewitt noted that it was Jenner's 'thoughtful common sense' that enabled him to succeed with vaccination.[72]

John Hunter merits less attention than Jenner here, although his accommodation into the great tradition invites inspection. Hunter, said Newman, pursuing some familiar themes of the inter-war years, was 'primarily and in the true sense, a naturalist' and an 'explorer of the unity of the human body' who relied on 'the recuperative forces of Nature.'[73] What had to be negotiated was the fact that Hunter was neither English nor a gentleman. This was done by making him a natural genius, a rough diamond that educational institutions would have corrupted. Horder described him as a 'pertinacious and persistent Celt, raw and rugged in body and in mind, but possessed of a "searching and impetuous soul," lit with a constant and consuming flame of inquiry after knowledge and more knowledge.'[74] It was to Hunter's advantage, recorded Newman, that 'not being a bookman', he was able to impress the next generation with the necessity of personal observation.[75] A genteel English education would have ruined him. 'Six weeks in Oxford were enough for John', wrote Sir Arthur Keith. Hunter 'saved his original genius by his timely escape.'[76] Suitably accommodated, however, the naturalist Hunter could stand in the great tradition. Concluding his chapter on Hunter and his contemporaries and pupils, Newman summarized the ways in which they had 'moved *English* Medicine forward.'[77]

The importance and insularity of this English medical historiography is, ironically, confirmed by one of its critics who in many other ways is easily accommodated among the patricians. Francis Crookshank, born in 1873, had appointments at various London hospitals and lived in Wimpole Street. His writings are packed with historical material and lament the rise of specialism in medicine and the disappearance of the 'whole' patient in the name of laboratory entities. Thus far there is nothing to distinguish him from other patrician physicians. But Crookshank was learned in French and German philosophy and literature. He introduced the psychology of Alfred Adler into Britain, and wrote a pamphlet, *Individual Psychology and Nietzsche*.[78] The unfamiliarity of his approach in the English context can be measured by his obituarist's remark that, 'he displayed unusual erudition and a subtlety of argument which more than occasionally defeated its own purpose.'[79] Rather than suffering from too much speculation, medicine for Crookshank was *not* sufficiently theorized to be a science. He said:

Such ordered knowledge of the phenomena of disease and the relations between them as would, in the terms of another celebrated definition, "constitute a true Science of Medicine" is not to be furnished by mere empirical observation: by "passive perceptions", that is however ordered and recorded; but by that process of reasoning concerning the "passive perceptions" in which alone, in the opinion of Plato, approved by Berkeley, does Science consist.

Historically this meant 'we arrive at the paradox ... that, when in the sixteenth century Medicine was, as we should say, less "scientific" than to-day, Medicine was indeed, as it now is not, a Science in very truth.' Crookshank denounced the philosophy that upheld 'the "reality" of causes, actions, forces and laws' with 'its staggering reliance on the something called Baconian or inductive logic.' He had no time for English empiricism (Bacon was much praised by the patricians). 'It is no paradox to say', he wrote, that 'just so far as Medicine has followed "the way pointed out by Bacon" and has freed herself from the "taint" of metaphysics, so far indeed has she ... ceased to remain a Science.' Medicine at present was 'a mass of empiricism, partly leavened by realist rationalisation.'[80] Anyone suggesting that medicine might proceed in this manner of course might be questioning the value of the labours of some of those central to the great tradition. This Crookshank was prepared to do. Although praising Sydenham, he condemned his reversion to 'scholastic realism' in his teaching 'that diseases are to be classified, as are the plants and flowers of the field.'[81] Crookshank owned that his own approach would 'admit in medical discussions the need for definitions – in John Hunter's opinion, of all things most damnable ... Yet, once the need for definition is admitted the whole airy edifice of a purely descriptive account of the Universe ... dissolves into the empyrean.' Crookshank's vision was remarkably relativist. He remarked of the ancients: 'They thought differently to us, truly. Did they think less adequately to their occasions than we do?' and he found space not only for Hippocrates in his discussion but for Galen also, a figure much traduced by writers such as Horder. 'We recognise Coans to-day amongst our wisest and best-loved physicians', said Crookshank, 'those whom we consult ourselves, as we would Hippocrates or Heberden. But our Cnidians and our Galens are amongst our most successful and renowned teachers.'[82] Ironically, Horder was renowned as possibly the greatest medical teacher of the age.

The great tradition in English medicine was kept alive for various purposes, most immediately the defense of the individual, generalist clinician. It had wider import too, in a world of cultural decay and social disintegration these men at the head of their profession said they had wider responsibilities to English society, in much the same way Leavis knew he had the responsibility for keeping his great tradition alive, not simply as good English literature but as part of a society which, if it valued that tradition, was, in some way, a healthy one. It is notable that the late youth of all the patricians (as was Leavis's) was spent in the era of gradualist reform spawned by New Liberalism.[83] It is their attachment to the gradualism, individualism and organicism of this creed which distinguishes them rather than any common allegiance to a political party, for their overt political sympathies varied quite widely, especially when Ryle's rather left-wing views are taken into account. The doctor's great tradition – at least when Jenner was summoned up – stipulated that medicine was best practised in a paternalist world of reciprocal duties and obligations, the doctor taking a wide role in setting moral examples and taking part in the wider life of society. The eighteenth-century doctors (including Jenner) described by Newman not only 'moved English Medicine forward' they made a 'contribution to culture and literature.'[84] In their combination of dedicated professional and civilized human being, the doctors declared themselves as successors not only to the medical tradition but to a priestly one. In the thirties Horder wrote that the doctor 'must needs be a priest as well as a physician... . [and] if the doctor was of necessity a humanist in former generations, it behoves him ... to be all the more a humanist to-day.'[85] 'The doctor', he noted in another address, 'is in the privileged position of the Almighty.'[86] The physician, said Ryle, is expected 'to combine in his person the attributes of scientist, healer priest and prophet.'[87] Similarly, Langdon Brown explained, the doctor was a very powerful figure, 'we cannot even observe a patient', he said, 'without altering him for good or evil.'[88]

The physician besides having an obligation to the patient had duties to society at large. This sense of the doctor's role was expressed by Horder in 1924: 'Medical men are citizens as well as doctors, and the medical profession has greater privileges and deeper obligations than are represented by the daily round of visits to sick persons.'[89] As Ryle observed in 1931: 'There is probably no servant of the community of whom a greater degree of omniscience is demanded, or upon whom a graver responsibility in respect of personal and sometimes social guidance is, from time to time, imposed.'[90] Two years later, Wilfred Trotter (a marginal patrician) said to University College Hospital students that this was a time when it was 'no longer possible to conceal the wholly unique importance of medicine for the very existence of social life.' An 'evolutionary course' had put medicine in the small class of professions that 'can still be called jobs for men.'[91].

These were not idle observations. These doctors *did* take seriously their perception that, as professionals, they carried the important burden of making and keeping English society healthy, literally and metaphorically. These men were active in all sorts of rationalist causes, speaking at meetings and lending their names to progressive movements. Horder, for example, was president of the Family Planning Association, the Smoke Abatement Society and the Cremation Society among others. Eugenics in particular claimed a great deal of their time (Horder had been President of the Society). Crookshank wrote a text on descent and race, *The Mongol in our Midst*, that went through at least three editions. With respect to eugenics the concerns of the patricians with the growth of mass culture appear in a rather different light. Although cinemas and places of popular entertainment provoked moralising of the Leavisite variety, they were also viewed by medical people and others as places were inappropriate liaisons were contracted, especially among the young. That is, they were foci for spreading venereal disease and contributors to national degeneration.[92] A major dimension of the patricians' activities was educational. They broadcast on the radio and spoke at working men's colleges. Educating the citizen in medical matters had wider consequences than an improvement of individual health. It promoted the 'public happiness', as Horder put it. Knowledge of the causes of heath would alert the citizen to the unhealthy dimensions of modern society. The patricians' sense of participatory citizenship, as described by Abigail Beach in her chapter, was marked, as was so much they pronounced upon, by, according to time, place and matter, a mixture of optimism, concern and disdain. Crookshank observed, 'nothing is more deplorable than the resort to our hospitals of young men and women, painfully eager for a diagnosis and a remedy, who, by spending less than they do on an evening's amusement at the "Pictures", could acquire a tooth-brush, a sufficiency of Epsom salts, and perfect health.'[93]

The patricians were not alone in the medical profession in considering they had a central role in the promotion of the public health and happiness, but other doctors who likewise perceived themselves to have similar duties saw the ends being achieved by rather different means. For instance, it was widely agreed in Britain in the first half of the century that the nutrition of the nation fell below all that might be desired. The attitude of Walter Morley Fletcher, former experimental physiologist turned Secretary of the Medical Research Council, was that fundamental research into the biochemistry of food was the solution. Fletcher recollected that in 1914 he met a government minister who observed 'well doctor I don't hold with research. If we want to stop disease we must give the people better grub and less dirt.' Fletcher said he agreed and added that he wished the minister 'could tell me what better grub was and what less dirt was – for I knew no way of finding out those two things except by persistent scientific research work.'[94] On the other hand, Horder who said he preferred 'the word "food" to "nutrition"' (shades of 'common sense') observed '[l]ook after the accessibility of food and nutrition will look after itself.'[95]

The patricians were the survivors of the collapse of many of the values and institutions of a liberal civilization. Put another way, almost everywhere they looked the free individual of bourgeois ideology seemed enslaved to forces beyond his control. Yet they were also the inheritors of scientific rationalism and regarded themselves as the custodians of a civilized way of life with a duty to sustain and enrich it. Their response to the crisis years in which they lived was a cocktail of despair and hope, faith in progress and nostalgia. Expressions of pessimism and optimism varied with the man, the occasion and the time. The England of doctor Jenner's jockey boots was the product of alarm and of utopianism. It embodied a general alarm about an imagined England disappearing under mass culture and also more tangible concerns about the threat to their patrician values and lifestyle and clinical individualism posed by a mechanizing medical world.

Acknowledgments

For comments on an earlier draft I should like to thank Michael Neve.

Notes

1 See for example D. L. LeMahieu, *A Culture for Democracy: Mass Communication and the Cultivated Mind in Britain Between the Wars*, Oxford, 1988; John Carey, *The Intellectuals and the Masses: Pride and Prejudice Among the Literary Intelligentsia, 1880-1939*, London, 1992; Francis Mulhern, *The Moment of Scrutiny*, London, 1979.

2 See Christopher Lawrence and George Weisz, 'Medical Holism: the context', in *Greater than the Parts: Holism in Biomedicine 1920-1950*, Christopher Lawrence and George Weisz (eds), New York, 1998, pp. 3–22.

3 Christopher Lawrence, 'A Tale of Two Sciences: Bedside and Bench in Twentieth-Century Britain' *Medical History*, 43 (1999): 421–49; Christopher Lawrence, 'Still Incommunicable: Clinical Holists and Medical Knowledge in Interwar Britain' in *Greater than the Parts*, Lawrence and Weisz (eds), pp. 94–111.

4 See Benedict Anderson, *Imagined Communities: Reflections on the Origin and Spread of Nationalism*, London, 1983; Robert Colls and Philip Dodd (eds), *Englishness: Politics and Culture 1880-1920*, London, 1986.

5 See Stephan Collini, *Public Moralists: Political Thought and Intellectual Life in Britain 1850-1930*, Oxford, 1993.

6 F. R. Leavis, *The Great Tradition*, London, 1973, pp. 11, 17.

7 Karl Mannheim, 'Conservative Thought', in *Essays on Sociology and Social Psychology*, London, 1953, pp. 74–164.

8 Typically found in 'Mass Civilization and Minority Culture' [1930] in F. R. Leavis, *For Continuity* [1933], New York, 1968, pp. 13–46.

9 Mulhern, *Moment of Scrutiny*, 32. On the elitism of the Scrutineers see Ian Mackillop, *F. R. Leavis, A Life in Criticism*, London, 1995.

10 Walter Langdon-Brown, *Thus We Are Men*, London, 1938, pp. 179–80.

11 For the historical and historiographical dimensions of this subject see E. P. Thomson, 'The Peculiarities of the English', in E. P. Thomson, *The Poverty of Theory*, London, 1978, pp. 35–92.

12 See Gareth Stedman Jones, 'History: the Poverty of Empiricism' in *Ideology in Social Science: Readings in Critical Social Theory*, Robin Blackburn (ed.), London 1972.

13 Collini, *Public Moralists*, 358.

14 Cited in John Harley Warner, *Against the Spirit of System: The French Impulse in Nineteenth-century American Medicine*, Princeton, 1998, 75.

15 Thomas Horder, 'The Approach to Medicine', *Lancet*, (1939): i, 913–917 at 916.

16   See John V. Pickstone, 'Past and Present Knowledges in the Practice of the History of Science', *History of Science*, 33 (1995): 203–24; *idem*, 'Ways of knowing: Towards a Historical Sociology of Science, Technology and Medicine', *British Journal for the History of Science*, 26 (1993): 433–58.

17   Samuel Gee, *Auscultation and Percussion*, London, 1893.

18   Samuel Gee, *Medical Lectures and Aphorisms*, London, 1902, 213.

19   Thomas Horder, 'The Influence of Radiology upon our Conceptions of Disease', *Proceedings of the Royal Society of Medicine*, 17, parts I & II (1924): 64–76.

20   Gee, *Medical Lectures and Aphorisms*, 209.

21   Henry Dale, 'Scientific Method in Medical Research', *British Medical Journal* (1950): ii, 1185–90 at 1187.

22   Gee, *Medical Lectures*, 4th edn, London, 1915, 363.

23   *Ibid.*, 1st edn, 232

24   'Clinical Aphorisms from Dr. Gee's Wards', collected and edited by Thomas J. Horder, in *Saint Bartholomew's Hospital Reports*, Samuel West and W. J. Walsham (eds), London, 1897, pp. 29–59.

25   Thomas Horder, 'Medicine and Old Ethicks', *British Medical Journal* (1924): i, 485–9 at 488.

26   Harold J. Cook, 'Good Advice and Little Medicine: The Professional Authority of Early Modern English Physicians', *Journal of British Studies*, 33 (1994): 1–31.

27   On the "Great", see Geoffrey Bourne, *We Met at Bart's: the Autobiography of a Physician*, London, 1963, 20.

28   See Christopher Lawrence, 'Incommunicable Knowledge: Science, Technology and the Clinical Art in Britain 1850-1914', *Journal of Contemporary History*, 20 (1985): 503–20.

29   Thomas Horder, *Health and a Day*, London, 1936, 30.

30   Eric Hobsbawm, *The Age of Extremes. A History of the World, 1914-1991*, New York, 1996, 106.

31   Langdon-Brown, *Thus We Are Men*, pp. 164–5. I am not agreeing with Keynes that in the pre-war years observers really did see a 'certain and permanent world', rather that, from the perspective of the thirties, it looked as though they did. Anxieties about European instability and the threat of the masses was often intense before 1914. See Daniel Pick, *War Machine: the Rationalisation of Slaughter in the Modern Age*, New Haven, 1993, especially chapters 9 and 10. Conversly the war itself was important nourishment of a vision of a previously arcadian England. See Paul Fussell, *The Great War and Modern Memory*, London, 1975.

32   Francis Crookshank, *The Mongol in our Midst*, 3rd edn, London, 1931, 35.

33   Langdon-Brown, *Thus We Are men*, 27.

34   Horder, *Health and a Day*, 70

35   Langdon-Brown, *Thus We Are Men*, 13.

36   Horder, *Health and a Day*, 69.

37   Crookshank, *Mongol in our Midst*, pp. 107, 179.

38   A. J. P. Taylor, *English History 1914-1945*, Harmondsworth, 1970, 383. In Germany, Georg von Bulow, drawing on Oswald Spengler's theories, observed "The West will decline when there are no more servants". Cited in Fritz K. Ringer, *The Decline of the German Mandarins: The German Academic Community, 1890-1933*, Cambridge, Mass., 1969, 223.

39   Langdon-Brown, *Thus we are Men*, 237–8.

40   Lawrence, 'Still Incommunicable'.

41   Sir George Newman, *Interpreters of Nature*, London, 1927, 151. Emphasis in original. On Newman see Steve Sturdy, 'Hippocrates and State Medicine: George Newman Outlines the Founding Policy of the Ministry of Health' in *Greater than the Parts*, Lawrence and Weisz (eds), pp. 112–34.

42   Horder, *Health and a Day*, 96. Emphasis in original.

43   Sir D'Arcy Power, *Medicine in the British Isles*, New York, 1930, 63.

44   Alexander George Gibson, *The Physician's Art*, Oxford, 1933, 28.

45   Horder, *Health and a Day*, 53.

46   Gibson, *Physician's Art*, 11.

47   John Ryle, *The Natural History of Disease*, London, 1936, 7.

48   Sir St Clair Thomson, 'Joseph Lister' in *British Masters of Medicine*, Sir D'Arcy Power (ed.), London, 1936, 138.

49   Power, *Medicine*, Preface (emphasis mine), pp. 59, 61.

50   See Philip Dodd, 'Englishness and the National Culture', in *Englishness*, Colls and Dodd (eds), pp. 1–28, 12.

51   Power, *Medicine*, pp. 45.

52   Ryle, *Natural History*, pp. 419, 8.

53   Gibson, *Physicians Art*, Title page, pp. 35, 37, 110.

54   Newman, *Interpreters*, chapter two title, emphasis mine, pp. 41, 46, 50, 66, 53, 51.

55   *Ibid.*, 120.

56   Sir Buckston Browne, 'Edward Jenner' in *British Masters of Medicine*, Sir D'Arcy Power (ed.), pp. 64–70 at 66.

57   F. Dawtrey Drewitt, *The Life of Edward Jenner*, London, 1933, 1. Slightly older than the other patricians, Drewitt (b.1848), a Fellow of the College of Physicians, retired early on a private income and devoted himself to natural history.

58   Sir William Hale-White, *Great Doctors of the Nineteenth Century*,

London, 1935, 1.

59 Buckston Browne, 'Edward Jenner', 66.

60 Drewitt, *Jenner*, 2.

61 Newman, *Interpreters*, 146.

62 Buckston Browne, 'Edward Jenner', 65.

63 Newman, *Interpreters*, 146, citing Edward Gardner in John Baron, *Life of Edward Jenner*, 2 vols, London, 1827, Vol. I, 15.

64 Drewitt, *Jenner*, pp. 4–5.

65 White, *Great Doctors*, pp. 4, 20.

66 Browne, 'Jenner', 66.

67 Horder, *Health and a Day*, 91.

68 Browne, 'Jenner', pp. 65, 66.

69 Hale-White, *Great Doctors*, 6.

70 Newman, *Interpreters*, 148.

71 Browne, 'Jenner', 65.

72 Drewitt, *Jenner*, 135.

73 Newman, *Interpreters*, 118, 119.

74 Horder, *Health and a Day*, 91.

75 Newman, *Interpreters*, 120

76 Sir Arthur Keith, 'John Hunter', in *British Masters*, Power (ed.), pp. 42–51, 45. Keith, formerly a practising physician, was for many years Conservator of the Hunterian Museum. He moved easily among the patricians.

77 Newman, *Interpreters*, 149. Emphasis mine.

78 Francis Crookshank, *Individual Psychology and Nietzsche*, London, 1933.

79 *Lancet*, (1933): ii, 1066.

80 Francis Crookshank, 'The Relation of History and Philosophy to Medicine', in Charles Green Cumston, *An Introduction to the History of Medicine*, London, 1926, pp. xv–xxxii at pp. xvii, xx, xxiii, xxvii.

81 Francis Crookshank, 'Science and Health' in *Science and Civilization*, F. S. Marvin (ed.), London, 1923, pp. 247–278 at 255.

82 Crookshank, 'The Relation', pp. xxii, xxx, xxxi.

83 Michael Freeden, *The New Liberalism: an Ideology of Social Reform*, Oxford, 1978.

84 Newman, *Interpreters*, 149

85 Horder, *Health and a Day*, 35.

86 *Ibid.*, 179.

87 Ryle, *Natural History*, 2.

88 Walter Langdon-Brown, 'The Return to Aesculapius,' *Lancet* (1933): ii, 821–22.

89 Horder, 'Medicine and Old Ethicks', 485.

90   Ryle, *Natural History*, 1.
91   Wilfred Trotter, *The Collected Papers of Wilfred Trotter*, Oxford 1941.
     Trotter acknowledged the traditional phrase now included women.
     He was marginal in that his commitment to medical science seemed
     to contain no hint of patrician nostalgia.
92   See Roger Davidson, *Dangerous Liaisons: A Social History of VD in
     Twentieth Century Scotland*, Amsterdam, 2000. No doubt Davidson's
     observations at this level of generality on the Scottish scene apply to
     England.
93   Crookshank, 'Science and Health', pp. 271–2.
94   Maisie Fletcher, *The Bright Countenance: A Personal Biography of
     Walter Morley Fletcher*, London, 1957, 179.
95   Horder, *Health and a Day*, 152.

4

'A combative sense of duty': Englishness and the Scientists

Anna-K. Mayer

... if he had been endowed with private means he would still have written copiously from a combative sense of duty and of the obligation laid on every man to proclaim the truth as far as he can see it.

One member of the intellectual aristocracy about another[1]

In the first half of the twentieth century, British scientists have repeatedly complained that they felt excluded from the narrow circle of a traditional liberal-humanistic élite. Thus, during the neglect-of-science-debate (1916–18), E. Ray Lankester led the battle against the humanist insistence that scientific subjects were not a suitable curricular staple for the development of 'personality' and the training of 'character', goals and achievements which it was the perceived task of English national education to foster.[2] G. H. Hardy observed one afternoon in the early thirties that 'when we hear about "intellectuals" nowadays, it doesn't include people like me and J. J. Thomson and Rutherford'.[3] In 1945, Joseph Needham felt he had to insist that an 'S' be included in UNESCO, for unless 'the word science appears in the title of the Organization', men of science would feel that the United Nations Educational and Cultural Organization had 'little to do with them.'[4] In the fifties, finally, C. P. Snow summed up the experience of decades in the expression 'the two cultures', which he made the theme of his notorious Rede lecture.[5]

With the older tradition of what Frank Turner has described as 'public science', such commentary and observations had two things in common: first, the perception that the scientific enterprise faced an uphill battle in a scientifically illiterate world and second, the expansionist hope for a greater influence of science in the world.[6] To take scientists' public statements about their enterprise at face value, however, does not necessarily make for good history, as David Edgerton has shown for the case of the relations of science and war.[7] Also, as he has repeatedly insisted, twentieth-century Britain was and is both a military nation and a scientific culture (indeed, many of the chapters in this book testify to this), and the British twentieth-century intelligentsia has at least in part recruited itself from the ranks of scientists.[8] By complaining that they felt excluded from an élite that refused to acknowledge the achievements of science as a contribution to true national culture, scientists may have been constructing their own instrumental myth.

One wants to wholeheartedly agree with Edgerton and yet there is no denying the historical fact that the relations between science and Englishness are complex. While the scientific giants of the seventeenth century – 'the century of genius' – have long held a place in national memory, it is also true that Britain has a tradition of both tacit and public denial that science and its practitioners contribute to that quintessential 'Englishness' which is said to sustain the country's national character. Englishness was commonly associated with the values and ideals of a liberal-humanistic education, which in turn has been linked to the political ideal of humanist republicanism and its conception of 'virtue' as an active component of public order.[9] In particular, Englishness has been associated with the notion that English national virtue is rooted in and incubated in country life. The celebrated 'English genius of liberty', that is, the maintenance of social peace through the exercise of individual virtue and compromise rather than excessive governmental force, was said to be embodied in a particular way of life; it was imparted, not in lessons, but in participation in that way of life, and if any form of education could claim to transmit it, this education was liberal-humanistic, for such education fostered the development of character.

In the decades between 1880-1920, much creative energy was dedicated to the invention of an Englishness epitomized by 'the rustic ideal', an ideal that invoked the wholesomeness of country ways, and with it all the personal and civic virtues embodied in village life.[10] From the onset of the First World War, science and technology became notoriously equated with Prussian statism and with modernism in general, while (it has been suggested) 'for the British this was a war to preserve a world', 'a war about values, about civilization, about sportsmanship, and especially about the relationship of the future to the past', indeed, 'a war to preserve and restore.'[11] On another note, to fare well (or to fare at all) in an Oxford common room in the twenties and early thirties, a scientist was required to display polymathic inclinations; adaptation, therefore, was one-sided and clearly favoured liberal-humanistic traditions.[12] In 1938, when private and public expenditure on scientific and industrial research already topped £10 million (and was steadily increasing), George Orwell was composing a declaration of love for traditional England.[13] In the same year, an assembly of fourteen luminaries from the intellectual élite produced *The English Genius. A Survey of English Achievement and Character.* There was not a single scientist among the contributors, whose statements largely summoned up images of an Englishness epitomised by life-in-the-country-parish. These images were constituted wholly by memory, a memory so highly selective that Britain's scientific achievement did not figure at all, while its industrial past assumed an episodic character: '[d]uring the last century transitory circumstances made England the workshop of the world, and we had to adapt ourselves to that not very congenial part ... But in reality we are neither very covetous nor very industrious ...'[14] In the traditional humanists' perception, none of these episodes, not even 'the post-war revolutionary upheavals', could change human nature, nor could they change true Englishness. Moreover, it was impossible for a scientist or engineer to dispute that the two were inextricably linked, for, in the eyes of the liberal humanist, scientific or technological professions did not qualify their practitioners to commentate on human nature, its fundamental needs or on the condition of the nation. Scientists, then, still competed for intellectual and moral authority in a culture which even in the judgement of A. J. P. Taylor remained morally Christian, and in which even those who favoured a social revolution maintained a highly critical attitude towards the numerous manifestations of a modern, scientific civilization.[15]

This chapter takes a look at scientists' relations to Englishness by examining how they reacted when confronted with élite preconceptions about both national character and the study of nature. I focus on a public incident that occurred at the annual meeting of the British Association for the Advancement of Science (BAAS) at Leeds in 1927 where the suggestion was made that mankind might profit from scientific research being discontinued for a decade. The Leeds incident gave scientists as a group an opportunity to articulate the relations of their enterprise to civilization and also to national culture. In Britain, the question of the social relations of science goes back to the nineteenth-century phenomenon of 'public science' briefly referred to above and beyond that to Francis Bacon and the foundation of the Royal Society.[16] However, a major phase of this concern began, as Neil Wood and William McGucken have argued, in 1931–2.[17] This phase is associated with the so-called 'social relations of science' movement in which key members of the scientific establishment opted to address the issue of whether science had a particular relevance for (potentially even a special duty towards) the social body as a whole.[18] The Leeds episode I am concerned with here pre-dates this movement. This paper, then, looks at attitudes displayed before it (briefly) became almost normal for scientists in general to reflect on their responsibilities towards the moral, social and political order within which they and their work were situated.

Of Moral Lags

On Sunday, September 4 1927, the famous rationalist anthropologist Sir Arthur Keith donned his doctor's gown and joined the civic procession to the parish church of Leeds, the town chosen for the annual meeting of the BAAS, to attend the Association Service. Flanked by Sir Oliver Lodge and Sir William Bragg (a predecessor and his successor in the presidential chair) and backed by 'leaders of science from all parts of the world', Sir Arthur occupied a place of honour in the crowded church. He was as yet unaware that fate was about to regale the Association with an opportunity to publicly dispute the place of science in civilization, for within less than an hour, science's assembled luminaries were told in the sermon that in order to save civilization, science must take a ten year holiday.

This suggestion came from a member of a class of men whose national irrelevance H. G. Wells had recently summed up with the pithy comment: 'the Bishops, socially so much in evidence, are intellectually in hiding.'[19] Essentially an invitation for bishops to take a permanent holiday in the name of human progress, Wells' observation also emphasized, in the rationalist manner, that such progress could be regulated automatically, that is, through the machinations of a meritocracy of scientific expertise. This debate itself was not new; and with it continued the controversy over the question of which professions were most intimately involved in determining the nature of genuine progress and, most importantly, which of them would be credited with the competence to bring it about. While no one would have disputed the contributions made by science and technology to material welfare, the idea that scientists truly personified human progressiveness by no means reflected the consensus of England's intellectual aristocracy as a whole, and the representatives of liberal educational ideals, Christians and secularists alike, found little incentive to go with Wells on this issue. In 1916, the Oxford classicist and educationalist Richard Livingstone had publicly disputed that scientists could be credited with any powers of moral judgement when he summed up 'science' as an enterprise that failed to 'make her followers good *guides* in regions outside her own confined kingdom', and (he argued) the biographies of scientific men confirmed this: a reader should not be 'amazed to find them uttering preposterous judgements on matters which lie outside [science]'.[20] At the time, none lesser than T. S. Eliot, one of the chief exponents of English literary criticism in inter-war Britain, supported this view, even though he cast it in the more subtle tones of the gently mocking critic: 'I do not deny the very great value of all work by scientists *in their own departments*, the great interest also of this work in detail and in its consequences. ... M. Durkheim, with his social consciousness, and M. Levy-Bruhl, with his Bororo Indians who convince themselves that they are parroquets, are delightful writers.'[21] To their mind, the classicist or the critic was better qualified for the task of arbitership and as such incidents as the earlier neglect-of-science-debate (1916–18) demonstrated, this conviction reflects holistic ideals of man and organicist tendencies generally associated with anti-modernism and its inherent antipathy to specialist knowledges.[22] In the eyes of the connoisseur, scientists across the board failed to qualify as genuine intellectuals because they could not be credited with the power of judgement.

Seen in this context, the mutual invitations, extended by Wells and the bishop, to retire for the benefit of mankind seem to indicate that the debate over the nature of human progress formed one of the key platforms for competition among those intellectual groups that asserted their public role by professing to have authoritative views on the issue. For all of them, to be intellectually in evidence was not separable from being socially in evidence. Rather, the intellectuals' conviction of their political importance was based both on the fact that they negotiated the moral, anthropological and social questions of the nation, and that they did so in public. Pulpits, ecclesiastic or secular, in the *Illustrated London News*, Leeds parish church or Alexandra Palace – all to the mind of the intellectual were important political sites in that they offered occasions for what was both an intellectual and social presence. The very combination constituted the intellectual's role in the steering of the ship of the nation. This battle of Englishness was (as ever) about moral authority.

The author of the ten year moratorium for science, Richard Livingstone's friend E. A. Burroughs, bishop of Ripon, fits the traditional humanists' description of an intellectual in every respect. His professional biography may serve as a genealogy of the scene enacted in Leeds parish church in 1927: Burroughs came up from

Harrow to Balliol in the same year as William Temple (the future archbishop), in 1900, and finished with a collection of prizes and a first in Classical Moderations and in Greats. At the time when Wells satirized the purple cloth in his *Soul of a Bishop* (1917), Burroughs was still a lecturer and fellow at Hertford College, Oxford, though he spent most of the war-years travelling and preaching to groups that in principle consisted of his peers and of former or future colleagues, namely officers of the British Expeditionary Force and staff and pupils of public schools.[23] Burroughs baffled his biographer by compiling, despite these constant engagements, a nearly 400 page strong 'plea for wholeness in thought and life', a tome which was published in 1916 and which went through numerous impressions. In this massive document of his spiritual war effort, Burroughs deplored the idea of the strong state and explicitly advocated those bonds of mankind which were 'independent of state control and would grow without state support.'[24] By then he had already proved himself a public moralist: the war was an essentially 'spiritual conflict', a 'holy war', in which the truly civilized defended traditional values against modernism in general and against its epitome – whose features had been measured in such compilations as Thomas Smith's vituperative *The Soul of Germany* – in particular. Burroughs also discovered for himself the English custom of using the centre page of the wartime editions of *The Times*, where he thundered about national sins under the *nom de plume* 'Oxoniensis'; and he consulted and mercilessly quoted governmental reports that quantified such sins, which (it was felt) manifested themselves in drunkenness, VD and 'war babies'. Those who knew him well agreed that Burroughs had the making of a prophet.[25] Soon, he displayed further signs of the kind of pessimism for which some of his contemporaries in the arts (not least of all the 'gloomy dean', W. R. Inge) achieved notoriety: by 1920, Burroughs could recommend the study of Latin Culture on the grounds that the corruption, under the influence of Greece, of the rustic morality of Ancient Rome embodied an important lesson in decline. In his eyes, there were deep analogies between the Roman Republic and a modern situation where science entered the educational system, spelling ruin for the Soul of England.[26]

Burroughs' extensive wartime activities displayed two chief features: continuous allusions to an idealist vision of the healthy society as a community that derived its well-being from the moral and spiritual soundness of its individual members; and a more dystopian theme which slowly gathered momentum – the spectre of modernity epitomised by Prussian state machinery which cast a shadow over the ideals of a voluntarist moral economy and the self-organising society, based on local ways of life and their specific nodes of authority (parish, public schools, Oxbridge colleges, *The Times,* eventually even Sunday radio). Along with many others who defended traditional liberal education as an embodiment of individualistic moral, intellectual and political values – public schools became his 'special sphere of influence' – Burroughs associated this spectre with science.[27] His activities in the twenties must be read in the context of this image: after he revealed himself as a prophet of spiritual reconstruction (even dropping his *nom de plume*), Burroughs steadily and substantially increased the extent to which he was 'socially in evidence' by successively taking up the office of Chaplain to the King, the canonry of Peterborough, the deanery of Bristol and lastly the bishopric of Ripon (1926). This latter appointment united Burroughs, prophet of Englishness, with a town much praised for its quintessential Englishness in the inter-war years, as Mike Bartholomew shows elsewhere in this volume.[28]

Facing Keith and his assembled BAAS members a year into his new office, Burroughs treated the crowded church to a sharpened version of his conjectures on the relations between science, religion and the evolution of civilization. Burroughs was convinced that science conflicted with the moral progress of mankind: to his mind, there was 'all the difference between knowledge and wisdom'; science, while it provided the former, had failed entirely to increase the latter. In other words, Burroughs diagnosed modern civilization as suffering from a 'moral lag', a gap between moral and scientific advance, for 'man's body had in effect gone on growing while his soul had largely stood still or gone back. And until the disproportion had somehow been rectified Man could not feel safe.'[29]

The inspirational source of this metaphor was the French critic of rationalism, Henri Bergson, who had used it in 1914 in a public lecture on the causes of the moral and social problems of his day, the war in particular.[30] By 1927, obviously, Burroughs' earlier misgivings about a potentially oppressive future society had matured into a full-blown abrogation of the sacred covenant between progress and mankind.[31] Far from decreasing the lag, science to his mind actively contributed to its increase in an alarming manner and, along with those who remained suspicious of modernist trends in church or society at large, he continued in the persuasion that the impact of science on religion and traditional ways of life was deeply corrosive and engendered a national decline as a matter of inevitability. Hence

Burroughs' plea for a ten year moratorium on scientific research as the sole effective measure to prevent us from careering towards an abyss. Rarely had a suggestion so perfectly epitomized the allegation that there was an innate antithesis between progress and morality.

Burroughs was by no means alone among British critics of modernity who maintained that science entailed a moral and political decline. Usually (and notoriously so) their misgivings chiefly focussed on industrialism and urbanization, and by the twenties formed the basis of an entire industry of fictional writing invoking an Arcadian image of England, as Mike Bartholomew shows in his chapter. Moreover, these misgivings gave rise to a culture of criticism which, in the case of literature, centred around such magazines as the *Adelphi*, the short-lived *Calendar* and later, *Scrutiny*. As Francis Mulhern put it, to counter the decline of humanistic values, exponents of this culture offered their services to administrate English literature as 'a new repository of moral values and, therewith, literary criticism as the privileged arbiter of social thought.'[32] Some of them also tapped into the ruralist strain in English culture and the tradition of lifting models of the ideal community from a world historically or geographically far removed from a problematic present. Charles Townshend has recently observed that 'as England became materially more urban, it became morally more rural' and thus characterized a period in late nineteenth-century history marked by the re-discovery of rural England. Typified, among others, by appeals to the whole-some piety and wise traditions of country life, this ideal was supplied with the topographical connotations of Southern England, more precisely Sussex, where such notables as Rudyard Kipling and Hilaire Belloc located ideal rusticity.[33]

Disgust with industrialism and urbanization blended well with dismay over science and scientific training. Liberal humanists tended to regard scientific education as a vocational training and hence as merely useful and not conducive to the growth of personality. Just before the Great War, E. G. A. Holmes, Chief Inspector for Elementary Schools and champion of Classical education, experienced a Sussex Damascus when, at the foot of the South Downs (where else?), he came upon a school with which he for once found nothing wrong; this school, to his mind, embodied the true lessons of an English education: kinship, indeed 'kinship with my kind'.[34] Two decades on Margaret Bondfield, member of MacDonald's cabinet, still told a gathering of educationists:

> Modern scientific education had enabled us to fill our streets with

noises and with smells and to plaster the countryside with glittering advertisements ... I do protest against such knowledge ... I wonder how far it is possible to grow up with a mechanical civilization and still retain the quietness of the countryside and the power to make use of our leisure.[35]

Statements such as these were as a matter of due course reported on exposed platforms such as *The Times*, and not only were they legion, they united a remarkable spectrum of views, including a Catholic tributary to this criticism of modern civilization, which championed a sympathetic re-examination of the achievement of the Middle Ages and criticized modernity as part of its campaign to rehabilitate medieval values. While the names that spring to mind here are scholars like T. E. Hulme, Christopher Dawson, Jacques Maritain and Etienne Gilson, the project was by no means confined to the élite citadels of learning, and in Britain it was led by those most active in the pursuit of the belief that science epitomized the downside of modernity. At the time of Burroughs' sermon, this included the group around G. K. Chesterton (who had converted to Rome in 1923) and Hilaire Belloc, whose combined controversial skill and zest made them sufficiently indistinguishable from one another as to cause G. B. Shaw to refer to them as 'Chesterbelloc'.[36] Initially not directed at natural science *per se*, but primarily at industrialism, Chesterbelloc's luddite fantasies were of long standing. Well over a decade before the Leeds sermon, they already concentrated their journalistic and monographic efforts on a reversal of modern trends, which they identified in the trinity of urbanization, consumerism and the increasing role of monopolistic and central political agencies.[37]

Chesterbelloc developed and published the ideal of 'distributism', an economic doctrine based on Christian social ethics as defined by Pope Leo XIII who had led the neo-scholastic revival of the late nineteenth century as part of a general call for a return to the true traditions of Western thought and action.[38] Arguing in favour of a co-operative ideal in the spirit of the medieval craft guilds, distributists demanded economics be based on specific Christian values. This constituted a condemnation of economic liberalism as at once Protestant, individualistic and 'de-Christianized',[39] and while this sounds like a head-on attack on English practices, Chesterbelloc remained the most English of intellectuals: they published regularly in the *New Statesman*, dominated the *Illustrated London News*, contributed to such ventures as the collection on *The English Genius* and were as a matter of due course invited by the BBC to comment on the state of the nation. Rather than end an English intellectual's career, entering into public combat with some strands of Englishness seems to have been constitutive of it.[40]

Much like Protestant commentators, however, Chesterbelloc fulminated against Prussianism; the Great War was a holy war, a life-and-death struggle between the forces of culture and barbarism.[41] In post-war England this affinity across the boundaries of religious beliefs continued and, indeed, it converged in the ruralist ideal of national character, among whose architects Chesterbelloc figured most prominently. The need for a remoralization of the modern condition emerged as a natural conclusion of such socio-ethical analyses. In books from *What's Wrong with the World* (1910) to *The New Jerusalem* (1921), Chesterton recommended the resettlement of the humane section of the population in rural communities; mankind, as he kept insisting, had the 'right to scrap its machinery and live on the land.'[42] Belloc, in turn, vociferously defended the unique importance of the 'free press' (i.e. the sectional or propagandist or fad press) for the maintenance of democracy. 'Sectionalism' or 'particularism', their specific brand of dignified individual resistance to modernity's industrializing, acquisitive, specializing and globalizing tendencies, supported the man who sold his bicycle and walked instead.[43]

Feudalism

Above all, however, what the Chesterbellocs and Burroughs' condemned was the notion that *laissez-faire* concerning science would result in progress; in this instance, they doubted the invisible hand of Providence. It is therefore not surprising that these denominations of Englishness also aligned *vis-à-vis* an issue brought to media attention by the Leeds meeting, namely Darwinism, the invisible hand of evolution.

A few days prior to Burroughs' sermon, Arthur Keith had discussed the theory of evolution in his presidential address to the Association, entitled 'Darwin's Theory of Man's Descent as it Stands Today'.[44] In this lecture, which was relayed by the BBC from the Majestic cinema, Leeds, at prime time (8:50 p.m.), Keith retold the story of Darwin's discovery of the animal ancestry of man in the language of military conquest.[45] The scientific evidence which had accumulated since Darwin, Keith asserted, proved 'that Man began his career as a humble primate animal, and has reached his present estate by the action and reaction of biological forces which have been and are ever at work within his body and brain.'[46] Especially with regard to the evolution of the latter organ, Keith admitted, our knowledge of such biological forces was still patchy. Why the human brain 'has made such great progress while that of his cousin the gorilla has fallen so far behind' or 'why inherited ability falls to one family and not to another, or why, in the matter of cerebral endowment, one race of mankind has fared so much better than another' were lags we could not yet fully account for.[47] Still, according to Keith the social relations between men could be explained in terms of the Darwinian principles of evolution.[48] Also, and perhaps more importantly, to Keith's mind we could assume that natural selection acted as a progressive force.

It was Oliver Lodge who made the link between Keith's discourse and the request for a ten year holiday for scientific research, when he responded to Burroughs in an evening lecture.[49] His qualifications to answer Burroughs' challenge were manifestly superior, for not only was he famous for his criticism of materialism, he had also recently delivered a course of public lectures on *Science and Human Progress*, and moreover, he had been appointed to this office by the Halley Stewart Trust, a body whose self-avowed central objective was 'Research for the Christian Ideal in all Social Life'.[50] In response to Burroughs' sermon, Lodge chided past scientists for their materialism and expressed regret that people were still piqued by the idea that they might be related to the lower animals.[51] Lodge's deduction that the bishop's remarks had been prompted by Keith's presidential address on evolution was not wholly far-fetched.[52] The address was front page news (Fig. 1) and not only did it cause a flood of letters to *The Times*, it also prompted Bede Jarrett, the Prior Provincial of the Dominicans in England, to make it the subject of the sermon he preached in the Catholic cathedral of Leeds on the very morning that Burroughs demanded the moratorium.[53] Jarrett's sermon was widely reported. The *New Statesman* even ran a two page article pitting Keith *vs* Moses.[54] The media, in short, were alive with the theme; Keith's address had started a Darwinism-fest.

As a well-known rationalist who had only recently delivered a lecture on *The Religion of a Darwinist* at one of the London ethical societies, Keith qualified as a worthy public enemy. But there was more. Following a suggestion Keith had originally made, the Association was celebrating the decision to support a movement to buy Charles Darwin's home and estate at Downe, Kent, and henceforth referred to it as a national shrine.[55] Some traditionalist guardians of the national heritage may have deemed this step

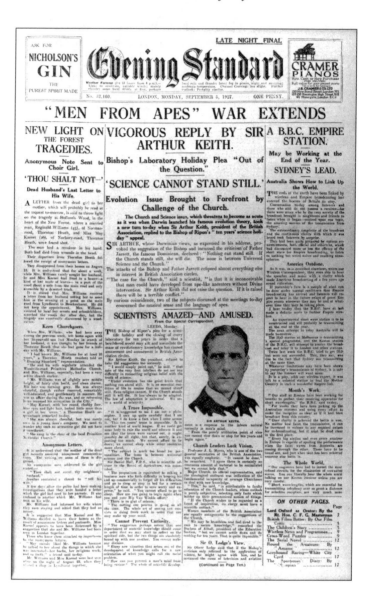

Figure 1

Title page of the Evening Standard, Monday 5 September 1927.
(By permission of Express Newspapers and the Syndics of
Cambridge University Library)

provocative, for to provide the scientific enterprise with the cultural and moral associations of Kentish rusticity was to enter into direct competition with those critics of modern civilization whose chief gesture consisted in pointing to an ideal of aesthetic and moral Englishness exemplified by the rural South.[56] Over a decade prior to Leeds, Keith had already planted his flag in the heartland of this England when he vouched for the authenticity of and thereby attached his name to the remains of what became known as 'Piltdown man', found in Piltdown, Sussex, in 1912.

Chesterbelloc rushed in to defend England and had since Piltdown taunted Keith into publicly defending evolution against its Christian critics. Ever ready to join into some Englishness-jousting, Keith had only a few months prior to the Leeds incident agreed to a request on the part of Richard Gregory (editor of *Nature*) to help support Wells in his latest ripostes to Belloc's continuous assaults on the *Outline*.[57] Keith reviewed both Belloc's books and Wells' *Mr Belloc Objects* for the magazine and subsequently engaged in an exchange with Belloc in its columns.[58] Chesterton eventually played umpire in their debacle and unsurprisingly, he came down on the side of his co-religionist.[59] Two years on, Keith and Chesterton explicitly discussed Burroughs' idea of a moratorium for the readers of the *New York Times Magazine*. Under the heading 'Should Science Take a Holiday?', Keith time and again referred his audience back to the context of the Seer of Downe, sprinkling his discourse with relics at once rustic and evolutionary:

> I have come into Darwin's country – in the County of Kent, England, to spend a week-end and write this message to The New York Times … I look across a meadow; beyond it is the "sand-walk" round which the seer of Downe used to perambulate as he meditated on the rigorous rules which regulate the affairs of the world – the laws of evolution … It is through Darwin's eyes that I seek to probe into the tide of human affairs and read the meanings of the portents which appear in our modern skies …[60]

Chesterton soon replied in the same organ, the title of his essay ('A Plea that Science Now Halt') already unambiguously supportive of the idea of a scientific holiday.[61]

The twenties debate over Darwinism clearly is part of the ecology of Burroughs' sermon and the entire notion of a holiday from what was perceived as the mad velocity of modern life. Yet judging from the surviving accounts of the sermon itself, there was absolutely nothing in it which would suggest, as Lodge hinted (and as was certainly true of the awesome Catholic duo), that Burroughs had any views on (let alone a quarrel specifically with) the idea that he might be related to the lower animals. Not a single one of the many letters *The Times* published in the aftermath of Keith's lecture referred to Burroughs or his sermon, nor did the Catholic press mention his name at any stage in its epic coverage of the debate on the descent of man. Keith did not list the bishop in his comprehensive accounts of his public opposition, published as *Darwinism and What It Implies* (1928) and *Darwinism and Its Critics* (1935). Moreover, Burroughs himself had referred only to physical and chemical laboratories and none of the examples of applied science he cited were even remotely related to biology. In an interview with the *Evening Standard*, he actually protested that his sermon had 'no reference whatever to Sir Arthur Keith's address' and that there was 'not a word from beginning to end that could be taken as a reference to Darwinism.'[62]

In effect, however, Burroughs did indeed have a quarrel with Darwinism, for he disputed that it was competition or rivalry which formed the springs of progress. At the time, the issue over Darwinism was not the animal ancestry of man, but a theory of society; the question was not whether man descended from the monkeys but whether the struggle for survival provided a viable and good model for social conduct, national and international. Keith followed diffusionist anthropology in the belief that cultural progress was the consequence of inter-tribal clashes, and Burroughs, while not taking direct issue, insisted on a rival conception of civilization and its advance.[63] He harked back to an old objection which was being rephrased at the time: Burroughs did not just take exception at the idea of a world conceived as mere matter working mechanically but explicitly endorsed the idealism of a master of Englishness, namely the (Scottish) physiologist and philosopher J. S. Haldane, who was just then delivering his Gifford Lectures on 'the sciences and philosophy'.[64] Since the closing decades of the nineteenth century, Haldane had propagated the view that the phenomena of life and of consciousness were not reducible to the laws of physics. He had done so on various professional occasions – in scientific papers, public addresses and in a booklet entitled *Mechanism, Life and Personality* (1913). Reprinted in 1921, this volume seems a likely source for Burroughs' Leeds sermon, where the bishop defended a vision of the universe conceived as organic, 'as personality, as spirit'. According to Burroughs, within such a cosmology, the road to progress lay in a holistic restoration and science fitted ill into this vision as it tended to 'eliminate personality ... for immediate practical purposes.' This conflicted with the very requirement of the hour, namely to put 'personality once more in the saddle, instead of letting things ride the world.'[65] Of all men, by the sound of it, the scientist resembled a Darwinistic animal the most.

The language used ('ruling motives', 'practical purposes', 'elimination of personality') indicates the general drift of Burroughs' argument: namely, that there was something wrong with 'the scientist' as such. Ten years had passed since Gregory, in his famous and still best-selling *Discovery, or the Spirit and Service of Science* (1916) had hoped to dismantle the notion of the scientist as a callous necromancer, ruled by ignoble motives, driven by short-sighted utilitarian considerations; and yet, the old complaints endured. For Burroughs, the scientist was a creature whose very essence consisted in habitually disposing of the one thing that made it human and a member of human communities: that is, personality. How momentous this kind of charge is, we know from such occasions as the earlier neglect-of-science debate, during whose course it had emerged that the idea of personality occupied a crucial position in Britain's liberal-humanistic educational philosophy. The argument for this was that England's political tradition of humanist republicanism was based on 'personality', the central function in the maintenance of social peace, in guaranteeing the future of the nation. 'Personality' (along with 'liberty') epitomised the quintessentially English answer to the 'spirit of the beehive' and the 'Prussianism' associated with it. Coming from one who had consistently opposed the idea that governmental agency could substitute for the health that a community derived through the moral and spiritual health of its members, Burroughs' remarks on the scientist and his methods amounted to a political denunciation, for he implied that neither contributed to the process by which social harmony was guaranteed on English soil. Somehow, the bishop had started with the universe and yet arrived at the scientist himself, whom he paraded as at once the symptom and the cause of the disease of modern civilization.

Burroughs conceded that scientists were endowed with mind (and therefore 'human'), for otherwise they would not be as successful. However, he insisted, they were nowhere near accounting for the phenomenon of 'mind', nor were they trying to. In targeting this characteristic of the scientist, the sermon stipulated the existence of an expert scientific culture that spread cancer-like and poisoned the wells of democracy. To the bishop's mind, the rules of the survival of the fittest did not guarantee the progress of civilization, but rather made probable a regress to barbarism. Chesterbelloc produced identical arguments. Not only had inventions produced 'murders of a moral and aesthetic sort, destroying the types and tradition by which civilizations live', also, we had 'in practice come back to ... feudalism.'[66] Belloc perpetually condemned industrialism as a new feudalism that subjected 'the masses of the people [to] the economic and the political control of a comparatively small number of industrial and financial barons', but more importantly, he accused 'the expert' of an irrepressible drive towards being 'a hierarch'.[67] Likewise, Chesterton intoned that 'Science means specialism and specialism means oligarchy';[68] in his *Eugenics and other Evils* (1922), he equated eugenics with 'scientific officialism' and the 'scientifically organised state' and he was thus well on the way to implicating specifically the natural scientist in the authoritarian crime of modernity.[69] As he saw it, an oligarchy of experts was taking it upon itself to rule mankind in the name of the machine, an oligarchy consisting not of an élite of men capable of moral judgment, but of 'men who dare not criticize', who 'did not know how to control [the scientific machine]', 'abnormal specialist[s]' who 'ha[d] ... no morality.' In Chesterton's nightmares, the scientist was ruled by 'the monomania that his own machine must be kept working and his own particular wheel continue to go round.' Both Belloc and Chesterton called upon a 'prehistoric and ancestral appetite', a 'wild tribal appetite which once used to be called democracy' to rise against the machine of scientific progress.[70]

Such antipathies to a rule of experts sporadically and repeatedly manifested themselves in British cultural life – most recently in the 1916-18 debate, where those who defended a humanistic education had argued against early specialization on the grounds that 'the political conditions of England [made] political and moral wisdom indispensable.'[71] Belloc spelt this out again for the readers of the *New Statesman*: expert knowledge was not only 'a different matter altogether from right judgement', but tended to be 'at conflict with right judgement.'[72] The specialist was regarded as inferior to the generalist humanist not only when it came to the important task of judging the educational needs of the next generation or the future moral requirements of the nation, he was useless even when it came to assessing what should be done with the fruit of his labour. These very same attitudes were being displayed in the public debates over Darwinism in the mid-twenties and thirties, when the critics of evolution defended not only 'the reasonable right of the amateur to do what he can with the facts which the specialists provide' (the unselfconscious shrug 'I'm not a scientist but ...' was a most common gesture), but also attempted to assert their greater authority in the adjudication of interpretative issues.[73] In keeping with this was the Rev. Jarrett's claim that Keith's references to the human mind meant not only that he was being unscientific, but that he was *trespassing*.

In contrast to humanistic authority, scientific authority was perceived as being necessarily limited to a specialism and invalidated when the individual endowed with it discussed matters outside this specialism. Moreover, liberal humanists believed that the scientist – *qua* scientist – was deprived of the ability to comment on matters non-scientific.[74] As Chesterton formulated it in his reflections on the 1930 meeting of the British Association, the scientists'

> lack of traditional philosophic balance, their ignorance of philosophic standards and their lack of philosophic anchorage, has left them at the mercy of the storm in a sea of error and unwisdom. They have fallen into the grave error and foolishness of assuming that because they discovered the how, they had simultaneously discovered the what as well as the wherefore and the why.[75]

At the time, philosophers such as A. N. Whitehead and E. A. Burtt were read as bolstering similar claims, *viz.*, that scientific judgement had very limited applications and moreover, that the world was waking up to this insight. Questions concerning both the ends of scientific applications and the desirability of progress, were to the humanist's mind not for the scientist *qua* scientist to answer. This disqualification entailed both the judgement that the civic functions of the scientific professions were best kept at a minimum and, of course, its opposite, namely that the scientist had to be brought to realize his civic obligation to humanize if the moral economy of a self-organizing society was to continue. While humanistic culture at large by no means shared the Catholic intellectuals' dreams of science based on a specific morality (i.e., along the lines laid down by Pope Leo XIII), it, too, faulted expert culture on moral grounds, doubting the scientists' capacity of judgement outside their narrow area of expertise.[76] True to nineteenth-century belief, humanistic intellectuals held that 'national character' was upheld through an ideal of conduct based on virtues acquired through liberal learning and through fellowship. Gentlemanly education was the condition for the 'gentlemanly' ideal of government which, assimilating liberal Anglicanism and romantic nationalism, constituted the national character and hence the moving force in history. With such a brief, how could scientists contribute to or represent essential 'Englishness'?

If you can't beat them, join them

Unlike the science correspondents of the daily press, scientists largely refrained from public speculation about Burroughs' apparent attitude to the animal ancestry of man. Instead, they hastened to extol the scientist's humanity. Eager to dispel the bishop's reservations, Lodge denounced the specialist as 'a man in blinkers' and, insisting that he himself 'had now got the blinkers off', he proceeded to include the scientist in the enclosure of human beings – and great ones as to that, namely 'poets and saints and philosophers and preachers.'[77] Lodge also admitted the difficulty of 'digesting the fruits culled by science in the past 20 years' and five years on, he could even on the airwaves 'agree with much that Mr Belloc said.'[78] J. L. Myres, one of the two general secretaries of the Association, conceded to Burroughs that 'there certainly is an enormous amount of material to be assimilated',[79] and within weeks of the Leeds sermon, Rutherford used the occasion of the opening of the new physics laboratory at Bristol university to confess that he had 'always been looking for a breathing space when, for a few years, no advances of consequence would be made; when I should gain an opportunity for studying in more detail ... the ground already won.'[80] Even *Nature* could not resist printing a suspiciously extensive comment on Sir Oliver's dancing which, the magazine surmised, had contributed to people gaining 'quite a different conception of the *human* side of the scientific members of the community from that usually held'.[81]

By the sound of it, some representatives of the scientific enterprise chose to empathize with Burroughs and joined in the chorus of complaints over the greater speed of modern life; some of them even accommodated Burroughs' point within the tradition of general complaints about 'over-specialization' as one of the appalling side-effects of modernity in general and professionalization in particular. With this, the scientists at Leeds endorsed the holistic ideals advocated by general educationalists who preached the need either for a return to a polymathic ideal or for a 'new synthesis' in education, knowledge and culture.[82] Indeed, in the twenties, even members of the younger generation of scientists – whom Lodge found particularly prone to a 'narrow outlook' – were making a name for themselves as intellectuals precisely by joining in the criticism of the numbing effects that 'the ever-rising tide of specialisation' had perpetrated on the empire of knowledge.[83] This *jeunesse dorée* counted Julian Huxley, A. S. Russell (the Oxford chemist, science broadcaster and journalist), Joseph Needham, and C. P. Snow among its ranks.

After the war the 'parliament of science' itself reassessed its function in the light of growing specialization. Since specialist scientific bodies did no longer require its assistance in establishing professional credentials, the British Association began to focus more on the task of transforming the public image of science and the related task of popularizing scientific knowledge.[84]

During the twenties, as Roy MacLeod and Peter Collins have observed, the Association became a platform for popularising scientific knowledge, and Keith's presidential address itself demonstrates how far this proselatizing zeal extended. Indeed, Keith gave priority to the successful communication of his talk to the 'wider audiences that heard his words by the wireless' (as opposed to the assembled scientists).[85] After Leeds, the presidents of the Association continued this shift to more general themes in the presidential addresses. In 1929 Sir Thomas Holland commented that 'the rapid specialization of science ... made it increasingly more difficult in recent years for any worker to express himself to his fellow-members' and proceeded to discuss how mineral exploitation affected the course of 'civilised evolution'. His predecessor, the crystallographer William Bragg, had already chosen to pass over the chance to give an exposition on his specialism; instead he 'release[d] his store of accumulated thought on the relationship of science to *craftsmanship* in a way which gave each specialized worker an opportunity to adjust his sense of relativity and proportion.'[86] As Keith's address showed, the specialized workers were only one of the audiences for the presidential addresses. With the choice of his theme – craftsmanship – Bragg picked a topic with obvious associations with the long history of opposition to the machine, an association which he found nonsensical: the health of a nation, he pointed out, depended on its craftsmanship; and science *was* craft. Noticeably enough, the presidential addresses after Leeds were at least in part dedicated to the task of alleviating the fears and of breaking down the resistance of those who were wary of the advance of science and technology.[87] Notably, General J. C. Smuts (who presided over the centenary meeting of BAAS in 1931) and Alfred Ewing (his successor) both acknowledged the problem of the lag, Smuts suggesting that ethics be linked to science to compensate for the ethical insufficiencies of society and Ewing suggesting that religion and science be considered co-operative factors in progress, with disaster being prevented by the guidance and restraint offered by religion.[88]

Overall, science's apologists proved to have learned their lesson from earlier occasions and made themselves at least compatible with

Englishness: they followed the established practice of outward conformity to liberal-humanistic discourse and they denied the inhumanity of the scientist. Bragg dedicated a presidential address to the issue and, honouring a tradition Gregory had revived in great glory in 1916, he explicitly confronted those who thought 'that science is inhuman', and who 'speak or write as if students of modern science would destroy reverence and faith'; surely the scientific worker was 'the last man in the world to throw away hastily an old faith or convention or to think that discovery must bring contempt on tradition'?

The accusation that the scientists made no moral contribution, however, they chiefly left alone. True, in that they acted as popularizers of scientific knowledge, scientists obeyed the moral imperative of educationalism. All the same, Horace Lamb expressed a standard attitude when asserting in his 1925 presidential address that science 'cannot fairly be asked to bear the responsibility for the use which is made of [its] gifts.'[89] Overall, it was taken for granted that 'the man of science has necessarily rather a narrow outlook'; even those who reflected on the phenomenon of specialization and its pitfalls at bottom accepted specialism as an inevitable concomitant of the progressive development of the scientific enterprise.[90] Scientists professed regret over expert culture, but they did not condemn it, least of all when it was that of their own profession. After all, scientific authority rested on increasingly specialized expert procedures.[91]

Scientists generally agreed with any English cassandra who maintained that the tremendous growth of scientific knowledge and the application of science constituted a problem. However, as other scholars have noted, the bulk of them had no difficulty in viewing themselves as moral while rejecting the idea of a responsibility for the administration of the fruits of science.[92] Part of this state of mind was the gospel of an essential distinction between pure and applied science, and at Leeds this was affirmed. Lodge was immediately quoted on the front page of the *Evening Standard* as saying that he would agree with the bishop if his 'criticism only referred to the application of science' and instanced 'the cases of television and aviation as being not really science but only its application.'[93] Russell remarked that science made 'its first appeal to those who are interested in truth for its own sake rather than to those who see in the applications of scientific knowledge a source of power over material things.'[94] That he echoed Gregory almost verbatim is not surprising in a former editor of the popular journal (*Discovery*) which was a spin-off of the 1916 debate and derived its name from Gregory's book.

Separating truth from power was to flirt with some Englishness in that it constituted a declaration of allegiance with the opposition to a rule of experts; but essentially it offered nothing beyond an affirmation of faith that the lag would sort itself out. What appears to have remained somewhat unclear was precisely how science would produce concrete models for the conduct of social life and methods to resolve the anarchy of politics, as rationalists and secular humanists, especially members of the British Science Guild, had long advocated for a reconstruction of Britain.[95] While, in the wake of the war, the editorials of *Nature* celebrated science as 'the only disinterested and effective agency in a cannibalistic and corrupt society', there evidently was no universal support for the application of scientific solutions to the current problems of society.[96] It was customary to lay the blame for this at the door of public opinion and its slowness 'in tolerating the changes or restrictions in its thoughts and habits which the results of ... experiments [in these fields] might demand.'[97] Yet this was only half the story, for the scientific establishment itself was reluctant to commit itself to specific plans for the promotion of a heightened social and political significance of science.[98] In fact, their views on this harmonized with the position maintained by traditional humanists, who held that university teachers in general had to 'conceive themselves ... as lovers, seekers, and preachers of pure knowledge for its own sake', as the master of Englishness, the Oxbridge historian and political theorist Ernest Barker reminded the BAAS in 1924. Nor did the scientific establishment appear to have a quarrel with the liberal-humanistic notion that scientists must be regarded as incurable specialists because science (in Livingstone's phrase) failed to 'make her followers good guides in regions outside her confined kingdom.'[99] Such claims Bede Jarrett was just emphasizing again in Leeds' Catholic cathedral, where he faulted Keith for transgressing the accepted boundaries of science: namely, for failing to stay 'within his province', for 'wander[ing] outside his sphere', for offering 'cheap philosophy' when he was 'not a philosopher' and so on.[100] Catholic intellectuals strenuously objected to the entire process of turning the BAAS into a public platform for the popularization of science and, though they were less public about it, more scholarly types thought along similar lines: Barker, for example, tacitly supposed that unlike history, government, economics or even modern languages, scientific subjects simply did not incline towards partisanship and the affairs of the world.[101]

In sum, scientists followed paths previously mapped out: they continued either the tradition of apologism and quoted the gospel of the spirit and service of science – if they could not constitute Englishness, they *served* Englishness. A few stuck to the aggressive scientism which in the neglect-of-science debate had resulted in the perpetrators' exclusion from the closure of the conflict. By midnight on Monday, the event was largely over, and while the *Evening Standard* printed an interview with Burroughs, the bishop left for his vacation.

Scientific Humanism and a New Englishness

There is, however, another side to the Leeds incident. Ultimately, the scientists, as Carroll Pursell has observed, got more mileage out of the incident than the critics of modernity, not least of all because they could claim that it was not they who had failed in the task of educating mankind towards a responsible use of science.[102] As Frank Crew (the eugenicist) pointed out accusingly, the bishop was 'more responsible than I for the development of the particular morality that makes any application of science to the betterment of the individual and the community and not to the deterioration of human affairs.'[103] The sermon backfired for Burroughs; indeed, it backfired so utterly that his biographer omitted any mention of it.

Burroughs, it must be noted, actually by no means despised the fruits of scientific labour if they aided his evangelical zeal: he used both telephone and aeroplane at least as early as 1916, he made free use of eugenic statistics to bolster his concept of 'national sin', he pioneered the use of wireless metaphors in his war-time sermons and he eventually even entered the history of the BBC as a pioneer in transatlantic and diocesan religious broadcasts.[104] Indeed, traditionalists within the church did not universally frown on the application of science in the creation of the radio – far from it, the new resource was used to disseminate the message of Christ and to counteract the degeneration of religion. As the High Church Anglican poet Alfred Noyes expressed it in 1925, by harnessing the radio waves 'science itself has revealed the whole universe to be an everlasting miracle.' Burroughs, like Noyes, obviously did not side with those who regarded the wireless as 'but one more symptom of the subjection of the modern world to mechanism.'[105]

That, his intellectual excellence notwithstanding, it made the bishop 'unhappy to be engaged in debate about what he held sacred' (as Temple pointed out) may account for a lot when it comes to explaining how the Leeds incident came about.[106] That 'he did not readily appreciate on what points his opponents would be sensitive' (same source) cannot have helped either. Burroughs was perhaps not ideally cast in the role of the 'combative intellectual'. Having met Keith twice over dinner on the previous Friday and Saturday and having decided that he was 'a delightfully humorous person', Burroughs was actually amazed by 'the seriousness with which he and others appear to treat my suggestion.'[107] To make matters worse, in his reply he assured the scientists that he 'was perfectly prepared to accept their verdict *in their own sphere*', a concession that was hardly designed to universally pacify, if one considers the previous history of two-culture-clashes during which the alleged superiority of humanistic studies had been defined precisely by arguing that scientists were constitutionally unfit for judgements outside their own sphere, and worse even, considering that this tradition had been revived by Jarrett only a day earlier.[108] By all accounts, such territorial rhetoric was used by the defence of humanistic culture for the purpose of asserting authority. That is, it was used in controversy and not really in an apologetic retreat. By joking about a moratorium, then, Burroughs had set himself up: Keith and many others who listened to the sermon gratified him 'by smiling more than once at places where they were intended to smile', but then they proceeded to turn a joke into an event.[109]

In this they were greatly aided by the daily press, for whose budding sub-profession of science journalism the Leeds incident proved an unexpected shot in the arm. The controversy provided *The Times*, but above all the *Manchester Guardian* and the *Daily Herald* (all of which had reported extensively on the Association meeting) with additional columns. What is more, it constituted front page news of greater interest even than 'the curing of shell shock by hypnotism and sex determination in eggs' (both topics whose moral ramifications secured them undisputed public attention).[110] Even the *Evening Standard*, for which the Association meeting had not been an absolute top priority, observed gleefully that the attacks of the bishop and Father Jarrett 'eclipsed almost everything else in [sic] interest in British Association circles.'[111] Well over a decade later J. G. Crowther, science correspondent of the *Manchester Guardian* between 1928-48, chose to paint a picture of scientists in extended outrage over Leeds, when he included the incident in his best-selling, at times semi-autobiographical *Social Relations of Science*. Leeds, he held, played a causal role in the rise of the social-relations-of-science-movement of the thirties.[112]

According to Chesterton, Keith's address already was a set-up, a performance staged both 'for the benefits of the newspaper reporters' and in aid of the scientific enterprise, for, as G. K. sarcastically commented, 'The Party was united; the flowing tide was with them; the cup was very nearly full...'[113] Burroughs' suggestion of a moratorium, then, helped stitch the matter up: not only did it provide scientists with an opportunity to publicly pull rank on those critics who, as had been noted, 'observe only the lack of ... control, and lay [the blame] at the door of science', and who, ever since the end of the war, had preached a 'gospel of despair' without ever confronting anyone in particular.[114] Also, the incident gave scientists a prime opportunity to unite in opposition to an alleged threat. Their collective protests were staggeringly repetitive, rendering Leeds a ritual performance in celebration of the scientific community: how could the church fail to 'realize that we can't take a rest – that nothing in this world can take a rest' (Keith); 'we must go forward, we can have no stagnation ... We must press forward towards the mark of our high calling in Christ Jesus' (Lodge); there was an 'inborn curiosity in man's mind' (Sir Daniel Hall, scientific advisor to the Board of agriculture, who clarified what was on the mind of many when associating the idea of a holiday with sloth – 'you cannot afford to go to sleep'); 'we cannot put the clock back' (Bragg); 'it cannot be done' (Myres, laconically).[115] The *Manchester Guardian* echoed this consensus in the headline 'NO MORE POSSIBLE THAN FROM MORALS'; and though he empathized with the Morrisites', Samuel Butler's and the Narodniki's reaction against machinery, young Needham soon told the first general conference of the Student Christian Movement that 'nothing can come from a mere backwards movement.'[116]

Overall, scientists were eager to display an optimism tempered by realism and they affirmed the values of a (scientific) humanism: scientists countered the spectre of a 'moral lag' with the Prometheus-argument, namely that it would be unnatural (and therefore morally wrong) to interfere with the progress of mind. In their collective homage to 'inborn curiosity' and the virtues of 'flexibility' and of 'seeing things as they really are', they retained central but extremely selective features of Matthew Arnold's famous statement of Victorian humanist Hellenism.[117] One of the goals of Arnold's programme had of course been to oppose the scientistic philosophies of his age, namely scientific naturalism, philosophical mechanism and utilitarianism. By adapting Arnold's Hellenism, scientists tapped into the tradition of English humanism while focusing on aspects of Englishness that were unproblematic for, even conducive to, the scientific enterprise. Loyalty towards tradition, complemented by the virtue of an innate 'dynamism', were key features of their rhetoric.[118] This aligned their language with the post-Arnoldian, reconstructed Hellenism of their own generation, a dynamic humanism which Frank Turner has called 'evolutionary' and which its idealist critics regarded as Darwinian.[119]

The scientists, in short, used Burroughs' taunt to shift the goalposts of Englishness. This overall strategy was also followed when they chose to point to the risks a moratorium would involve. This meant to explicitly deploy the forces of a utilitarian morality to cast a moral shadow over the idea of a scientific holiday. Unsurprisingly, the spectre of Malthus – the widening gap between the production of foodstuffs and population growth, itself the result of moral debility – was ushered in on a number of occasions. The goalposts of Englishness could be shifted both by rearranging English humanism and by reappointing icons of the English past that had been neglected or even vilified by the enemy. One aspect of this procedure was to discredit idealistic doctrines of national and international order that relied chiefly on the power of persuasion and on the idea of voluntary co-operation and altruism. British science had previously been no stranger to the idea of a rationalised imperialism and while the experience of the war generally inspired a vogue of political and intellectual internationalism, we also know that old habits die hard.[120] In the twenties, the heritage of social Darwinism, transmitted through the lasting impact of Karl Pearson, the foremost scientific apologist for a rationalised imperialism, continued to furnish the argument in favour of a vision of national survival masterminded by scientific expertise. Ever in the front line, Keith queried if it was conceivable that we could have both peace and progress: Burroughs' '10 years truce [was] another kind of world league'; its multiple ifs and buts ('If we could get somebody to rule the world *and* educate it *and* see that the truce were carried out ...') proved that rather than a solution, it was an illustration of the problems that confronted mankind.[121] It was escapist, for if Darwin was right in thinking that competition or rivalry were the springs of progress, 'could we still hope to progress when we have eliminated from nations and nationalities their present rivalries?'[122] Barely a month after Leeds, Keith answered this question for the readers of the *Evening Standard*:

Schoolmasters, statesmen, and philanthropists cry out against the spirit of competition, and would gladly welcome its eradication from

91

human nature. ... [Yet] so deeply is the spirit of competition – the desire to struggle – engrafted in human nature, and so essential is it for the zest of life, that the People which resolves to dispense with it becomes a certain loser.[123]

With this, Keith claimed that the patrician, Christian-humanist ideal of conduct and the idea of 'Englishness' it embodied conflicted with the interests of the race. As Rhodri Hayward shows in his chapter, Keith viewed national survival as depending, not on traditional Englishness, but instead on those savage features of man which liberal-humanistic culture worked so hard to erase.

While only a few scientists publicly agreed with Keith on this, they still unanimously associated the idea of a scientific holiday with civilizational regress. The two arguments were intimately connected in the minds of many, not least of all due to the ambiguity of the term 'civilization', which easily could substitute for 'nation'.[124] Keith, of course, insisted that 'we cannot sleep while other countries move ahead.'[125] Bragg advised against following Burroughs' advice, arguing that to 'hinder the growth of science in any way [was to] hinder the growth of craftsmanship', and as 'the state of a nation's craftsmanship was an index of its health', a moratorium would produce another lag: for what was true about individuals was obviously true about civilizations, namely that 'those who failed to recognise the principle will be left behind by those who do not.'[126] Keith especially pressed the point that England could not afford to follow Burroughs. A terrible fate had befallen all those civilizations – 'Egypt, Palestine, Mesopotamia, India, Tibet, China and Greece' – which, at some point, had decided 'to send science on a holiday and simply mark time.' A civilization was 'a live thing; it must either grow or decline. It declines if science goes on holiday.'[127]

That an arrest of scientific progress entailed a civilizational regress had of course long been made explicit by J. B. S. Haldane, the son of the Gifford Lecturer of 1927/8. Using an undergraduate essay from before the war to entertain a gathering of the Cambridge Heretics, the younger Haldane pointed out that the advocates of an arrest belonged to a most peculiar class of persons typified by Chesterton, whom he suspected of favouring a return to the Middle Ages.[128] Within a month of Burroughs' sermon, Haldane entertained the readers of the *Evening Standard* with an article whose subtitle says it all: 'Will Man Return to Barbarism or Live Forever and Colonize the Stars.' In the same series (on 'The Destiny of Man') Julian Huxley likewise made it clear that man had to progress towards 'efficiency', unless he wanted to set in motion a spiral of degeneration that would either 'affect the whole of human stock; or nation after nation may rise to a certain pitch only to fall at the hands of one rising from barbarism, and the process continue indefinitely, each nation degenerating with civilisations becoming purged again in adversity.'[129] Huxley followed William James in the quest for human activities that would substitute for war, and accordingly he condemned blind competition. Still, Keith had no qualms about reading Huxley as saying that 'unless the advice of scientific men is followed – the riding of the jockeys rationalized and the hereditary "make up" of the mounts improved – this momentous race [i.e. Humanity's "Grand National"] ... will prove a fiasco ...'[130]

In fact, between the mid-twenties and the mid-thirties, rationalist scientists in particular spent considerable energy on the public refutation of all those who disputed the universality of the theory of evolution. While the patent reason for Darwinists to engage in these disputes may have been that they objected to the notion of sharing their authority in matters biological with lay-people, the overall context of the debates suggests that a far more comprehensive authority was concerned, namely the authority of determining the shape of things to come.[131] This obviously puts these quarrels in a straight line of descent from the Victorian conflict between naturalism and traditional world views, in which, as MacKenzie (*pace* Turner) has pointed out, what was at stake was '*who* should have authority to pronounce on the cosmos, society and people, and who would gain the very worldly advantages that flowed from possession of that authority.'[132] In inter-war Britain, this conflict endured.

Conclusion

In the aftermath of the Great War, 'progress' remained a key issue in the intellectual pulpits. In one contemporary reading of current affairs, a tension had been building up between progress and morality, resulting in a moral lag of such desperate proportions that it threatened the existence of civilization. Critics of science contrasted what they perceived as a recent development with a vision of an enduring England, an England whose morality was essentially rural and whose order was maintained through the exercise of individual virtue and compromise. Within this vision, England required science at the most in medicinal doses; ideally, science was only to develop applications that were approved by the connoisseur and that formed a welcome tool for the task of preserving existing English institutions and reviving 'the English spirit'. In sum, to the mind of the liberal-humanistic intellectual, spiritual goals were to take precedence over material goals. Not by coincidence did the author of *English for the English* (1921), a key document in the post-war movement to install English literature in a central position in British education, propose 'immaterial communism' as the new programme of national regeneration and moral rearmament.[133]

While a powerful image, the notion of a moral lag had a twin in the spectre of Malthus which again resonated with the considerations of Imperial leadership. To allude to Malthus and also to a serious game that went by the name of 'humanity's Grand National' was to tap into a heritage as quintessentially English as nostalgic ruralism. The virtues of competitiveness were, after all, far from unfamiliar to those who, independently of whether they eventually became scientists or bishops, had struggled all the way up the ladder of public school and university. This experience was shared on all sides: the representatives of the 'old humanities' had long been prepared to sacrifice what has been termed 'a holocaust of undergraduates every year' to produce in each generation just one outstanding classical scholar. William Osler, who reminded them of this, also reminded them that this was 'Nature's method': did it not 'cost some thousands of eggs and fry to produce one salmon?'[134] Those involved in constructing a non-Darwinian evolutionism and in building it, as Peter Bowler has phrased it, 'into a wider opposition to materialism', had been baptized in the tradition of competitive examinations whether their names were Burroughs, Haldane (J.S.) or Lodge.[135]

Post-World War I debates on social evolution in general and the Leeds incident in particular revealed that scientists' attitudes both to Englishness and to science's potential to reinvent Englishness comprised a wide spectrum. 'National culture', insofar as it manifested itself through Burroughs' sermon and its reception, at any one time evidently was not just one monolithic structure; rather, it was a function of competing notions. While Britain was well on its way to becoming (or continuing as) a military and industrial nation, rival concepts of what made the nation *cohere* were reasserting (or continuing to reassert) themselves. In this struggle, scientists did labour under a handicap in that their expertise seemed alien to a particular (and seemingly culturally dominant) conception of Englishness, and in that, consequently, it was not obvious how science and its practitioners could be taken to represent the mythical core of national identity. By contrast, English literature and art, for example, undeniably had a vast potential for articulating and symbolizing varying moods of national culture. However, scientists were also able to turn their handicap to their advantage. Prior to their fling with the notion of a social responsibility of science, the British scientific establishment shrugged off ideas of directing science towards particular 'social' ends, on the grounds that this would be alien to the scientific enterprise and, in effect, unEnglish: for them, planning was not just incompatible with creativity (as such critics of national planning as Michael Polanyi or J. R. Baker were soon to emphasize);[136] planning was incompatible with individualism, that is, with the very root of national virtues like dynamism and self-regulation and the spring of what was conceived as civilizational advance as such. The professedly rationalistic and secular-humanistic wing of the scientific enterprise, on the other hand, employed the issue of science's responsibility to expand the older argument that traditionalistic Englishness kept the nation back; for them, to fail to embrace a more efficient Englishness was to fail both one's patriotic duty and, again, one's duty towards civilization as such. While their ideal of Englishness differed dramatically from that of the bulk of the scientific establishment, rationalists proved just as keen to claim a place for their enterprise within the national heritage.

In sum, a decade before it began to seem appropriate to argue that scientific research should be geared towards the solution of social problems and to embark on a discourse on civic duties that were peculiar to the scientist, scientists were by no means uninterested in the idea of associating their enterprise with the ideological fabric of the nation. Rather, when opportunity presented itself, they used it to disabuse their public of the perception that the scientific enterprise was alien or even harmful to a truer England. They emphasized the extent to which 'science' stood for the enduring values it was allegedly destroying, or mapped out vistas of a reinvented yet authentic Albion. They worked with, rather than against, what was presented as cultural precept and native tradition. Most important of all, perhaps, they engaged in public debate and thus displayed that combative sense of duty which, according to the liberal humanistic word-smiths of Englishness, still counted as the all-important outer mark of the inner (English)man, as Oxbridge dons from Barker to Herbert Butterfield were keen to emphasize even after the Second World War.[137]

Notes

1 Douglas Woodruff, 'Hilaire Belloc', *Dictionary of National Biography* (1951-60), 88.

2 On the importance of 'personality' for the sound social body, see also

Matthew Thomson's contribution to this volume. On the neglect-of-science-debate, see A.-K. Mayer, 'National Education, Science, Morality: a Debate and its Context', paper delivered at the conference on *Humanism, Citizenship and Science in the Inter-war Years*, Wellcome Institute, London, 16 February 1996.

3 Quoted after C. Snow, 'The Two Cultures', *New Statesman*, 6 October 1954, pp. 413–4 at 413.

4 This, Needham alleged, had happened to UNESCO's inter-war predecessor, the League of Nations' International Institute of Intellectual Co-operation. J. Needham, 'The Place of Science and International Scientific Co-operation in Post-War World Organization', *Nature*, 10 November 1945, pp. 558–61 at 559.

5 Snow, 'The Two Cultures'; *idem, The Two Cultures and the Scientific Revolution*, Cambridge, 1959.

6 On 'public science', see F. M. Turner, 'Public Science in Britain, 1880-1919', *Isis*, 71 (1980): 589–608.

7 D. Edgerton, 'British Scientific Intellectuals and the Relations of Science, Technology and War', in *National Military Establishments and the Advancement of Science and Technology. Studies in Twentieth Century History*, Paul Forman and J. M. Sánchez-Ron (eds), Dordrecht and London, 1996, pp. 1–35.

8 D. Edgerton, 'Science in the United Kingdom: A Study of the Nationalization of Science', in *Science in the Twentieth Century*, J. Krige and D. Pestre (eds), Amsterdam, 1997, pp. 759–76; *idem, Science, Technology, and the British Industrial 'Decline', 1870-1970: the Myth of the Technically Determined British Decline*, Cambridge, 1996; *idem, England and the Aeroplane: an Essay on a Militant and Technological Nation*, Basingstoke, 1991.

9 As has been argued, most recently by Charles Townshend, in the nineteenth century the British state became a kind of republic in spite of its monarchical trappings. It was set on a new footing through the 'counter-mobilization of the respectable' when the Chartist movement was stifled by middle-class solidarity, in what G. M. Young called a 'triumphant vindication of the English way'. See Charles Townshend, *Making the Peace: Public Order and Public Security in Modern Britain*, Oxford, 1993, 1.

10 *Englishness. Politics and Culture 1880-1920*, R. Colls and P. Dodd (eds), London, New York and Sydney, 1986; *Patriotism: the Making and Unmaking of British National Identity*, Raphael Samuel (ed.), London and New York, 1989. For the decades between 1920-40, see Bill Schwarz, 'The Language of Constitutionalism: Baldwinite Conservatism', in *Formations of Nations and People*, 1984, pp. 1–18;

Patrick Wright, *On Living in an Old Country: the National Past in Contemporary Britain*, London, 1985, chs. 1–3; Malcolm Chase, 'This is no Claptrap: This is our Heritage', in *The Imagined Past: History and Nostalgia*, C. Shaw and M. Chase (eds), Manchester, 1989, pp. 128–46; Chris Waters, 'J. B. Priestley', in *After the Victorians. Private Conscience and Public Duty in Modern Britain. Essays in Memory of John Clive*, Susan Pedersen and Peter Mandler (eds), London and New York, 1994, pp. 209–26.

11   Modris Eksteins, *Rites of Spring: the Great War and the Birth of the Modern Age*, New York, 1989.

12   J. B. Morrell, 'The Non-Medical Sciences, 1914-1939', in *The History of the University of Oxford*, vol. 8, *The Twentieth Century*, Brian Harrison (ed.), Oxford, 1994; *idem, Science at Oxford 1914-1939. Transforming an Arts University*, Oxford, 1997, esp. pp. 54–9.

13   George Orwell, *Coming up for Air*, London, 1939. See also Bernard Crick's introduction to Orwell's *The Lion and the Unicorn: Socialism and the English Genius*, 1982 (first published 1941).

14   W. R. Inge, 'Religion', in *The English Genius. A Survey of English Achievement and Character*, Hugh Kingsmill (ed.), London, 1938.

15   A. J. Taylor, *English History 1914-1945*, Oxford, 1965, ch. 5 'Normal Times: 1922'.

16   W. McGucken, *Scientists, Society and State; the Social Relations of Science Movement in Great Britain, 1931-1947*, Columbus, 1984, 3.

17   *Ibid.*; Neil Wood, *Communism and British Intellectuals*, New York, 1959, 121.

18   McGucken, *Scientists*; Peter Collins, *The BAAS and Public Attitudes to Science 1919-1945*, Ph.D. thesis, University of Leeds, 1978.

19   H. G. Wells, *The Soul of a Bishop*, London, 1917.

20   Livingstone, *A Defence of Classical Education*, London, 1916, 53.

21   T. S. Eliot, 'Euripides and Professor Murray', reprinted in *The Sacred Wood*, London, 1920; Stefan Collini, "On Highest Authority': The Literary Critic and Other Aviators in Early Twentieth-Century Britain', in *Modernist Impulses in the Human Sciences 1870-1930*, Dorothy Ross (ed.), Baltimore and London, 1994, pp. 152–70.

22   Of course, the entire notion of gentlemanly government was associated with liberal learning as opposed to trained expertise. Ernest Barker, the historian and political theorist, bracketed these values with 'Englishness' per se and thus represented them as an embodiment of both personal and national character. See Julia Stapleton, *Englishness and the Study of Politics. The Social and Political Thought of Ernest Barker*, Cambridge, 1994.

23   Burroughs, *A Faith for the Firing Line*, London, 1915; *The Fight for*

the Future, London, 1916; World-Builders All. The Task of the Rising Generation, London, 1917.

24   Burroughs, *The Valley of Decision. A Plea for Wholeness in Thought and Life*, London, 1916.

25   H. G. Mulliner, *E. A. Burroughs. A Memoir*, London, 1936; introduction by Temple, Archbishop of York.

26   Burroughs, *The Latin Culture*, London, 1920.

27   *World-Builders All* was dedicated 'to the masters and boys at Eton, Uppingham, Wellington, and Weymoth', whom Burroughs visited in the capacity as the Archbishop's messenger in the National Mission of Repentance and Hope. During one of those visits, Burroughs met the young author of *The Heart of a Schoolboy*, a reply to attacks on the Public School system such as Alec Waugh's famous *The Loom of Youth* (1917). Burroughs introduced the MS. to C. J. Longman, who published it in 1919.

28   A version of this chapter is also published as 'Englishness: the case of H. V. Morton', in *The Representation and Reality of War: Essays in Honour of D. G. Wright*, K. Dockray and K. Laybourn (eds), Stroud, 1999.

29   Sermon as reported in *Times*, 5 September 1927. Various versions of the sermon appeared in other national newspapers.

30   Bergson, *La Signification de la Guerre*, Paris, 1915. Note that from the beginning of the war and beyond, the image of Germans as scientific giants but moral pygmies was a common one. See D. Edgerton, 'British Scientific Intellectuals', pp. 6–7.

31   There are obvious parallels with contemporary futuristic fiction: see I. F. Clarke, *The Pattern of Expectation 1644-2001*, London, 1979. Replications of the theme were J. B. S. Haldane's run-ins with Bertrand Russell and the first Lord of Birkenhead. Russell, *Icarus, or the Future of Science*, London, 1924; Haldane, *Daedalus, or Science and the Future*, London, 1924; Lord Birkenhead, *The World in 2020*, London, 1930; *Haldane's Daedelus Revisited*, K. R. Dronamraju (ed.), Oxford, 1995.

32   Francis Mulhern, *The Moment of Scrutiny*, London, 1981, 18.

33   See C. Townshend, *Making the Peace*; Alun Howkins, 'The Discovery of Rural England', in *Englishness*, Colls and Dodd (eds), pp. 62–88.

34   See Ian MacKillop, '*Women in Love*, Class War and School Inspectors', in *D. H. Lawrence. New Studies*, Christopher Heywood (ed.), London, 1987, pp. 46–58.

35   *New York Times Magazine*, 7 September 1930.

36   *Catholic Authors. Contemporary Biographical Sketches, 1930-1947*,

M. Hoehn (ed.), Newark, 1948.

37 See e. g. Jay Corrin, *G. K. Chesterton and Hilaire Belloc: the Battle against Modernity*, Ohio, 1981. Belloc's *The Servile State* (1912) already predicted the erosion of personal liberty of the mass of the people.

38 Pope Leo XIII's encyclical *Aeterni Patris* (1879) recommended a renewal of interest in patristic and medieval philosophy and theology; part of the philological movement were Jacques Paul Migne (1800–1875), who made the texts available, and the theologians Matthias Joseph Scheeben (1835–1888) and John Baptiste Frazelin (1816–1886). By 1927 the continental Catholic Revival had for half a century presented medieval thinking as the historical matrix of the best in modern thought, including modern scientific thought (e.g. Gilson 1913, *La Liberté chez Descartes et la théologie*). Leo XIII had however also launched an attack on what he regarded as the twin evils of monopolistic capitalism and socialism with his encyclical *De Condicione Opificium*, popularly known as 'The Worker's Charter' (*Rerum Novarum*, 5 May 1891).

39 See e.g. H. Somerville, 'How the Reformation de-Christianized Economics', *The Month*, 148, August 1926; Donald MacLean, 'Catholic Economics', *The Month*, 150, December 1927; G. O'Brien, *The Economic Effects of the Reformation*, London, 1923. Also R. H. Tawney, *The Sickness of the Acquisitive Society*, London, 1920 and *Religion and the Rise of Capitalism. A Historical Study*, London, 1926.

40 George Santayana, in his *Soliloquies in England* London, 1922, concluded that the national character was Protestant through and through and maintained that '[a]n Englishman who becomes a Catholic ceases to be an Englishman.' Even Dean Inge, however, went through the ritual of calling this observation 'overstated' (*English Genius*, Kingsmill (ed.)). While this perception did of course stick, this did not mean that Catholics were excluded from the task of defining national character. On the contrary, the contributors of *The English Genius* counted Catholic intellectuals such as Belloc and Woodruff and sympathizers such as the poet Alfred Noyes.

41 Corrin, *Battle*; Belloc's *Europe and the Faith* (1921) interpreted the Great War as a clash between the forces of materialism (i.e. Prussia) and the forces of European and Christian civilization.

42 Armytage, *Heavens Below. Utopian Experiments in England 1560-1960*, London, 1961.

43 Belloc, *The Free Press*, London, 1918. Armytage, *Heavens Below.*

44 Keith, 'Darwin's Theory of Man's Descent As It Stands Today' in

Report of the British Association for the Advancement of Science (Leeds)
1927, pp. 1–15.

45 *Radio Times*, 16 (No 204), 26 August 1927.

46 Keith, 'Darwin's Theory', 4.

47 Keith, 'Darwin's Theory', 11. On the central role and status of the
brain in Keith's political imagination, see Rhodri Hayward's
contribution to this volume.

48 Keith, 'Darwin's Theory', pp. 12f.

49 *New York Times*, 6 September 1927; also *Times*, 5 September 1927;
Daily Herald, 5 September 1927; *Manchester Guardian*, 5 September
1927.

50 Lodge, *Science and Human Progress*, London, 1927.

51 *Times*, 5 September 1927; *New York Times*, 5 September 1927;
Manchester Guardian, 5 September 1927, 6 September 1927; *Daily
Herald*, 6 September 1927.

52 *New York Times*, 6 September 1927; *Daily Herald*, 6 September
1927.

53 On the victory fantasies of the opposition to Darwinism, see Peter
Bowler, 'The Humanists' Opponents: Science and Religion in Inter-
war Britain', paper presented at the Wellcome Workshop on
'Humanism and Citizenship in the Inter-war Period', 16 February
1996. *Times* printed 15 letters on 'Darwinism Today' between
September 2–10. For Rev. Bede Jarrett's service, see *Daily Herald*, 5
September 1927; *Manchester Guardian*, 5 September 1927. Jarrett
keenly supported the Dominican tradition of linking the order with
the old universities and it was he who took the Dominicans back to
Oxford after centuries of exile, where he founded Blackfriars, Oxford.

54 'Keith *vs* Moses', *New Statesman*, 10 September 1927, pp. 672–3.

55 *Nature* 120, 10 September 1927; Keith, 'Should Science Take a
Holiday?', *New York Times Magazine*, 7 September 1930. For the
idea that Downe was a 'shrine', see e.g. F. O. Bower, 'Size and Form
in Plants', in *Report of the British Association for the Advancement of
Science (Bristol) 1930*, pp. 1–14 at 1.

56 Howkins, 'The Discovery'. On the pastoralism of the recent past of
British science, see Simon Schaffer, 'Physics Laboratories and the
Victorian Country House', in *Making Space for Science*, J. Agar and
Crosbie Smith (eds), Basingstoke, 1997. For the rural (in contrast to
urban) setting of nineteenth-century English science (in contrast to
German science), see Soraya de Chadarevian, 'Laboratory Science
versus Country-House Experiments. The Controversy between Julius
Sachs and Charles Darwin', *British Journal for the History of Science*,
29 (1996): 17–42.

57 Gordon McOuat and Mary Winsor, 'J. B. S. Haldane's Darwinism in its Religious Context', *British Journal for the History of Science*, 28 (1995): 227–31; Armytage, *Sir Richard Gregory*, London 1957; also Vincent Brome, *Six Studies in Quarrelling*, London, 1958; David C. Smith, *H. G. Wells. Desperately Mortal. A Biography*, New Haven and London, 1986, pp. 245–67.

58 *Nature*, 15 January 1927; 19 February 1927; 19 March 1927; 9 April 1927.

59 Chesterton, *The Thing*, London, 1929, esp. 'The Mask of the Agnostic' and 'The Outline of the Fall'. Chesterton continued to engage in the issue over evolution. Barely a year before his death he got involved in the 1935 media-debate between the creationist scientist Ambrose Fleming (the president of the Victoria Institute, an evangelical think-tank), Keith, the Catholic convert Arnold Lunn, the psychologist C. E. M. Joad and others. One of the upshots of this debate was the Evolution Protest Movement. Keith, *Darwinism and Its Critics*, London, 1935.

60 *New York Times Magazine*, 7 September 1930.

61 *New York Times Magazine*, 5 October 1930. It has been suggested that public interest in the Leeds incident on the other side of the Atlantic should be read in the context of the recent trial of Thomas Scopes for teaching evolution (the so-called monkey trials of 1925). Carroll Pursell, '"A Savage Struck by Lightning": the Idea of a Research Moratorium, 1927-37', *Lex et Scientia*, 10 (1974): 146–61.

62 *Evening Standard*, 6 September 1927.

63 On diffusionism, see Henrika Kuklick, *The Savage Within: the Social History of British Anthropology, 1885-1945*, Cambridge, 1991.

64 On the construction of a non-Darwinian evolutionism into a wider opposition of materialism, see Peter J. Bowler, 'Evolution and the Eucharist: Bishop E. W. Barnes on Science and Religion in the 1920s and 1930s', *British Journal for the History of Science*, 31 (1998): 453–67 at 454.

65 *Times*, 5 September 1927. The metaphor is originally Emerson's. R. W. Emerson, 'Ode inscribed to W. H. Channing', in *The Portable Emerson*, ed. Mark van Doren, New York, 1956, 323.

66 Chesterton, 'A Plea'.

67 MacLean, 'Catholic Economics', *The Month*, 150, December 1927; Belloc, 'Bad News for the Expert', *New Statesman*, 19 July 1930.

68 S. L. Jaki, *Chesterton, a Seer of Science*, Urbana, 1986.

69 Chesterton, 'A Plea'.

70 Belloc, *New Statesman*, 19 July 1930; Chesterton, 'A Plea'.

71 Livingstone, *Defence*.

72 Belloc, 'Expert'.

73 Chesterton, *The Everlasting Man*, London, 1925. Bowler, 'The Humanists', has also noted that all the critics of evolution 'defended the right of the well-read amateur to analyze scientific issues which raised religious or philosophical questions'. For Chesterton playing umpire, see *The Thing*, 1929.

74 *Manchester Guardian*, 5 September 1927.

75 Chesterton, 'Saner Science', *G.K.'s Weekly*, 20 September 1930.

76 See note 38.

77 *Times*, 5 September 1927; *Manchester Guardian*, 5 September 1927.

78 *New York Times*, 6 September 1927; *Evening Standard*, 6 September 1927.

79 *Evening Standard*, 5 September 1927.

80 'Study and Research in Physics', *Nature* 120, 10 September 1927.

81 *Ibid.*

82 See e.g. the educationism of the positivist educationalist F. S. Marvin, from his programmatic utterances in *The Living Past: a Sketch of Western Progress* (Oxford, 1913) to *The Nation at School* (London, 1933). See also A.-K. Mayer, 'Moralizing Science: The Uses of Science's Past in National Education in the 1920s', *British Journal for the History of Science*, 30 (1997): 51–70.

83 *Manchester Guardian*, 5 September 1927. J. Needham, 'Mechanistic Biology and the Religious Consciousness', in *Science, Religion and Reality*, J. Needham (ed.), Cambridge, 1925, pp. 219–57.

84 Peter Collins, *The BAAS*; *idem*, 'The British Association as Public Apologist for Science, 1919-1945', in *The Parliament of Science: the British Association for the Advancement of Science 1831-1981*, P. Collins and R. MacLeod (eds), Northwood, 1981, pp. 210–36. R. MacLeod, 'Retrospect: the British Association and its Historians', *ibid.*, pp. 1–16.

85 *Discovery*, 8 (No. 94), October 1927. See also letter to the *New Statesman*, 17 September 1927, whose author admitted that until he realized that Keith was addressing a wireless audience, he was mystified as to how 'such palpably second-hand and shallow utterances' could be 'coming from an authority'.

86 Holland, 'The International Relationship of Minerals', in *Report of the British Association for the Advancement of Science (South Africa) 1929*, pp. 22–37; Bragg, 'Craftsmanship and Science', in *Report of the British Association for the Advancement of Science (Glasgow) 1928*, pp. 1–20.

87 Collins, *The BAAS*.

88 Smuts, 'The Scientific World-Picture of To-day', in *Report of the*

British Association for the Advancement of Science (London) 1931, pp. 1–18 at 13; Ewing, 'An Engineer's Outlook', in *Report of the British Association for the Advancement of Science (York) 1932*, pp. 1–19, esp. 16–19; *idem*, 'Allied Forces for Progress', *Discovery*, 15 (April 1934): 101–2.

89   Lamb, 'Presidential Address', in *Report of the British Association for the Advancement of Science (Southampton) 1925*, pp. 1–14 at 4.

90   *Manchester Guardian*, 5 September 1927. Needham explicitly stated that the tendency towards scientific specialization was 'quite inevitable and can only be partially controlled'; Needham, 'Mechanistic Biology'.

91   For a slightly different context, David Hollinger has argued that the rise of secular scholarship and science relied on a strategy of 'justification by correct cognitive conduct'; Hollinger 'Justification by Verification: the Scientific Challenge to the Moral Authority of Christianity in Modern America', in *Religion and 20th Century American Intellectual Life*, M. J. Lacey (ed.), Cambridge, 1989.

92   E.g. Edgerton, 'British Scientific Intellectuals', 7; Gary Werskey, *The Visible College: A Collective Biography of British Scientists and Socialists of the 1930s*, London, 1978; J. G. Crowther, *The Social Relations of Science*, London, 1941.

93   *Evening Standard*, 5 September 1927. Note that Lodge exempted the wireless.

94   Russell, 'The Dynamic of Science', in *Adventure. The Faith of Science and the Science of Faith*, B. H. Streeter (ed.), London, 1927.

95   Collins, *The BAAS*; William McGucken, *Scientists*, esp. pp. 15f.

96   *Nature* 106, 23 September 1920.

97   Russell, 'Dynamic'.

98   Collins, *BAAS*; McGucken, *Scientists*.

99   Barker, 'The Nature and Conditions of Academic Freedom in Universities', in *Report of the British Association for the Advancement of Science (Toronto) 1924*, pp. 247–55.

100 As reported in *Manchester Guardian*, 5 September 1927.

101 Chesterton in *G.K.'s Weekly*, 17 September 1927; and 'Saner Science', *ibid.*, 20 September 1930. Barker, 'Academic Freedom'.

102 Pursell, 'A Savage'.

103 *Daily Herald*, 6 September 1927; *New York Times*, 6 September 1927. Even such enthusiastic supporters of the application of science to human affairs as Crew, however, did not expect scientists to fashion policies for human betterment; Crew had an advisory capacity in mind, and thus an ideal scenario in which specialist scientists had the ear of those skilled in statecraft. Crew in

'Symposium: Professors of Foresight', *The Listener*, supplement, December 1932.

104 *Ripon Diocesan Gazette*, April 1934; *Yorkshire Post*, 21 May 34. See also Kenneth M. Wolfe, *The Churches and the British Broadcasting Corporation 1922-1956. The Politics of Broadcast Religion*, London, 1984.

105 Alfred Noyes, 'Radio and the Master Secret', in *Radio Times*, 18 September 1925, pp. 549–50 at 550.

106 Temple, in Mulliner, *Burroughs*.

107 *Evening Standard*, 6 September 1927. Years later, an exasperated Burroughs still protested that his suggestion of a moratorium had been uttered in jest; see his letter to the U. S. physicist Robert Millikan, 25 March 1930, quoted by Pursell.

108 *Manchester Guardian*, 5 September 1927.

109 Burroughs in *Evening Standard*, 6 September 1927.

110 *Daily Herald*, 6 September 1927.

111 *Evening Standard*, 5 September 1927.

112 Crowther, *Social Relations*.

113 Chesterton in *G.K.'s Weekly*, 17 September 1927.

114 A. E. Heath, 'Science and Education', in *Science and Civilization*, F. S. Marvin (ed.), Oxford, 1923, pp. 221–46 at 226.

115 For Keith, see *Daily Herald*, 6 September 1927; *Manchester Guardian*, 6 September 1927. For Lodge, see *Daily Herald*, 5 September 1927; *Manchester Guardian*, 5 September 1927. For Hall, see *Evening Standard*, 5 September 1927; on general education, *Times Educational Supplement*, 11 January 17. For Bragg, see Bragg, 'Craftsmanship'. For Myres, see *Evening Standard*, 5 September 1927.

116 Needham, 'Religion in a Scientific Age', *Nineteenth Century*, (November 1931): 580–93; also published as 'Religion in a World Dominated by Science', in Needham, *The Great Amphibium*, London, 1931, pp. 9–50 at 28.

117 On Victorian Hellenism and in particular the famous Arnoldian notion, see Frank M. Turner, *The Greek Heritage in Victorian Britain*, Yale, 1981, pp. 17–36.

118 Among ideologues of dynamism were educators such as A. E. Heath and Percy Nunn and such notables as Richard Gregory and William Bragg. Heath, 'Science and Education'; Nunn, 'Science', in *The New Teaching*, John Adams (ed.), London, 1918, pp. 154–98; Gregory, *The Spirit and Service of Science*, London, 1916; Bragg, 'Craftsmanship'.

119 Turner, *Heritage*, pp. 61–76; Percy Gardner, preface to Adolf Michaelis, *A Century of Archaeological Discoveries*, tr. B. Kahnweiler, London 1908, pp. viii–ix; cited after Turner, 70.

120 On the imperialism of 'public science', see F. M. Turner, 'Public
     Science'; D. MacKenzie, *Statistics in Britain, 1865-1930. The Social
     Construction of Scientific Knowledge*, Edinburgh, 1981; also H.
     Kuklick, *Savage*; Edgerton, 'British Scientific Intellectuals'. On inter-
     war thought and debate of political internationalism, see *Thinkers of
     the Twenty Years Crisis. Inter-war Idealism Reassessed*, D. Long and
     Wilson (eds), Oxford, 1995.

121 *Evening Standard*, 5 September 1927 (my italics).

122 *New York Times Magazine*, 7 July 1930.

123 Keith, 'The Last Chapter of Life. Humanity's "Grand National" and
     the Type of Man who will win it', *Evening Standard*, 14 October
     1927, pp. 7, 9.

124 There is an historical precedent for the somewhat paradoxical
     combination of Englishness and internationalism in scientific
     propaganda. As Rob Iliffe suggests, members of the early Royal
     Society proposed a co-operative, international experimental
     philosophy and simultaneously argued that it was peculiarly English.
     For the Royal Society and its propagandists, 'the future of natural
     philosophy rested on persuading others of the unique fertility of
     English experimentalism.' At the same time, 'xenophobic comments
     … also served to bolster philosophical internationalism.' Rob Iliffe,
     'Foreign Bodies: Travel, Empire and the Early Royal Society of
     London Part 2. The Land of Experimental Knowledge' in *Canadian
     Journal of History*, 34 (1999): 23–50.

125 *Evening Standard*, 5 September 1927.

126 Bragg, 'Craftsmanship'.

127 Keith, 'Should Science'.

128 Haldane, *Daedalus*. For details about the genesis of the book, its
     sales figures and its impact, see *Haldane's Daedalus Revisited*,
     R. Dronamraju (ed.).

129 Huxley, 'The World with Mechanism Enslaved. How the Race of the
     Future may live', *Evening Standard*, 12 October 1927 pp. 7, 9.

130 Keith summing up his predecessors in the *Evening Standard* series,
     'The Last Chapter'. The series counted J. B. S. Haldane, 'The
     Golden Age – and then! Will Man return to Barbarism, or live
     forever and colonize the Stars?', *Evening Standard*, 10 October 1927,
     pp. 7, 9; Dean Inge, 'The World Frozen Out. An Ice Age Vision,
     with a Robot Inferno as the Last Civilization of all', *Evening
     Standard*, 11 October 1927, 7; J. Huxley, 'The World'; and the
     ethicist C. Delisle Burns, 'Saving Mankind from the War. Will
     World Security be Achieved by Co-operative Government?', *Evening
     Standard*, 13 October 1927, pp. 7–8.

131 I do not have the space here to deal with this issue, but it should be
     noted that English or British concern with national identity and
     future direction clearly mirrors contemporary debates elsewhere. For
     the German context, for example, see Jeffrey Herf, *Reactionary
     Modernism. Technology, Culture, and Politics in Weimar and the Third
     Reich*, Cambridge, 1984.

132 MacKenzie, *Statistics*, ch. 4: 'Karl Pearson'; F. M. Turner, *Between
     Science and Religion: the Reaction to Scientific Naturalism in Late
     Victorian England*, Yale, 1974; *idem*, 'Rainfall, Plagues, and the
     Prince of Wales: a Chapter in the Conflict of Religion and Science',
     in *Journal of British Studies*, 13 (1974): 46–65; *idem*, 'The Victorian
     Conflict between Science and Religion: a Professional Dimension',
     Isis, 69 (1978): 356–76.

133 George Sampson, *English for the English*, Cambridge 1923; *The
     Teaching of English in England* (Report of the Newbolt Committee),
     HMSO, 1921. On the cultural and political mission of the Newbolt
     Committee and its report, see Chris Baldick, *The Social Mission of
     English Criticism, 1848-1932*, Oxford, 1987; Stephen Ball, Alex Kenny,
     David Gardiner, 'Literacy, Politics and the Teaching of English', in
     Bringing English to Order: the History and Politics of a School Subject, I.
     Goodson and Medway (eds), Falmer, 1990, pp. 47–86 at 52.

134 William Osler, 'The Old Humanities and the New Science. The
     Presidential Address delivered before the Classical Association at Oxford,
     May 1919', in *British Medical Journal*, 5 July 1919, pp. 1–7 at 4.

135 On the intrinsic competitiveness of liberal education in nineteenth-
     century Oxbridge, see Sheldon Rothblatt, 'Failure in Early
     Nineteenth-Century Oxford and Cambridge', *History of Education*,
     11 (1982): 1–21; *idem*, 'The Student Sub-culture and the
     Examination System in Early 19th Century Oxbridge', in *The
     University in Society*, Lawrence Stone (ed.), vol. 1, pp. 247–303;
     Andrew Warwick, 'Exercising the Student Body. Mathematics and
     Athleticism in Victorian Cambridge', in *Science Incarnate. Historical
     Embodiments of Natural Knowledge*, Christopher Lawrence and
     Steven Shapin (eds), Chicago and London, 1998, pp. 288–326.

136 McGucken, *Scientists*, pp. 265–306.

137 See Douglas Woodruff's obituary of Belloc, as cited in note 1; also
     Barker, *National Character*, London, 1927; *idem*, 'An Attempt at
     Perspective', in *The Character of England*, Oxford, 1947, pp.
     550–75. Butterfield, *The Englishman and His History*, Cambridge,
     1944; *idem*, 'Reflections on the Predicament of Our Times',
     Cambridge Journal, 1 (1947): 5–13.

5

'The shell of a prosperous age': History, Landscape and the Modern in Paul Rotha's *The Face of Britain* (1935)

Timothy Boon

The new documentary forms of the inter-war years embodied particular approaches to the social sphere and to national identity. This is especially true of documentary films. Not just contemporaries, but historians too, have written at length on the importance of these approaches for documentarists.[1] Much recent literature has focused on a small canon of 'classic documentaries', and, as a result, certain ways of addressing and representing social themes, present in the work of some directors, have been under-represented in the historiography of the documentary. The key example is the work of Paul Rotha (1907-1984). Many of the films he produced and directed have significance for the themes of this book, as they are concerned at various levels with themes of nationhood and citizenship. This chapter examines the film that most explicitly addressed these themes, *The Face of Britain* (made 1934-5). Rotha's Britain was not, as would be typical of the period, Britain in name only, but England in fact. *The Face of Britain*, as an account of nationhood, combines aspects of Englishness and Scottishness, conveyed visually through urban and rural landscapes with a pastoral-technological account of national history. Rotha's account uses arguments about the necessity of planning, presented within a commentary which is recognisably modernistic both in its language and in the overall structure of its argument. I explore the relation of these aspects of the film's vision of nationhood to contemporary arguments in print and to recent historical work. In particular I compare Rotha's vision with that of J. B. Priestley and the architect Arthur Eden. I argue that, if we are to grasp the totality of ways in which nationhood was understood in the past we must look to all representational media.

Paul Rotha: Films and Film Making

Although this chapter focuses on Rotha's work, this should not be taken to signal an auteurist interpretation.[2] But in this case, where evidence is sparse, the film itself and Rotha's papers provide the main sources of my reading.[3] I have argued elsewhere that authorship of films should be seen to extend beyond the director towards the whole range of people involved – the 'interest group'. Films could not be made without the financial, practical and intellectual contributions of people other than film directors, and such people often had a major influence on how the subjects of the films were represented.[4] Rotha himself expressed something similar in a letter to Eric Knight in 1933. He noted, 'only one man can write a script of a film and that is the director and the cutter ... But that does not include content. The subject, theme and even narrative situations can be suggested (not written) by outside sources and adapted as thought fit.'[5] Later in his career, however, several collaborators did go as far as writing sections of scripts.[6] So, individuals other than film makers often had a strong impact, if not on a film's framework, then certainly on the subject and its associations. A shared ideology was the key to the intimacy of these collaborations. This chapter explores the ideas shared among Rotha, his intellectual sources and his collaborators.

Paul Rotha, along with John Grierson, was one of the two most prominent figures in British documentary film. Rotha's father was C. J. S. Thompson, first curator of the Wellcome Historical Medical Museum. Rotha trained at the Slade School of Fine Art (where he adopted his surname from his mother's side), worked briefly as an art director for British International Pictures, before publishing *The Film Till Now* (1930), an influential textbook on the history of film.[7] In the same year, after 6 months working with John Grierson at the Empire Marketing Board Film Unit, he branched out on his own. In 1932–3, with support from Shell Petroleum and Imperial Airways, he made his first substantial documentary, *Contact*, on the subject of international air travel. During the thirties he directed or produced another nineteen films, including *Shipyard* (1935).[8] This film related the construction of a liner at Barrow-in-Furness to cyclical unemployment in the town.[9] But his influence was as much via his prolific written work as through his films. His *Documentary Film* (1936) was the first book-length justification of the genre in Britain.

For Rotha, as for many others, documentary was not simply the British school of Grierson, and *Documentary Film* is a lengthy argument about the distinctiveness of the genre. Rotha's arguments were framed, not within the philosophical idealism of Grierson, but within dialectical materialism.[10] An anonymous reviewer in *The Times* picked this up, 'Mr Rotha elaborates [his definition of documentary] by tacking onto it a frankly materialist view of social evolution. This is not surprising, for the aesthetic left in the cinema is also ranged on the left politically.'[11] Rotha presented documentary as a serious-minded antidote to the frivolity of Hollywood: 'not only does the story-film today spend its time in reflecting the least important aspects of capitalistic society but it is often made to do so in a cynical or unintelligent fashion.'[12] Using a conventional Marxist base/superstructure metaphor he argued:

> we must not forget that it is to the advantage of a dominant class to produce and perfect a form of indirect propaganda for the preservation of its interests. All institutions, whether political, sociological or aesthetic, fundamentally reflect and assist in the maintenance of the predominating influences in control of the productive forces in their particular era. To this the cinema is no exception.[13]

He berated British and American Feature films not just because he saw them as frivolous, but because in his view they failed to adopt a suitably cinematic technique:

> the story-film has followed closely in the theatrical tradition for its subject-matter; converting, as time went on, stage forms into film forms, stage acting into film acting. The opposite group of thought … proceeds from the belief that nothing photographed, or recorded on to celluloid, has meaning until it comes to the cutting-bench; that the primary task of film creation lies in the physical and mental stimuli which can be produced by the factor of editing.[14]

Elsewhere he was more blunt. In 1933 in a review of Vsevolod Pudovkin's *Film Technique* he stated that most story films had been produced 'upon basically wrong principles'.[15] Rotha's argument, couched in the language of citizenship, rested on the notion of an appropriate response to the modern world. In *Documentary Film* he wrote: 'Civilisation today, in fact, presents a complexity of political and social problems which have to be faced by every thinking person … it rests with the ordinary person to act not merely as a passive voter but as an active member of the State.'[16] He did, however, concede in passing at the end of the book that his model of documentary 'presupposes, from a propagandist point of view, a greater social and political consciousness among the people than actually exists.'[17]

Graham Greene, reviewing *Documentary Film*, stated that 'The first part of Mr Rotha's book, so admirable when it reaches the actual making of documentaries, is rather tiresomely Marxist.'[18] I now turn to this 'admirable' section. It is only here that Rotha made a clear series of distinctions between documentary and other types of film making. He believed that the Russian directors and theoreticians, Sergei Eisenstein, Alexander Dovjenko, and particularly Pudovkin, had developed a definitive film construction technique.[19] He criticised films which did not marry technique to purpose, extending this criticism to all aspects of technique, including acting, photography ('technique must come second to content') and editing ('the aim of cutting is to stir the emotions of the audience so that it will be receptive of context without the cutting itself becoming prominent').[20] After separate discussion of the visual and aural components of films, he turned to how a film's themes should be treated. He stressed the importance of the social engagement of the documentary film-maker, arguing that: 'Before [the director] can create, before he can become in any way significant in his work, he must be able to understand the social relationships contained in his theme and be dynamic in his social analysis.'[21]

Rotha defined two styles of documentary: the descriptive, *reportage* or journalist approach, which he said aimed to be

> an honest effort to report, describe or delineate a series of events, or the nature of a process, or the workings of an organisation on the screen ... The less your journalist director sensationalises his material, the better is his purpose served, because by dramatisation he would sacrifice exactness for impressionism.[22]

The other style, the 'impressionistic', 'demands', he wrote,

> just such an exacting understanding of material as the reportage method, but it selects only those elements of the subject which are capable of dramatisation. It aims to produce a general emotional effect and not a detailed literary description. It aims to disturb the audience emotionally, to make it feel for itself the social or other references contained in the subject.[23]

The Face of Britain belongs to this category. Finally, discussing structure and scenario, Rotha stated a preference between the two, and committing himself to a dialectical method in impressionistic documentary. His argument for the impressionistic style was partially founded on the nature of the cinema audience: 'We must make allowance for a tolerant and mildly uninterested audience, upon whom our films must create emotional effect as well as persuade to a certain way of thinking.'[24] Gingerly, he introduced the idea of dialectic as a means of structuring films. Quoting Marx from the *Critique of Political Economy*, that 'the mode of production in material life determines the general character of the social, political and spiritual process of life', he proceeded to recommend the classic Hegelian principle of thesis/antithesis/synthesis. He wrote:

> The dialectic as drama is conflict and must dictate the structure of the film. The pattern-of-three arises again and again during production: in the fundamental composition of the film strip (the conflict between frame and frame, shot and shot, etc.), the building up of symphonic movement (comparative rhythms), the imagistic use of sound (two motives expressed simultaneously giving rise to a third idea), the structure of sequences and, indeed, quite possibly in the structure of the film as a whole.[25]

Rotha was deeply involved in the technicalities of film construction, to the extent that when the Film Society, an organisation established in 1925 to show art and experimental films, had a copy of Pudovkin's *A Simple Case*, Rotha borrowed it and analysed the close detail of how it achieved its montage effects.[26]

'The Face of Britain'

In *Documentary Film* Rotha described *The Face of Britain* as 'a film of the natural and scientific planning of Britain with reference to the respective power of coal and electricity.'[27] It is striking that the film's title should specify Britain rather than England. Study of the Rotha archive reveals that early drafts went under the title *The Face of England* and imply no intention to film north of the border. It is perhaps little surprise to learn that it was a Scot, Inverness-born and Glasgow-educated Hugh Quigley (1895–1979), who introduced the Scottish element to the film. Quigley was Chief Statistical Officer of the Central Electricity Board, but his interests extended very broadly, into literary criticism, history and topography, as his publications show.[28] In a letter in June 1934, responding to the script Rotha had sent him, he said 'I would suggest that we should change the title to "The Face of Britain" instead of "The Face of England", because you will probably have a certain infusion of Scottish scenery in it.'[29] The copy of this version of the script in the Rotha archive has 'England' in the title crossed-out and replaced with 'Britain'. Quigley's book of Highland topography, without reference to his role in its production, commented that *The Face of Britain* 'would have been more accurately called "The face of the Scottish Highlands and Industrial England".'[30] Quigley's intervention was decisive, not simply in the inclusion of Scotland, but in the manner in which it is shown. Philip Dodd argues that, in an influential tradition deriving from Matthew

111

Arnold, the culture of the Celtic nations was held to be peripheral to the metropolitan culture of England. Furthermore, the 'autonomous contribution of the Celts to Civilisation was confined to the past.'[31] However Quigley's version of Scotland, as we shall see in more detail below, contained a modernistic ambition to provide the hydro-electric power to transform the entire nation. Quigley's view implies not that Scotland was included in England as a nation, but that it was part of a British one.

The Face of Britain is divided into four sections dealing with pre-industrial Britain, the industrial revolution, hydro-electric power and 'the new age'. It was initiated in May or June 1934, while Rotha was regularly crossing the country to Barrow-in-Furness to record the construction of the liner Orion for his film *Shipyard*. It was shot between July and November and edited between August 1934 and spring 1935.[32] The precise origins of the film's contents and arguments are obscure. Two of his previous films had been concerned with the role of industry in the early thirties. *Roadwards* (1933) was ostensibly a promotional film for Daimler. Rotha described it in a letter to Knight displaying a vulgar-Marxist, anti-boss sentiment coupled to a conventional urban/rural distinction in what David Matless has called the 'motoring pastorale' style.[33]

> Straightforward handling with a strong labor bias in the cutting which the big bugs of the motor business cannot see. I've tried briefly to tell the story of the wide stretching roads which have flung themselves across the face of England since the War – how the wide arterials lead to the country hedgerows and beyond to the real country scene, how to get there you must first go to the industrial scene – with belching chimnies [sic] and sweating workers.[34]

Rotha's next film, *Rising Tide* (1934), included more on English industry in its treatment of the trade between England and South Africa. Rotha envisaged it as: 'A vast industrial survey of England, the transport by rail of freight to the [Southampton] docks, the loading, the departure ... the long voyage across the Atlantic down the coast of Africa ... then Capetown and the reloading of the ship with raw products from the South and back again to England.'[35] This 'vast industrial survey' involved filming paper mills, cotton, glass and steelworks in Lancashire, and a steelworks in Sheffield.[36] Colls and Dodd have argued that documentary film makers were part of the social reporting tradition which dated to the late nineteenth century and the 'Into Unknown England' writings that included George Sims' *How the Poor Live* (1883) and Lady Bell's *At the Works* (1907).

Colls and Dodd quote Grierson speaking of the documentarists' need 'to travel dangerously into the jungles of Middlesborough and the Clyde.'[37] John Baxendale and Chris Pawling, discussing the journey narratives of the thirties, write of 'the way in which the documentary film movement and Mass Observation articulate a felt need on the part of progressive middle-class intellectuals to move out of the metropolis and discover the "provinces".'[38] Rotha, the southern and metropolitan artist, could be taken as an example. He expected to travel into the 'foreign land' of the industrial north to discover the authentic face of industrial capitalism. The architectural writer Arthur Eden similarly spoke of 'the wilderness of a northern industrial town' and 'the desolation of its suburbs'.[39]

Rotha's autobiography suggests that it was simply fortuitous that he was able to gain support for *The Face of Britain*. He presents it as a project inspired by intellectual sources including Priestley's *English Journey* (1934), which he had just read.[40] We may take it that Priestley's views on the state of the nation both challenged and confirmed Rotha's presuppositions, helping him to form the precise vision which is articulated in *The Face of Britain*. Rotha's autobiography also states that he had 'been interested in a series of articles about the changing pattern of the English countryside in the *Architectural Review.*' The only items which fit the description are Eden's series on 'The English Tradition in the Countryside' published between March and May 1935, with stills from Rotha's film.[41] Even though publication occurred rather late in the editing stage of *The Face of Britain*, for stills from an unreleased film to be used as illustrations, Rotha must have been moving in the same social circles of architects as Eden. This is worth examining because in *The Face of Britain* architectural modernism has a prominent place. We have evidence for Rotha's membership of architectural circles at this time. He was certainly associated with the architect Basil Ward by early 1936. Ward was a member of Connell, Ward and Lucas, a practice most closely identified with the introduction of continental Modernism into Britain. Connell's 'High and Over' in Amersham, commenced in 1929, was one of the first Modern Movement buildings in the country.[42] A cartoon by Rotha in the *Architectural Review* in 1932 is taken by one recent writer to refer to houses designed by this practice at Saltdean.[43] Early in 1936, when he established his trade organisation, Associated Realist Film Producers, Rotha made Ward one of six advisors from outside the film trade.[44] In 1936 Rotha was advising the public relations committee of RIBA, of which Ward was a member, on a programme of films.[45] Ward and

Connell appear amongst thirty of Rotha's friends in a spoof historical sequence in his 1938 film *New Worlds for Old*.[46]

Rotha's politics, associations and reading were informed by an emotional response to the Depression that he shared with many Left intellectuals. He wrote to Knight whilst he was in Scotland filming sequences for the film in July 1934:

> On the way here everything was marked by tragedy. All through the industrial Midlands and Lancashire, the terrible slums of Glasgow and the Clyde Valley, you could see the scarred mess that greedy men have made of this lovely country. And so much of it is now disused. Great slabs of countryside littered with rusting factories and crumbling chimneys, refuse from another age when men trampled upon everything to get rich.[47]

Whatever the sources of his thematic concerns, Rotha also had to build support for making the film. First he persuaded Bruce Woolfe, managing director of Gaumont-British Instructional, to which he had been attached since *Contact*, to agree to the project.[48] Woolfe agreed to pay for footage on condition that Rotha find sponsorship.[49] Rotha turned to Quigley, who had already published on *Electrical Power and National Progress*, and provided an introduction and conclusion for Ismay Goldie's *Housing and Slum Clearance in London* (1934), both of which conveyed a rationalist, planning-based response to social problems, not unlike Rotha's.[50] In his introduction to the latter work, for example, Quigley argued that the 'planned city ... is taken as an absolute necessity of the modern world; it takes the place of an economic scheme based on *laissez-faire*, which has been unequal to the task of maintaining the population, absorbing its natural increase and creating a higher standard of living.'[51] The advocacy of corporatist, planning solutions instead of *laissez-faire* is a familiar trope in reformist writings in the inter-war period.[52] But Quigley was more active a member of the Left than this may imply. He was a member of the XYZ Club which 'provided an intelligence service on City activities' to the Labour Party and 'helped shape [its] thinking on financial policy.' Hugh Gaitskell and Hugh Dalton were amongst its members.[53] Another mark of Quigley's commitment to planning solutions was his membership of the committee of Political and Economic Planning which produced the 1936 report on electrical supply.[54] Like Rotha, he had published in the *Architectural Review*.[55] Just months before Rotha approached him about *The Face of Britain*, he wrote a letter supporting the work of the GPO Film Unit to Stephen Tallents, the government official in charge, during one of the Treasury's periods of scepticism about the Unit's value.[56]

It is not entirely surprising that the CEB should fund Rotha's film, because in addition to Quigley's support for documentary, he had previously employed Bruce Woolfe's company, among others, to make thirteen films. Low describes these as 'silent films that were in fact little more than lantern lectures, with long, informative titles replacing the lecture.'[57] Quigley's letter to Tallents had drawn a contrast between the quality of the documentary film *Industrial Britain* and those made by Woolfe's companies. From 1934, following a minor coup in which the CEB came to exert greater control over the Electrical Development Association (EDA), the production of publicity films seems to have been delegated from the CEB to this organisation.[58] Films, which spear-headed a reinvigorated publicity drive in the campaign against the gas industry for domestic users, were intended to be populist and included titles such as *Plenty of Time for Play*, *The Wizard in the Wall*, and *Well, I Never!* These films were fundamentally different in kind from *The Face of Britain*, the release of which is not mentioned in the *EDA Bulletin*.[59] Quigley also clearly saw it as different because in a letter to *The Times* promoting the CEB's use of films only the month after its release, he made no explicit reference to it, discussing instead *Power* and *Electricity: From Grid to Customer*, the two earlier films made by Gaumont-British Instructional's predecessor company, British Instructional Films.[60]

Rotha recalled in his autobiography that he and Quigley 'at once saw eye to eye about a film on the possibilities of replanning Britain, both industrial and rural, based on the flexible power of the national grid.'[61] Quigley took an active part in *The Face of Britain*, making extensive suggestions for places to film and loaning Rotha some books.[62] In correspondence Quigley deliberately pointed Rotha to both English and Scottish scenery: his list of proposed landscapes to illustrate this section of the film included the top of Auchnotroch in the Clyde valley, as well as more familiar English sites such as Wenlock Edge. Quigley met Rotha in Scotland, perhaps also accompanying him on an inspection of pithead baths in July 1934, during one of his filming sorties.[63] This is rather less surprising when we learn that Quigley, already the author of several volumes of topography, was to publish in March 1936 his volume for the Batsford *Face of Britain* series, *The Highlands of Scotland*.[64] The choice of Arthur Cummings, Liberal political columnist of the *Daily Chronicle* to speak the commentary for *The Face of Britain* may also have been at Quigley's suggestion, given Cummings' authorship of

The Moscow Trial, an account of the trial of Metropolitan-Vickers engineers on spying charges, although his book rather took the side of the Soviet courts.[65]

The Face of Britain was unlike other films of the period in its intellectual ambitions; as an early outline explained that the 'conception of this film is unusual. Documentary in style and approach, it sets out in three acts a dialectic which argues the effect of the mechanisation of industry on our social lives and, after a survey of the chaos produced by unplanned industry, suggests the urgent necessity for a planned and organised future.'[66] This description provides the key to understanding the relationship between the form the film took and the theoretical argument of *Documentary Film*, composed at the same time as Rotha was editing *The Face of Britain*.[67] Dialectic here refers both to the Marxist historiography and to the dialectical montage (editing) used to structure the film, theory of film construction, which, as we have seen, was derived from the Soviet school of Eisenstein and Pudovkin. We can see that Rotha's commitment to Marxist theory was not without reservation. He wrote to Knight in October 1933 'Good God, Knight, isn't there some middle way? I know all the Marxist stuff – thesis, antithesis equals synthesis – but somehow I'm not convinced. I know that all art is governed by economics – by the social system – that there's no such bunk as art for art's sake – but somehow I'm not satisfied.'[68] By the time he was doing his first rough edit of a section of *The Face of Britain* in August 1934, he was more bullish, although he confessed to having drunk 'too much beer' when he wrote:

> I believe, but god what modesty, that this Face of Britain is taking up where Ten Days that Shook the World left off with ideological documentary. It is the first pure dialectic documentary to be attempted in this country. It is no longer just simply building something – tracing a thing from its beginning to a logical conclusion – it [is] stating a definite dialectic argument and asking the intelligent answer from the audience.[69]

Ten Days that Shook the World was the title of the edited version of Eisenstein's *October* circulated outside the Soviet Bloc in the interwar period. David Cook explains Eisenstein's model of Marxist dialectical montage:

> This dialectic is a way of looking at human history and experience as a perpetual conflict in which a force (thesis) collides with a

counterforce (antithesis) to produce from their collision a wholly new phenomenon (synthesis) which is not the sum of the two forces but something greater than and different from them both ... Eisenstein maintained that in film editing the shot or 'montage cell', is a thesis which when placed into juxtaposition with another shot of opposing visual content – antithesis – produces a synthesis (a synthetic idea or impression) which in turn becomes the thesis of a new dialectic as the montage sequence continues.[70]

This was what Rotha had in mind and we can see in *The Face of Britain* that he was employing precisely this model both at the microscopic and at the macroscopic level. The more microscopic use is particularly visible in a sequence in 'The Smoke Age' section where Rotha intercut other material with a workman stoking a kiln; rhythmically, at the end of the shovel's swing, he intercut first several views of the industrial landscape of The Potteries, then a graveyard. The synthesis comes when the rhythmic soundtrack – *musique concrète avant la lettre* – ceases, with a shot showing a graveyard's funerary statue in the foreground and smoking factories in the distance.

Historiography and *The Face of Britain*

The remainder of this chapter is devoted to three aspects of the film: the periodisation of its historical structure; the landscape-based idea of nationhood it encodes; and the particular account of modernity it purveys. The latter two themes are present in different degrees throughout the film, lending weight and colour to the overall historical account. This makes simple thematic discussion difficult, so, after a short historiographical account, this chapter follows the sequence of the film.

The Face of Britain, as we have seen, is structured as a historical dialectic, despite Rotha's concession that 'by some modern authorities it is considered an out-of-date method when applied to history.'[71] 'Heritage of the Past', first of the four sections, and analytically the film's thesis, paints an idyllic view of Britain's landscape and community before industrialisation. 'The Smoke Age' provides the antithesis, describing the impact of the industrial revolution on the land and people of Britain. The synthesis is achieved jointly by 'The New Power' which introduces hydro-electric generation, and 'The New Age' which demonstrates the planning of Britain, which the film argues electrification permits.[72] Historical contextualisation had not previously played so important a role in any documentary film, but following *The Face of Britain* it became a common feature in the late thirties.[73] The dominant model, as introduced here by Rotha, was of a national British history with industrialisation as the key event. This model tallies in the most general sense with Dodd's analysis of English culture, but not with its detail. Dodd argues that 'during 1880-1920 the conviction that English culture was to be found in the past was stabilised. The past cultural activities and attributes of the *people* were edited and then acknowledged, as contributions to the evolution of the English national culture which had produced the present.'[74] The historical model of *The Face of Britain* differed in two important respects from that discussed by Colls and Dodd. First, the conception of historical process was not the smooth transitions of Whig history, but the dynamic and continuing change of historical materialism.[75] For Rotha, the character of the nation was not now stable, or perhaps slowly evolving, rather the dynamic of history was continuing to forge new versions of it. Second, he located nationhood mainly within a historical account attached to national geography rather than people. Rotha's was not the history of English *people*, either dominant or subordinated, and their 'single and continuous history' of Englishness which had been 'appropriated by and bec[o]me the responsibility of certain narrowly defined groups and their institutions.'[76]

Colls and Dodd have extended their analysis to documentary films and they find in several examples, including Grierson and Robert Flaherty's *Industrial Britain* (1933), Alberto Calvalcanti and Grierson's *Coalface* and Arthur Elton and Edgar Anstey's *Housing Problems* (both 1935), the same sense of nationhood in terms of the class relations between the *people* of Britain.[77] More recently K. and P. Dodd gave greater stress to the documentarists' development of a new sense of masculine national identity which, it is argued, the film makers found by abandoning the south east for the geographical peripheries of the industrial north and coastal fishing villages, a trope also discussed by Baxendale and Pawling.[78] But although this analysis is useful, *The Face of Britain* does not sit entirely comfortably within it. The dominant visual images are of English and Scottish places, and there are few shots within which people are the main focus.[79] Nor was Rotha's type of 'national past' purveyed by the Historical Association, which by 1918 had developed two principal 'tendencies', both political-historical. First a stress on the imperial aspect of Britain's national past and second a stress on Britain's standing relative to the European nations. The significance of the Celtic countries had been discussed in Historical Association circles, but they were to be subordinated within the history of Great Britain and 'the world-wide Commonwealth'.[80]

The co-existence of these various accounts of nationhood suggests not just that national identity was constructed in historical terms in the sixty years before the Second World War, but that culturally prominent individuals and groups of different persuasions held to and purveyed different historiographies of nationhood. Here the encapsulation of particular historical accounts within films can be seen to be particularly significant in a period in which it was widely agreed that cinema had particular persuasive force with general audiences.[81] Symptomatic of this perception is the fact that the Historical Association was actively debating the historical accounts presented in films at the time when *The Face of Britain* was released.[82]

Rotha's vision of national identity was conveyed by a montage of different places in England and Scotland; rural areas for the period before industrialisation, industrial scenes for the 'smoke age' and modern architecture or infrastructure for 'the new age'. So conventionalised is the technique of filming rural or industrial scenes in the *present* to represent the *past*, that the representational leap that is being taken may pass unnoticed. We might ask in what sense harvesting practices in interwar England bear much relation to pre-industrial practice, just as we might question the closeness of the shots of Depression-era Stoke on Trent to scenes at the height of the industrial revolution. But this representational convention is eloquent about interwar intellectuals' attitudes to the relationship between the present and the past; in a sense the past is only accessible via the politics of the present.

Rotha's cinematic convention compares interestingly with the literary tropes in Priestley's vision. In the final chapter of *English Journey*, Priestley portrayed himself as stuck in a London fog on the Great North Road and reflecting on the three Englands he had encountered. For him, there was the Old England; then 'the nineteenth-century England of coal, iron, steel, cotton, wool, railways'; and finally modern England 'with Woolworths as its symbol'. He commented: 'as I looked back on my journey I saw how these three were variously and most fascinatingly mingled in every part of the country I had visited. It would be possible, though not easy, to make a coloured map of them.'[83] In Priestley's view, England's rural and industrial pasts co-habit with its tawdry present. The different historical archetypes he employs – which we may exemplify as the Cotswolds' village, the industrial town of Shotton and the suburban sprawl of London – must, in his view, be added together to make a sum which is 'England'. Arthur Eden's articles on the English tradition in the countryside, Rotha's other stated source for the film, also contained an implicit periodisation. His subject was similarly divided into three parts which map onto Rotha's and Priestley's. Each was the subject of a separate article; 'Making of the Tradition', 'The World of Make-Believe' and 'The Re-birth of Tradition'.

The periodisation of *The Face of Britain* shared features with those of Priestley and Eden, but did not derive simply from either. Rather, we may say, all three have a common ancestor. At first glance, this periodisation seems reminiscent of Lewis Mumford's into eotechnic, palaeotechnic and neotechnic phases of the history of technology, presented in his *Technics and Civilisation* published in September 1934 in Britain.[84] We know that when Rotha read *The Culture of Cities* soon after it came out in 1937, he was inspired to make a film based on it, a film which he said 'will tell how Everytown, 1938, England grew up; just how housing and public services have been related, or in so many cases unrelated, to the needs of the community. This ... is something that I've wanted to do for years, something for which *The Face of Britain* was a notebook.'[85] The implication is that there was something of Mumford in the conception of *The Face of Britain*. It seems unlikely, however, that if Mumford had been the immediate source of Rotha's periodisation, his name or his terminology would have been so completely absent from the not insubstantial archive papers relating to the film's production. But Mumford's scheme was, of course, also a codification of existing historical accounts. Rotha's periodisation must derive from sources encountered earlier in his educational and political development. These could have included Patrick Geddes' *Cities in Evolution* (1915) which had been the basis of Mumford's periodisation.[86] Ultimately, the Left film-maker (Rotha), the middlebrow journalist (Priestley), the modernist aesthete (Eden) and the urban theorist (Mumford) seem to have derived their sense of history and their particular location within it from an older model, that of the catastrophic interpretation of industrialisation.

Cannadine associates the development of the catastrophic account of industrialisation with the revival from the 1880s of the 'condition of England question', with the Booth and Rowntree surveys and works such as Andrew Mearns' *The Bitter Cry of Outcast London*. This is essentially the same tradition within which, as we have seen, Colls and Dodd place documentary film.[87] Arnold Toynbee put the notion on the historical map with his introduction of the term 'industrial revolution'.[88] He wrote:

There were dark patches even in [Adam Smith's] age, but we now approach a darker period, – a period as disastrous and terrible as any through which a nation ever passed; disastrous and terrible, because, side by side with a great increase of wealth was seen an enormous increase of pauperism; and production on a vast scale, the result of free competition, led to a rapid alienation of classes and to the degradation of a large body of producers.[89]

Cannadine sees the 'symptom of a desire to locate the historical origins of contemporary social conditions in the Industrial Revolution' as being equally strong with Fabian historians such as the Hammonds, especially in *The Village Labourer* and *The Town Labourer*, and the Webbs, including Beatrice's *My Apprenticeship*. These works associated the social problems of industrialisation with unbridled *laissez-faire* and looked to greater state intervention and stronger trades unions as means of improving the lot of the urban proletariat. For these writers on the Left, as well as those less politically engaged who took up the interpretation, the industrial revolution was 'nasty, mean, brutish and fast', was caused by a series of technical inventions exploited by *laissez-faire* capitalists and occurred 'around 1780'.[90] We may note that this was precisely the type of periodisation, hinging on industrialisation, which Rotha expressed in *The Face of Britain*, and which Priestley and Eden also assumed in their written works. The fact that the 'LSE school' of Fabian social historians – the Webbs and Hammonds – 'can best be described as left-wing Liberal', rather than as members of the Marxist Left, as Rotha styled himself, helps explain the pervasiveness of the catastrophist view.[91] There is another aspect of the catastrophist account which is worthy of note: the industrial revolution is portrayed within it as the middle term, with a preceding rural 'golden age', and a succeeding aftermath requiring organised response, usually of a collectivist nature, a model which evidently appealed to many of those who were influenced by catastrophism.[92]

Parallel with social impact, other commentators perceived the industrial revolution as an aesthetic catastrophe. This was particularly visible in Ruskin, here writing in 1859:

From shore to shore the whole island is to be set thick with chimneys as the masts stand in the docks of Liverpool; that there be no meadows in it; no trees; no gardens; only a little corn, grown upon the house tops, reaped and threshed by steam ... Under these circumstances ... no designing or any other development of beautiful art will be possible. ... Beautiful art can only be produced by people who have beautiful things about them, and leisure to look upon them; and unless you provide elements of beauty for your workmen to be surrounded by, you will find that no elements of beauty can be invented by them.[93]

As we shall see, this tradition was also powerful in shaping the views of Rotha and his contemporaries.

'Heritage of the Past': Nation and Landscape

The Britain represented in *The Face of Britain* is a landscape and built environment seen as the product of historical forces – notably industrialisation – which was amenable to modification by the planning of town and country. The heritage theme is introduced in the first section of the film. Rotha described the intended tone and pace of this section in an early version of the script: 'Sentiment, peace, nature, romance characterise this first part. It must flow smoothly with poetry and charm.'[94] In service of this aim, one and a half minutes of music and birdsong accompany shots of harvesting before the commentary: 'Most of us, at some time in our lives, have looked back to the time when the face of Britain was beautiful and the natural products of the soil were harvested so that man might eat and live.' (Fig. 1) Church bells and organ music, combined with slow cutting between shots of Cuddington, a Buckinghamshire village, introduce the next passage of commentary:

> Most of us have longed for a return to that epoch of serenity, when, in the quiet villages each cottage and house stood in its garden, in groups around the church. In those villages, men lived and died with little thought outside the life of their self-contained community, loving and knowing only the things that belonged to the soil, which was their livelihood.

This is very like the preservationist notion of the village conveyed by Vaughan Cornish, author of *The Scenery of England* (1932), when recalling his Suffolk upbringing: 'Few things that mattered much in our daily life were beyond the horizon of the parish, and everything within that horizon entered into our life.'[95] This may partly be what Graham Greene had in mind when he spoke of the film's 'faults of simplification and sentimentality'.[96] Similarly Priestley's *English Journey* noted:

> There was, first, Old England, the country of the cathedrals and minsters and manor houses and inns, of Parson and Squire ... There are people who believe that in some mysterious way we can all return to

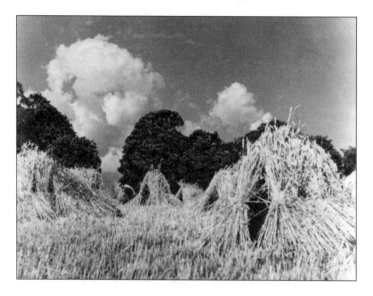

Figure 1
Accompanying commentary:
"Most of us, at some time in our lives, have looked back to the time when
the face of Britain was beautiful and the natural products of the soil were
harvested so that man might eat and live."
Heritage of the Past from *The Face of Britain*
BFI Films, Stills and Designs, courtesy Viewtech Film and Video

this Old England; though nothing is said about killing off nine-tenths
of our present population, which would have to be the first step.[97]

A crucial difference between Priestley's and Rotha's accounts is
that while *English Journey* is geographically explicit, with chapters
devoted to particular localities, such as Bournville or Shotton,
The Face of Britain took the opposite approach. Rotha wrote:

> The material for the film is unconnected in place but closely
> associated by ideas but it is not desirable to show places which are at
> once recognised by the mass of the audiences for such recognition of
> familiar places will distract attention from the thematic purposes to
> which the places are being put.[98]

We may see here an analogy with Rotha's comparison of the use
of dramatic characters in the Russian cinema. Rotha observed,
'Eisenstein's *October* was the dialectic of the mass; Pudovkin's *St*

123

Petersburg was the dialectic of the individual expressing the mass.'[99] In *The Face of Britain*, Englishness is not personified in recognisable places. Instead, the viewer is presented with the mass of English landscape, not its separate individual characteristics. This deliberate blurring of specificity is also analogous to the level of generalisation in Eden's articles. One sign of this is the drawings by Robert Austin which accompanied these articles of an ideal-typical English scene from primeval forest to '1930: the triumph of the mining camp'.[100] The first of Eden's pieces, which maps onto Rotha's 'heritage of the past', is likewise concerned to establish a long rural history of England before industrialisation. Eden argued that: 'Throughout the centuries the work of man in the landscape has been a process of bringing under control and reducing to a human order the apparently chaotic manifestations of the non-human world.' And again, 'the tradition of the English countryside is a tradition of improvement rather than of preservation.' Finally, in Eden's view, during the eighteenth century, of the two motives for changing landscape – the economic and the ornamental – it was the latter which, for the first time, provided the 'essentially English features of our landscape, the hedges, the hedgerow trees and the decorative, but not rigidly formal plantations.'[101] This sense of a landscape deliberately created by human activity is clearly present in Rotha's narrative:

> Thus, as man first made it, the framework of Britain was a pattern of hedges and fields and trees and hamlets which had been handed-down from generations of unceasing effort and knowledge deep-rooted in the land. That pattern stood first and foremost for work, and while men laboured at sowing and at the harvest, the face of the land remained beautiful.

English and Scottish landscapes, urban as well as rural, appropriate to each section, provide most of the visual material for the remainder of the film. Industrial and especially urban landscapes feature in the second section, Scottish rural scenes in the third, whilst the last section is illustrated with modern English urban and rural landscapes.

'The Smoke Age':
Industrialisation and Catastrophe

The Face of Britain represented the industrial revolution as both an aesthetic and a social catastrophe. Rotha described his cinematic intentions for this section: 'in direct contrast with the first sequence, the character of this is violent, powerful and aggressive, most of it being swiftly cut and intercut with conflicting movements.'[102] The film presents industrialisation, following the discovery of the six coalfields, as a storm; speeded-up cloud movements, trees bending in the wind and underexposed footage of landscape, intercut with smoking chimneys, symbolise the intemperate arrival of industry.[103] In contrast with the sunlit harvest and village shots of the first section, the audience is told: 'The sun was hidden behind the smoke cloud of furnace and factory', introducing explicitly a series of dark and light metaphors to the film. The narrative argues, 'without plan or order, without thought for future decades, industry was developed as fast as men could work and build.' We have already met this representation of industrialisation as rampant *laissez-faire* in the Fabian historians and in Quigley's work. Here uncontrolled industrialization is in contrast both with the 'pattern' (for which read 'order') of the past and with the town and country planning suggested in the film's synthesis. The disorder of industrialisation had direct aesthetic consequences: 'There grew up huge centres of manufacture and countless small buildings uglier still to house the servants of industry. Meadow and field were blotched with giant tips for slag. The power of steam and coal dominated the land.' This follows on the *musique concrète* sequence described above, ending on its graveyard and industrial scene. (Fig. 2) The social impact is spelled out in a contrast in the next block of commentary; industrialisation, it states:

> gave Britain a new place in the sun. It gave her industrial, economic and political power, but at how terrible a price in the degradation and destruction of human life. And so today we endure this heritage of the industrial revolution, spreading its congestion of factories and slums over the face of the land, leaving for new generations the shell of a prosperous age.

The meaning of this last phrase is clearer in Priestley, who spelled out the cliché: 'You cannot make omelettes without breaking eggs, and you cannot become rich by selling the world your coal and iron and cotton goods and chemicals without some dirt and disorder. So much is admitted. But there are far too many eggshells and too few omelettes about this nineteenth-century England. What you see looks like a debauchery of cynical greed.'[104]

Priestley's list-style journalism reached new lengths in his description of the period parallel with Rotha's 'Smoke Age':

125

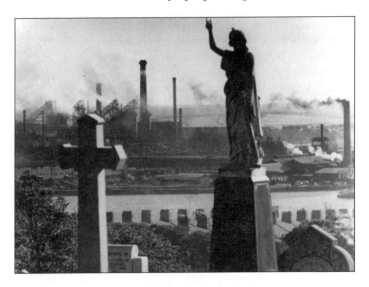

Figure 2
Accompanying commentary:
"Today we endure this heritage of the industrial revolution, spreading its
congestion of factories and slums over the face of the land, leaving for new
generations the shell of a prosperous age."
The Smoke Age from *The Face of Britain*
BFI Films, Stills and Designs, courtesy Viewtech Film and Video

there is the nineteenth-century England of coal, iron, steel, cotton,
wool, railways; of thousands of rows of little houses all alike, sham
Gothic churches, square faced-chapels, Town Halls, Mechanics'
Institutes, mills, foundries, warehouses, refined watering-places, Pier
Pavilions, Family and Commercial hotels, Literary and Philosophical
Societies, back-to-back houses, detached villas with monkey trees,
Grill Rooms, railway stations, slag heaps and 'tips', dock roads,
Refreshment Rooms, doss-houses, Unionist or Liberal Clubs,
cindery waste ground, mill chimneys, slums, fried-fish shops, public
houses with red blinds, bethels in corrugated iron, good class
draper's and confectioners' shops, a cynically devastated countryside,
sooty dismal little towns, and still sootier grim fortress-like cities.[105]

This list, like Rotha's commentary, concentrated on the visual. It
is entirely possible, of course, that contemporary audiences, with the
aural and visual perceptions specific to their time, might have
assumed more in certain words and phrases than is present on the

surface of the text here.[106] In particular, as Alan Mayne has argued, the term 'slum' was a highly negative figure of speech, especially, we may suspect, in the era of anti-slum crusades, which dominated public health policy in the interwar period, a subject dealt with in Elizabeth Darling's chapter.[107] As Chris Waters has suggested, however, Priestley felt sufficiently out of tune with the 'age of the mass' that he stressed what he perceived to be positive aspects of the industrial era. For example, he held the 'solid lumps of character' who peopled the factories of the last century in high esteem. He imagined a sense of working-class community, which he attached nostalgically to his turn-of-the-century Bradford childhood.[108]

For both Rotha and Priestley there was continuity between the impact of industrialisation in the past and its effects in the present. The commentary for 'The Smoke Age' starts and ends in the present tense: 'but under this lovely face of Britain, in six great areas there lies coal' to 'and so today we endure this heritage'. But the bulk of this section is in the past tense, for example: 'so a new type of work arose and disfigured the face of the land'. The footage illustrating the words, however, was of industrial areas of Britain (especially the Potteries and Shotton) in the present. Likewise, in Priestley's *English Journey*, the 'England of the dole' overlaps with nineteenth-century England: 'For generations, this blackened North toiled and moiled so that England should be rich and the City of London be a great power in the world. But now this North is half derelict, and its people, living on in the queer ugly places, are shabby, bewildered, unhappy.'[109] Eden, too, saw the industrial revolution as pivotal in the nation's history: 'the main point that affects us here is the sudden expansion of industry, and therefore of urban population, in a country which had hitherto had a rural population three times that of the towns.' He refers in passing to the 'crowded and insanitary conglomerations of shoddy houses and factories' which constituted the industrial towns. Yet his main focus was aesthetic:

> The tragedy of the nineteenth century, in the visible world at least, was that the leaders of thought and artistic expression allowed themselves to be repelled by the grimness of the new towns ... The machine had created bad towns. Therefore the machine was bad. It could not be abolished, however, and the only course open to those who disapproved was to ... escape from the ever-present material realities into a world of make-believe of their own creation.[110]

An early draft of *The Face of Britain* had incorporated a more explicitly architectural statement than occurs in the final version:

VISION	SOUND
Sound Steel works exteriors	'Architects left Industry to the Engineers ...'
Public Buildings, Town Halls	'and served the gallant art of self-respect.'[111]

In his second article, Eden explained his term 'the world of make-believe', as the intellectuals' flight from 'the grim realities of the incomprehensible present into the known and intelligible past', it was 'solace from the uncertainty of the changing human scene in the seemingly eternal certainties of nature.' Pugin was the chief villain here, but Cowper was also to blame, with his aphorism, 'God made the country, and man made the town.'[112] Man, as Eden had already established, made both:

> It never occurred to the government departments, local health committees and builders of the time that the provision of light and air and drains was intimately connected with the question of design ... Design was a matter which only affected churches and town halls, and consisted in the application of ... ornament ... It was not concerned with the housing of the working classes, nor with the construction of reservoirs ...[113]

For Eden, the catastrophe of industrialisation was therefore overwhelmingly aesthetic and only minimally social.[114] Here his prose was very close to Rotha's: 'Slag heaps towered over the miserable cottages of the workpeople, and mounds of waste material from the mines were spread over heath and pasture.'[115] Rotha wrote (as cited earlier): 'There grew up huge centres of manufacture and countless small buildings uglier still to house the servants of industry. Meadow and field were blotched with giant tips for slag. The power of steam and coal dominated the land.' But for Rotha, the catastrophe was equally social and aesthetic and he juxtaposed 'Britain's ... new place in the sun' with the 'terrible ... price in the degradation and destruction of human life.'

The screen is occupied, after the storm sequence, with a series of industrial landscapes, generally cut together in rapid sequence: steelworks, the potteries, Shotton. Here, Quigley once again gave explicit direction: 'The prize slum areas are undoubtedly to be found in Sheffield and the Potteries.'[116] Priestley also devoted a chapter to the area, and it was his treatment of Shotton which drew Rotha there; both men were affected by the squalor of the mining town dominated by a giant slag heap: 'the atmosphere was thickened with ashes and sulphuric fumes; like that of Pompeii, as we are told, on the eve of its destruction.'[117]

'The New Power and The New Age': Modernity and Modernism

Rotha worked hardest on the dialectical structure of what eventually became the last two sections of the film. Earlier drafts cover this territory in as few as one and as many as four sections. It is the addition of sections depicting hydro-electric power and the electrical grid in the sixth generation of the script – the one sent to Quigley – that made the crucial difference between Rotha's first notions and the final form of the film. None of these scripts is dated, but it is reasonable to assume that the expansion of the coverage of electricity from one passing sentence in the earlier scripts to a whole section was the product of Rotha's first discussions with Quigley who returned the compliment by alluding to the film in his book of Highland topography:

> The Grampian [hydro-electric] scheme, one of the largest of its kind in Europe, has been carried out with sufficient care of the amenities, particularly in the construction of dams, runways and power stations, to ensure that those developments should not conflict with the landscape itself. The best evidence of this is a film prepared by Paul Rotha and entitled *The Face of Britain*.[118]

The 'New Power' section starts in the same lyrical mode as the first, with birdsong and water sounds slowly replaced by electrical whines. Shots of Highland streams and lochs are intercut with images of high voltage electrical apparatus (filmed at Metropolitan-Vickers). 'It will be seen', Rotha wrote, 'that the sequence works up from comparative peace and calm to a climax of flashing light.' The narrative states:

> So electricity is born to bring back the sun to Britain. A Nation plan is formed to carry power and light into the furthest corners of the land. Lochs are dammed to make giant reservoirs of energy. Waterfalls are harnessed, rivers diverted along new manmade channels. Tunnels are bored and aqueducts constructed so that turbines may turn to create the great new driving power ...[119]

Here Rotha attaches his light metaphor to a 'nation plan', in an instance of what Bill Luckin has described as 'techno-arcadian' visions of the capacity of the grid to transform the rural economy.[120] Rotha wrote: 'At this point the mood alters slightly. From an impressionistic construction sequence we merge now into a more graceful, almost lyrical treatment. The music also changes and a special "March of the Pylons" must be written.'[121] There is no sign that the film used anything other than library music and this sequence of fast cutting between shots of pylons filmed from a variety of angles is instead accompanied by an electronic whine increasing in pitch in steps: 'From the sources of this energy to North, South, East and West, the pylons carry their living load, over mountains, fields and rivers, never checking in their stride as they carry the new power to the waiting cities and eager countryside.' (Fig. 3) Both Luckin and Matless have shown that the aesthetic impact of pylons was the main object of contention as the grid was constructed from the late twenties onwards. Rotha might have come anywhere on a spectrum of attidudes to this issue, although with the growing favour shown towards pylons from the early thirties, his paean is not unconventional.[122] Matless argues that in Peach and Carrington's *The*

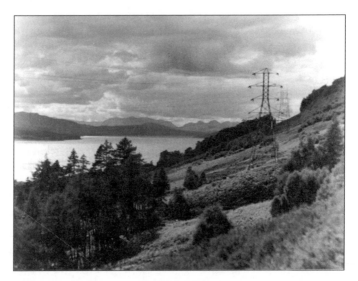

Figure 3
Accompanying commentary:
"From the sources of this energy to North, South, East and West, the pylons carry their living load, over mountains, fields and rivers, never checking in their stride as they carry the new power to the waiting cities and eager countryside."
The New Power from *The Face of Britain*
BFI Films, Stills and Designs, courtesy Viewtech Film and Video

Face of the Land (1930) 'pylons stood out as fit for their purpose and in harmony with the landscape, shot in perspective to convey a composed march of power over the land.'[123] In *The Face of Britain*, fitness for purpose – the modernist definition – is the yardstick of aesthetics. This is seen in the version of the script Rotha sent to Quigley:

> The new age has brought efficiency, comfort, health, and a mechanised environment. But have we lost the Beauty which makes the past so attractive to us? Is there no beauty in the modern world just as there was in the past? A pylon on a Yorkshire Moor is no more of a desecration than Stonehenge on Salisbury Plain; The one is of today; the other of the past.[124]

Quigley, inevitably an enthusiast for the grid, advised Rotha about particularly picturesque sites for the filming of pylons.[125] For him, the hydro-electric scheme and pylons made a positive contribution to the Highlands; he talked of the appropriateness of 'contemporary machine civilisation' to the landscape:

> The purist, looking at Schiehallion across the transparent waters of Loch Rannoch, may turn round and gaze with amazement and perhaps repulsion at the line of towers gliding over the moors, and proclaim aloud the desecration of the landscape. But is it desecration? Is it not rather the first clear sign of new life which will change the landscape so radically that it will no longer be an uninhabited sterile wilderness but a rich country, alive and happy with human activity.[126]

This can be seen as an example of modernistic preservationism, 'a movement for the planning and preservation of landscape which sought to ally preservation and progress, tradition and modernity, city and country in order to define Englishness as orderly and modern', as David Matless has put it.[127] This view is echoed in the commentary which closes the power section of the film: 'the heavy smoke clouds of the past can be dissipated for ever. But a plan for power is only part of the greater plan to make Britain a land designed for living in, to make a New Age possible. A great new world lies ready to be created. There is much to be done.'

Quigley's modernism was completely in line with the CEB's and the EDA's main public relations strategy that stressed the modernity of electricity in relation to other sources of power.[128] The last two sections of *The Face of Britain* conformed with this line. 'The new age' section argues that planning, married to electrical power, can

131

provide the solution to 'the ghastly squalor, brought about by the uncontrolled spread of industry.' It returns to both the aesthetic and the public health aspects: 'Not only must slums be cleared, but we must see that nothing ugly takes their place. The new communities must be planned in whole and in detail with a full understanding of the cultural and practical needs of a new society.' Priestley and Rotha parted company most clearly in their attitude to this 'new age'.[129] For Priestley:

> The third England ... was the new post-war England, belonging far more to the age itself than to this particular island. America, I supposed, was its real birthplace. This is the England of arterial and by-pass roads, of filling stations and factories that look like exhibition buildings, of giant cinemas and dance-halls and cafés, bungalows with tiny garages, cocktail bars, Woolworths, motor-coaches, wireless, hiking, factory girls looking like actresses, greyhound racing and dirt tracks, swimming pools, and everything given away for cigarette coupons.[130]

Priestley was as disdainful as any aesthete of this age; we may compare, for example, Anthony Bertram, author of the Penguin Special *Design*, complaining of 'bungaloid growths' and 'the abominable Tudoristic villa of the By-pass road'.[131] Priestley complained:

> I cannot help feeling that this new England is lacking in character, in zest, gusto, flavour, bite, drive, originality, and that this is a serious weakness. Monotonous but easy work and a liberal supply of cheap luxuries might between them create a set of people entirely without ambition or any real desire to think and act for themselves, and perfect subjects for an iron autocracy.[132]

Rotha found himself more at home in this England. Describing his intentions for 'The New Age' section, he stated: 'an orderly march of progress, firm and dominating, a building up towards prosperity and optimism characterises this final sequence. It must be impregnated with an urgency to get these things done or else England will return to the chaos of the Victorian era of dirt and smoke.'[133] Here his language became more explicitly modernist: 'Strange new architectures arise to meet the demands of a changing civilisation, shapes and forms of simple beauty, dictated only by the purpose which they are meant to serve. Out of steel, glass and concrete, the architects and engineers must transform the face of Britain.' (Fig. 4) Fitness for purpose is here combined with the stress on expertise which typified those advocating planning-based responses to national problems. He continued: 'New sources of power, new means of communication, new methods and new processes are here for the service of man. This is an age of scientific planning, co-operation and collective working.'

The final version of the film is notable for its generalising and direct advocacy of modernist planning. Earlier drafts contained more about the downside of modernity, saying, for example, that 'for all the attempts at Olde Worlde petrol stations and Tudor roadhouses, we cannot put back the clock.'[134] Fitness for purpose, especially with regard to petrol stations which modernists saw as symbols of the new age, was of prime importance. Inappropriate design of them also

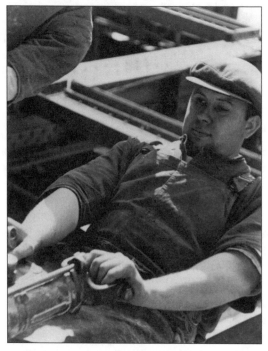

Figure 4
Accompanying commentary:
"Not only must slums be cleared, but we must see that nothing ugly takes their place. The new communities must be planned in whole and in detail with a full understanding of the cultural and practical needs of a new society."
The New Age from *The Face of Britain*
BFI Films, Stills and Designs, courtesy Viewtech Film and Video

incurred the wrath of the authors of *The Face of the Land*; 'Shamness' was to be avoided at all costs.[135] Here, apparently, Priestley seems close to Rotha, in that they shared a dislike for the tawdriness of the modern age. But Priestley, while he could, in passing, ask why there had been no plan for the 'England of the dole', in the end looked towards the 'inner glowing tradition of the English spirit', rather than to the corporatist planning and expertise favoured by Rotha and Eden, to save the nation.[136]

Rotha's vision for 'The New Age' was closer to Eden's third article which was devoted to the rebirth of the English tradition in the countryside. Here Eden stated the problem as being 'how to reconstitute a balance between the claims of town and country.' This could 'only be solved by a general return to the improving tradition of the English landscape – the tradition which was for the time being swamped by the developments of the nineteenth century.'[137] This also was the view of the architect and designer John Gloag, summarised by Matless as: 'The Georgian and the Modern stand apart like town and country with a Victorian mess in between; the preservationist task was to sweep away the clutter and connect to an earlier age of English design.'[138] Throughout, Eden preached an unblinking acceptance of the necessity of change that he believed the modern world demanded. For example: 'The English village was almost perfect for the purposes for which it was built, but its purpose having changed, the village must change too. Its planning will have to be related to the changed conditions in agriculture, and it will be governed also by considerations of modern transport, modern hygiene, and modern social ideals.'[139] The modernistic implication is clear; this village is a machine for living in.

The Face of Britain closes with an appeal to citizenship, which is entirely typical of thirties' documentary:

> Britain has tremendous wealth of human material and physical resources. She is now at a turning point in her civilisation. If her citizens will realise alike the opportunity and their own responsibilities, they can make this ancient land a well-ordered and gracious heritage where the sun will always shine on the children of the future.

The use of the citizenship motif in the hands of the historical materialist Rotha bears a different cargo from that found in the more politically centrist documentarists. Just as the dynamic of history was, for Rotha, forging new versions of nationhood, so the urgency of citizenship rhetoric was not for citizens to sign-up to how things were, but to become an active and engaged force in how they should become. This echoes Eden's sense of active preparation for a planned future; his series saw 'the present not only in relation to the past, but also as the threshold of the future.'[140]

In the closing moments of the film, accompanied by the last quoted block of commentary, we see the completion of the cycle of light metaphors with which Rotha nuanced both the commentary and the visuals of the film. At this point the audience sees a couple walking on the crest of a hill. As the final words are spoken, the man points at the scenery with outstretched hand. This was a contemporary visual trope seen, for example in Ellis Martin's covers for the Popular and Tourist editions of Ordnance Survey maps, which show a map-user on a hill overlooking a valley. Here is a metaphor of 'literal and metaphorical overview' which Matless argues 'was central to preservationists' self-styled authority.'[141] Authority is both the subject and the implied question at the end of the film. A summary, perhaps prepared as a press release, stated that the film 'tries to use the documentary form for the expression of a dialectical purpose – to set out an argument plainly and simply yet allow the audience to draw their own conclusions.'[142] It is clear, however, that the only conclusions available to the audience were to support the technocracy it proposed.

To generalise, we may characterise these final sections of the film as expressing a brand of 'scientific modernism'. Calinescu defines modernity as 'a stage in the history of Western Civilisation – a product of scientific and technological progress, the industrial revolution, of the sweeping and social changes brought about by capitalism' and modernism as an aesthetic response to those changes.[143] In the Weberian tradition, modernity is typified by rationalisation, the various processes by which culture in all its aspects has become subject to calculation, measurement and control, epitomized by the growth of state bureaucracy and administration. Frankfurt School theorists saw aesthetic modernism as a negative response, as a rebellion against such rationalisation and codification.[144] John Carey's *The Intellectuals and the Masses* similarly portrays literary and artistic modernism as a way that some intellectuals kept art sacred and unavailable to the mass by making it incomprehensible: 'machine civilisation' was often associated with the malign influence of the mass.[145] And there certainly was a conservative tradition of revulsion against modernity, which is seen as much in the patrician physician Thomas Horder as in the literary critic F. R. Leavis, as Chris Lawrence has shown.[146] But modernism is not just about the discontents of modernity, and modernists were not necessarily obscurantist nor disdainful of mass society. There is a prominent aesthetic modernism, of gleeful response to the modern age. Le Corbusier is only the most obvious example, with his paeans to ocean-going liners and aeroplanes and his prescription that a house be a machine for living in.[147] There is also, as Marshall Berman has suggested, a strand of aesthetic modernism which originates explicitly in Marx and which proposes in historical materialism a mechanism which not only made past and present, but which also determines how the future may be made.[148]

Rotha's modernism was in the Left tradition which Berman describes. *The Face of Britain* is not alone amongst Rotha's films in carrying the message of scientific rationalisation as a means to revolutionary and positive change in society. Here Weber's rationalisation is inverted because rationalisation is willed and promoted as the way to a better society. This is not unlike the view of Otto Neurath, one of the stars of Viennese Logical Positivism, who proposed that planned science and the Modern design of the Bauhaus promised a 'new form of life'.[149] In Peter Galison's formulation: 'Anyone wanting to "enter the promised land" liberated from the past "will seize upon the formation of the new form of life as a technical achievement".'[150] Perhaps it is little surprise to discover that when Neurath came to Britain during the Second World War, it was not long before Rotha, excited by his advocacy of scientific planning, collaborated with him, animating ISOTYPE diagrams for propaganda films.[151]

The Face of Britain straddles the fence of modernity and modernism; it represents modernity – and the history of its arrival via industrialisation – and it uses modernist technique to do this. The film might, in this double sense, have been seen by contemporaries as scientific. First, it argued that science, technology and architectural Modernism provide the means to ameliorate the problems created by industrialisation. Second, Rotha aestheticised his account via the dialectical montage of Eisenstein and Pudovkin. For many, Russian montage theory was considered to be a rigorous and scientific approach to film construction; Ivor Montagu's preface to the English edition of Pudovkin's *Film Technique* (1933) compared its impact on film to that of Mendel's genetics on plant breeding.[152] The film's association of electricity with a socially transformative force may also have been read in some quarters as Leninist, recalling the equation that 'Communism is Soviet power plus the electrification of the whole country.'[153]

Conclusion

This chapter presents *The Face of Britain* as a contingent cultural artefact which encapsulates a particular selection of contemporary views of history, nationhood and modernity. The point may be emphasised by brief discussion of a very different contemporary film with national concerns. Bruce Woolfe's film, *England Awake!* (1932), part compilation, part new shooting, was envisaged by its 'devisers', Woolfe and the novelist John Buchan who was on the board of British Instructional Films as a morale booster at the height of the Depression in 1931.[154] It commences with a crowd protesting outside the Duke of Wellington's house a century before, in 1831, that the new prosperity promised after Waterloo had not materialised. Its leader, brought before Wellington, is told by him that the officer class has not forgotten its duty. The remainder of the film is narrated by Wellington, sometimes shown in a ghostly double exposure. A sequence follows of 'great inventions' acted out in short vignettes: Faraday and electromagnetic induction, Stephenson and his Rocket, Brunel trying to persuade non-believers of the future of steamships. This is followed by images of imperial possessions (Canada, Australia and South Africa) explored by 'courageous Englishmen' and takes in the contributions of British Engineers to the development of these countries. British products, including textiles, mechanical engineering and coal are praised as 'the finest in the world'. This sequence culminates on the eve of the First World War with the statement that 'peace and prosperity lay on the land like a benediction.' The war is depicted as the occasion after Waterloo on which the English had saved Europe. 'But again,' Wellington intones 'we shall have our reward if we show ourselves worthy of it.' A final tour of England and the Empire concludes with the English countryside, a quotation from Shakespeare and *Land of Hope and Glory*.[155] This conservative picture of English history (literally Conservative in the case of Buchan who was a Tory MP between 1927 and 1935) is markedly different from Rotha's *The Face of Britain*. Industrialisation in *England Awake!* is a benediction, not a shadow, and engineers are representatives of the officer class, not of the professional scientists, architects and engineers with social consciences in Rotha's vision.

By studying films in terms of their constituting context we may gain a sense of the close dynamics of cultural history. *The Face of Britain* is a very particular expression of a complex of ideas concerning nation, history, landscape, aesthetics, politics and cinema circulating in the inter-war period. In the network of associations upon which it was contingent, if we consider Quigley, Priestley and Eden in addition to Rotha, we have a cross section of Liberal and Left opinion in the mid thirties. The film, seen by us today, is like a single frame of a cinema film, visible to close study, but divorced from its proper context. This chapter has seen the film as the product of its environment, preserved at its point of closure, when no other influences could mould its form. But we also need to know what happened when this artefact came to be seen, examined and used. If we consider how audiences, specialised and general, might have responded to it, we must also recall that the concerns it represented would have been read in terms of the audience's existing assumptions about nation, history, landscape, aesthetics, politics and cinema. One passing example is the National Smoke Abatement Society, which gave favourable coverage both to the film and to Mumford's *Technics and Civilisation*.[156] If such an organisation could understand these cultural artefacts in the light of their own interests, then so could any viewer.

Acknowledgements

Viewing copies of both *The Face of Britain* and *England Awake!* are held at the National Film and Television Archive, 21 Stephen St, London W1P 2LN. I should like to thank the staff there for access to both. For permission to reproduce the stills, I thank BFI Films, Stills and Designs, and Viewtech Film and Video, which holds copyright on the film. I acknowledge with pleasure the permission granted by by the executor of the Rotha estate and UCLA to reproduce quotations from the Rotha archive (see note 3). I thank staff at the RIBA, Science Museum, and Wellcome Institute Libraries. I gratefully acknowledge my debt to my employers, The Science Museum, London, and to my family.

Notes

1 See, for example J. Baxendale and C. Pawling, *Narrating the Thirties: a Decade in the Making, 1930 to the Present*, Basingstoke, 1996; S. Hall, 'The Social Eye of Picture Post', *Working Papers in Cultural Studies*, 2 (1972): 71–120; I. Aitken, *Film and Reform: John Grierson and the Documentary Film Movement*, London, 1990. The key work on documentary and nationhood is R. Colls and P. Dodd, 'Representing the Nation: The British Documentary Film, 1930-45', *Screen*, 26 (1985): 21–33. For contemporary sources see J. Grierson in *Grierson on Documentary*, F. Hardy (ed.), London, 1966; P. Rotha, *Documentary Film*, London, 1936. See also *Speak for Yourself: a Mass-Observation Anthology, 1937-1949*, A. Calder and D. Sheridan (eds), Oxford, 1985.

2 See the discussion in *The Cinema Book*, P. Cook (ed.), London, 1985, pp. 114–206.

3 Rotha's papers are held in the Department of Special Collections, Charles E. Young Research Library, UCLA, Los Angeles, CA 90095–1575. This paper uses two parts of the archive; Box 26, Rotha's letters to Eric Knight (hereafter, 'Rotha to Knight, date'), and Box 12, Item 3, production papers for *The Face of Britain* and *Shipyard* (hereafter, '*Face of Britain* documents').

4 T. M. Boon, 'Films and the Contestation of Public Health in Interwar Britain', Ph.D. thesis, University of London, 1999; '*The Smoke Menace*: Cinema, Sponsorship, and the Social Relations of Science in 1937', in *Science and Nature (BSHS Monograph 8)*, M. Shortland (ed.), Oxford, 1993, pp. 57–88; 'Agreement and Disagreement in the Making of *World of Plenty*', in *Nutrition in Britain: Science, Scientists and Politics in the Twentieth Century*, D. Smith (ed.), London, 1997, pp. 166–189.

5 Rotha to Knight, April 1933.

6 A particularly egregious example is provided by the nutrition scientist John Boyd Orr who suggested scenarios for a 1936 nutrition film, and entirely rewrote the last third of Rotha's *World of Plenty*, Boon, 'Agreement and Disagreement', pp. 177–9.

7 For a useful discussion of the nature of this book, see D. L. LeMahieu, *A Culture for Democracy: Mass Communication and the Cultivated Mind in Britain between the Wars*, Oxford, 1988, pp. 218–222.

8 Figures from P. Marris, *Paul Rotha (BFI Dossier 16)*, London, 1982, pp. 96–9.

9 The main biographical source is his autobiography, P. Rotha,

Documentary Diary, London, 1973, which is usefully supplemented by Marris, *Paul Rotha*.

10   For Grierson's film-making philosophy, see Aitken, *Film and Reform*.

11   Anon, 'The Cinema and Society: Documentary Films' (review of Rotha's *Documentary Film*), *The Times*, 4 February 1936.

12   Rotha's rejection of Americanisation was conventional amongst British intellectuals in this period; see LeMahieu, *Culture for Democracy*, pp. 118–121. For Priestley's attitude see below.

13   Rotha, *Documentary Film*, 44.

14   *Ibid.*, pp. 76–7.

15   P. Rotha, 'Pudovkin on Film Technique' (review), *Sight and Sound*, Winter 1933, 140.

16   Rotha, *Documentary Film*, pp. 48–9.

17   *Ibid.*, 236.

18   *Spectator*, 24 January 1936, reproduced in *Mornings in the Dark: the Graham Greene Film Reader*, D. Parkinson (ed.), London, 1995, 489.

19   LeMahieu states that Rotha's coverage of film theory in *The Film Till Now* 'leans heavily on Pudovkin's' *Film Technique*, see *Culture for Democracy*, 220.

20   The 'Continental Realists' such as Ruttman, director of *Berlin* for example; Rotha, *Documentary Film*, pp. 161, 193, 200.

21   *Ibid.*, 223.

22   *Ibid.*, 225.

23   *Ibid.*, 226.

24   *Ibid.*, pp. 232–3.

25   *Ibid.*, pp. 234–5.

26   Rotha to Knight, May 1933. For The Film Society, see Arts Enquiry, *The Factual Film*, Oxford, 1947, pp. 154–5.

27   Rotha, *Documentary Film*, 255.

28   Hugh Quigley was born in Stirling and graduated from Glasgow University in French, German and Italian in 1919. He was economist in the research department of Metropolitan-Vickers, 1922-1924, and head of the statistical department of the British Electrical and Allied Manufacturers' Association, before going to the CEB in 1931 (until 1943). See *Who Was Who 1970-1979*. His publications included, in addition to those listed in note 50: *Italy and the rise of a New School of Criticism in the 18th Century, with Special Reference to the Work of Pietro Calepio*, Perth, 1921; *A Plan for the Highlands. Proposals for a Highland Development Board*, London, 1936; *Republican Germany. A Political and Economic Study*, London, 1928.

29   Quigley to Rotha, 26 June 1934, *Face of Britain* documents.

30   H. Quigley, *The Highlands of Scotland*, London, 1936, 11.

31 P. Dodd, 'Englishness and the National Culture', in *Englishness: Politics and Culture 1880–1920*, R. Colls and P. Dodd (eds), London, 1986, pp. 1–28, at 12–13.

32. There is a gap in Rotha's letters to Knight at this point, but the spring 1935 issue of *Cinema Quarterly* states that Rotha was 'at present directing *The Face of Britain*', whilst the summer issue includes a plate of stills from it, described as his new film, implying that it was completed in the spring.

33 D. Matless, *Landscape and Englishness*, London, 1998, pp. 63–7. See below for discussion of urban and rural themes in *The Face of Britain*.

34 Rotha to Knight, 3 September 1933.

35 Rotha to Knight, October 1933 (This is Rotha's tentative date, presumably added to this undated letter when he was writing *Documentary Diary*).

36 Rotha to Knight, January 1934.

37 Colls and Dodd, 'Representing the Nation', pp. 22–3.

38 Baxendale and Pawling, *Narrating the Thirties*, pp. 12–3.

39 W. A. Eden, 'The English tradition in the countryside: III. The Re-Birth of Tradition', *Architectural Review*, 77 (1935): 193–202 at 193 (hereafter, Eden, 'Re-Birth of Tradition').

40 Rotha, *Documentary Diary*, 102; J. B. Priestley, *English Journey: Being a Rambling but Truthful Account of what one Man saw and heard and felt and thought during a Journey through England during the Autumn of the Year 1933*. It was serialized in the *Daily Herald* and published as a book in April 1934.

41 W. A. Eden, 'The English Tradition in the Countryside. I. Making of the Tradition', *Architectural Review*, 77 (1935): 85–94 (hereafter, Eden, 'Making the Tradition'); 'The English Tradition in the Countryside: II. The World of Make-Believe', *ibid.*, 142–52 (hereafter, Eden, 'World of Make-Believe'); and Eden, 'Re-Birth of Tradition'. Eden qualified at the Liverpool School of Architecture, and after the War became Historic Buildings Surveyor to the London County Council and Greater London Council. He was author of *The Process of Architectural Tradition*, London, 1942. He died in 1975; see *The Times*, 17 April 1975, 18.

42 *Modern Britain 1929-1939*, J. Peto and D. Loveday (eds), London, 1999, pp. 19, 128.

43 This is reproduced in D. Dean, *The Thirties: Recalling the English Architectural Scene*, London, 1983, pp. 16, 19.

44 See Boon, '*The Smoke Menace*', pp. 74–5.

45 T. Haggith, '"Castles in the Air": British Film and the

Reconstruction of the Built Environment, 1939-51', Ph.D. thesis, University of Warwick, 1998; *Memorandum for the Production of a Programme of Documentary and Instructional Films on Architecture*, 1 February 1936, RIBA archives.

46   Rotha, *Documentary Diary*, 226.

47   Rotha to Knight, 18 July 1934. Rotha modified the text when he quoted it in his *Documentary Diary*, 103.

48   Strictly speaking, *Contact* was made under the auspices of Woolfe's previous company, British Instructional Films. Rotha describes the transition in *Documentary Diary*, pp. 96–7.

49   *Ibid.*, 102.

50   H. Quigley, *Electrical Power and National Progress*, London, 1925; H. Quigley and I. Goldie, *Housing and Slum Clearance in London*, London, 1934.

51   Quigley and Goldie, *Housing and Slum Clearance*, 11.

52   Matless, for example, argues that 'preservationists argued that in the nineteenth century an attitude of *laissez faire* had destroyed the town, and in the twentieth century was destroying the country', *Landscape and Englishness*, 28.

53   B. Pimlott, *Labour and the Left in the 1930s*, Cambridge, 1977, 37.

54   L. Hannah, *Electricity Before Nationalisation*, London, 1979, pp. 250–1.

55   H. Quigley, 'Economic Background', *Architectural Review*, 74 (1933): 160–1.

56   Quigley to Tallents, 9 March 1934, PRO T160/742, Swann *The British Documentary Film Movement*, Cambridge, 1989, 62.

57   R. Low, *Films of Comment and Persuasion of the 1930s*, London, 1979, pp. 141–3.

58   B. Luckin, *Questions of Power: Electricity and Environment in Inter-War Britain*, Manchester, 1990, 25.

59   See Anon, 'The E. D. A. film campaign', *EDA Bulletin*, December 1934, pp. 3–6. See also the issues for January and March (both pp. 3–4).

60   H. Quigley, 'Films of Fact: Work of the Grid' (letter), *The Times*, 26 November 1935, 10.

61   Rotha, *Documentary Diary*, 103. The implication of the sequence of scripts is rather different from Rotha's account; see below in the *'Heritage of the Past'* section.

62   Quigley to Rotha, 26 June 1934, *Face of Britain* documents. The books were: an exhibition catalogue 'of drawings and models of London and the provinces', *The Face of Scotland*, London, 1933 and *The Face of England*, London, 1932.

63 *Ibid.* The letter suggested Rotha meet him on a tour of pithead baths and coal mines; expenses claims for the shoot include 'July 11th, Glasgow, Refreshments for Mr. Quigley', *Face of Britain* documents. But there are no shots of pithead baths – popular amongst social reformers – in the film, though the BFI stills department does hold, amongst Rotha's originals from *The Face of Britain*, a still photograph from a pithead bath.

64 H. Quigley, *The Highlands of Scotland*, London, 1936.

65 *The Moscow Trial*, London, 1933. For a review of the book, see *Times Literary Supplement*, 20 July 1933, 487. For Quigley, see footnote 30. Amongst Cummings' other books are: *The Press: And A Changing Civilisation*, London, 1936; *This England*, London, 1944. See *DNB*, 1950-1959, pp. 278–9. In 1939 Cummings lent support to the documentarists in the debacle over British films for the New York World's Fair; Rotha, *Documentary Diary*, pp. 105, 237–8.

66 *Face of Britain* documents. The Rotha archive contains at least six generations of script, which from internal evidence run in a sequence, with the first four describing a three section film. The versions are: 1. 'THIS IS ENGLAND! Rough notes of a possible film subject'; 2. 'THE FACE OF ENGLAND'; 3. an exact copy of 2 with handwritten additions; 4. 'THE FACE OF ENGLAND' with hand-written notes typed up and a descriptive paragraph added; 5. is a five section version in outline; 6. is a full draft script in visuals and script, and the version sent to Quigley. All these were produced between 8 April 1934 when Rotha proposed *Shipyard* to Woolfe (7pp document commencing 'This report has as its reference the consideration of film productions ...', dated 8 April 1932 – the year is surely a typographical error) and 26 June when Quigley wrote to Rotha about this last version of the script. There are also draft and final commentaries, and a précis written after the film's completion.

67 This timing is clear from his letters to Eric Knight. The commission for the book is mentioned in Rotha to Knight, 29 January 1934, and progress, for example in that of 8 August 1934, 3.

68 Rotha to Knight, 7 October 1933.

69 Rotha to Knight, 8 August 1934.

70 D. A. Cook, *A History of Narrative Film*, New York, 1981, 170.

71 Rotha, *Documentary Film*, 235. There is no indication of which authorities he is referring to here.

72 Alternatively, the film may be seen as having a rolling dialectic in which the fourth section is a second synthesis to 'The Smoke Age' as a second thesis and 'The New Power' as a second antithesis.

73 Grierson and Wright's *Conquest* (1930) had given a crude historical

account of the conquest of North America; R. Low, *Documentary and Educational Films*, London, 1979, 53. See Swann, *British Documentary Film Movement*, pp. 114–5. This contextualisation is seen in later films produced and directed by Rotha, including *Today we Live* (1937) and *World of Plenty* (1943), but also in John Monck's *Health for the Nation* (1939), which was made on behalf of the Ministry of Health.

74   Dodd, 'Englishness', 22. Emphasis mine.

75   See R. Colls, 'Englishness and the Political Culture', in *Englishness*, Colls and Dodd (eds), pp. 29–61.

76   Dodd, 'Englishness', pp. 19, 21.

77   Colls and Dodd, 'Representing the Nation'.

78   K. and P. Dodd, 'Engendering the Nation: British Documentary Film, 1930-1939', in *Dissolving Views: Key Writings on the British Cinema*, A. Higson (ed.), London, 1996, pp. 38–50.

79   One exception is that reproduced here as plate four. It is interesting to note that earlier treatments for the film (those which I have numbered three and four) include lists of 'characters' – the labourer, farmer, steel worker, miner, electrician, architect – parallel to 'materials' which are mainly types of places and buildings, but these characters are not dominant visual features of the final film.

80   K. Robbins, '*History*, the Historical Association and the "National Past"', *History*, 66 (1981): 413–25 at 423.

81   According to the *Health Education Year Book*, London, 1939, 'the value of the Film as an impressive visual medium of education needs no emphasis', 111.

82   Anon, '"Historical" films: Concern at False Ideas', *The Times*, 3 January 1936, 14. This followed an earlier Historical Association enquiry into the use of films in history teaching, published as F. Consitt, *The Value of Films in History Teaching*, London, 1931. See R. Low, *Documentary and Educational Films of the 1930s*, London, 1979, pp. 9–12.

83   Priestley, *English Journey*, pp. 368–90 at 380.

84   Anon, 'Man and Machine' (review of Mumford's *Technics and Civilisation*), *Times Literary Supplement*, 11 October 1934, 687. It was available from at least April 1934 in America.

85   Rotha to Knight, 20 December 1938. For a brief account of the fate of this project, see Rotha, *Documentary Diary*, pp. 228–9.

86   Patrick Geddes, *Cities in Evolution*, London, 1915.

87   D. Cannadine, 'The Present and the Past in the English Industrial Revolution', *Past and Present*, 103 (1984): 131–172 at 133–4.

88   The historical etymology of the term 'industrial revolution' has been

exhaustively explored by Donald Coleman, who attributes it not to Toynbee, but to Engels whose first lengthy statement, *The Condition of the Working Class in England* (published in German in 1845), memorably included close description of the living and working conditions of Manchester textile workers. This was not translated into English for over forty years. See D. Coleman, *Myth, History and the Industrial Revolution*, London, 1992, pp. 1–42.

89   A. Toynbee, *Lectures on the Industrial Revolution in England*, London, 1884, 84.

90   Cannadine, 'Present and Past', pp. 135–8.

91   J. Kenyon, *The History Men: The Historical Profession in England Since the Renaissance*, London, 1983, pp. 238–9.

92   Toynbee's, for example, was by no means a rosy view of the pre-industrial age, but his text includes such expressions as: 'On the whole, the agricultural labourer, at any rate in the south of England, was much better off in the middle of the eighteenth century than his descendants were in the middle of the nineteenth', *Lectures*, pp. 69, 71.

93   From Ruskin's *The Two Paths* (1859), quoted in *Industrialisation and Culture, 1830-1914*, C. Harvie *et al.* (eds), London, 1970, 311.

94   Fourth version of script (see note 66).

95   Quoted in Matless, *Landscape and Englishness*, 43.

96   *Mornings in the Dark*, Parkinson (ed.), 489.

97   Priestley, *English Journey*, 372.

98   Fourth version of the script (see note 66).

99   Rotha, *Documentary Film*, 233.

100   The full sequence is in the second article, Eden, 'World of Make-Believe', pp. 147–9.

101   Eden, 'Making the Tradition', 94.

102   Sixth version of script (see note 66).

103   We may compare Charles Beard's description of the industrial revolution coming '"suddenly from the sky", creating a system in which "the horrors of the industrial conditions under unrestrained capitalism" were likened to slavery or the reign of terror', quoted in Cannadine, 'Present and Past', 138.

104   Priestley, *English Journey*, 374. The proverb is quoted as having been in use from at least 1859 in J. Simpson, *The Concise Oxford Dictionary of Proverbs*, Oxford, 1982, 168.

105   Priestley, *English Journey*, 373.

106   I mean to imply something akin to Michael Baxandall's notion of 'period eye', describing the types of period-specific knowledge which the viewer of a painting might have had in the past, as elucidated in his *Painting and Experience in Fifteenth Century Italy*, Oxford, 1988.

107   A. Mayne, *The Imagined Slum*, Leicester, 1993, pp. 1–4.

108   Priestley, *English Journey*, 378; C. Waters, 'J. B. Priestley 1894-1984: Englishness and the Politics of Nostalgia', in *After the Victorians: Private Conscience and Public Duty in Modern Britain*, S. Pedersen and P. Mandler (eds), London, 1994, pp. 209–26 at 212–6.

109   Priestley, *English Journey*, pp. 380, 383.

110   Eden, 'World of Make-Believe', pp. 143–4.

111   Sixth version of the script (see note 66).

112   Eden, 'World of Make-Believe', 144.

113   *Ibid.*, 151.

114   The 'captains of industry … without the imagination which might have made their contribution to the scene an improvement rather than a catastrophe … created a new type of man-made landscape which still remains a fitting memorial to their greed', *ibid.*, 145.

115   *Ibid.*,

116   Quigley to Rotha, 26 June 1934, *Face of Britain* documents.

117   Priestley, *English Journey*, 316; Rotha, *Documentary Diary*, 104.

118   Quigley, *Highlands of Scotland*, 11.

119   Sixth version of the script (see note 66).

120   Luckin, *Questions of Power*, esp. pp. 73–90.

121   Sixth version of the script (see note 66).

122   Luckin, *Questions of power*, pp. 100–1.

123   Matless, *Landscape and Englishness*, 52.

124   Sixth version of the script (see note 66).

125   Quigley to Rotha, 26 June 1934, *Face of Britain* documents.

126   Quigley, *Highlands of Scotland*, 11.

127   Matless, *Landscape and Englishness*, 14.

128   This modernistic sentiment is seen particularly clearly in the Electrical Development Association's 1935 film, *Plenty of Time for Play*, which looked forward to the electrified world of 1955 in which the need for work had been drastically curtailed and domestic drudgery almost eliminated. For competition with gas, see Boon, 'The Smoke Menace', pp. 71–4.

129   Priestley, *English Journey*, 376. Rotha's 'The New Power' may be the third part of the film's dialectic, but it is not presented as a separate period, but more as the antithesis to coal.

130   Priestley, *English Journey*, 375.

131   A. Bertram, *Design*, Harmondsworth, 1938, 61.

132   Priestley, *English Journey*, 379.

133   Fifth version of the script (see note 66).

134   Sixth version of the script (see note 66).

135   Matless, *Landscape and Englishness*, pp. 59, 49.

136 Priestley, *English Journey*, 385.

137 Eden, 'Re-Birth of Tradition', 194.

138 Matless, *Landscape and Englishness*, 54.

139 Eden, 'Re-Birth of Tradition', 197.

140 Eden, 'Making the Tradition', 87.

141 Matless, *Landscape and Englishness*, pp. 38, 75–7.

142 'The Face of Britain', two page summary with credits, *Face of Britain* documents.

143 Calinescu, quoted in Z. Bauman, *Modernity and Ambivalence*, Ithaca (N.Y.), 1999, 3, n. 1.

144 A. Rabinbach, *The Human Motor: Energy, Fatigue, and the Origins of Modernity*, New York, 1990, 85.

145 J. Carey, *The Intellectuals and the Masses*, London, 1992.

146 C. Lawrence, 'Still Incommunicable: Clinical Holists and Medical Knowledge in Interwar Britain' in *Greater than the Parts: Holism in Biomedicine 1920-1950*, C. Lawrence and G. Weisz (eds), New York, 1998, pp. 94–111.

147 Le Corbusier, *Towards a New Architecture*, London, Architectural Press, 1927.

148 M. Berman, *All That is Solid Melts Into Air: The Experience of Modernity*, New York and London, 1988.

149 On Otto Neurath (1882-1945), see wG. A. Reisch, 'Planning Science: Otto Neurath and "The International Encyclopaedia of Unified Science"', *British Journal for the History of Science*, 27 (1994): 153–176.

150 P. Galison, 'Aufbau / Bauhaus: Logical Positivism and Architectural Modernism', *Critical Enquiry*, 16 (1990): 709–752 at 716.

151 See list in: J. Edwards, M. Twyman, *Graphic Communication through ISOTYPE*, Reading, 1975, 45.

152 V. Pudovkin, *Pudovkin on Film Technique: Five Essays and Two Addresses* (Ivor Montagu, Translator), London, 1933.

153 This view had been popularised in Britain at the International Congress of the History of Science and Technology, in 1931; see especially: M. Rubinstein, 'Electrification as the Basis of the Technological Reconstruction of the Soviet Union', in *Science at the Cross Roads: Papers Presented to the International Congress of the History of Science and Technology, Held in London from June 29th to July 3rd, 1931, by Delegates of the U. S. S. R.*, G. Werskey (ed.), 2nd edn, London, 1971, pp. 115–45.

154 Low, *Documentary and Educational Films*, 23.

155 "'Nought shall make us rue / If England to itself do rest but true'" – King John. Recent work on Elgar's reputation after 1918, has shown

that he retained a level of popularity, despite not writing any new large scale works. *Land of Hope and Glory*, on the other hand, had had its greatest popularity during the first world war, and may have sounded rather old fashioned to a 1932 audience. See J. Gardiner, 'The Reception of Sir Edward Elgar 1918 – *c.*1934: A Reassessment', *Twentieth Century British History*, 9 (1998): 370–395.

156 Anon, '"The Face of Britain": A Film to See', *Journal of the National Smoke Abatement Society*, May 1936, 41. Anon, 'Smoke in its True Perspective: An Appreciation of "Technics and Civilisation"', *ibid.*, May 1935, pp. 33–7. For the NSAS, see Boon, '*The Smoke Menace*'.

6

'Enriching and enlarging the whole sphere of human activities': The Work of the Voluntary Sector in Housing Reform in Inter-War Britain

Elizabeth Darling

In recent years, historians have come to recognise that to account fully for the ideology which underlay the practices of the British Welfare State in the decades after 1945, an awareness of the philosophy of social welfare developed by all strands of the voluntary sector, both before and after 1918, is crucial.[1] Much of this work has focused on a reassessment of the sector's role in areas such as social work, but little attention has been paid to the sector's involvement in debates about social housing.[2] This is surprising since the provision of state-subsidised housing would become one of the most significant areas of activity within the Welfare State and it can be argued that it was the approach to social housing developed by voluntary housing associations in the twenties and thirties, rather than that of central governments in the same period, that was more influential on post-war housing policy. To begin the process of revising the origins of Welfare State housing policy is, then, one of the aims of this paper. I discuss both the voluntary sector's theory and practice of housing which were developed as a distinct critique of government policy. They also owed much to the sector's ideological roots in debates about citizenship and the concept of social reform as a means to a higher good: a philosophy summarised neatly by Elizabeth Denby's words at the head of this chapter.[3]

The concept of 'enriching and enlarging the whole sphere of human activities' will be explored through an evaluation of two of a series of exhibitions called 'New Homes for Old' that were held in London between 1931 and 1938 and organised by a group of women drawn from several of London's many voluntary housing societies. They sought, through the use of models, photographs, posters and films, to demonstrate the existence of slum conditions and the work being done to replace them by voluntary societies in London. Their intention was to raise both the public's and government's awareness of the housing conditions in which nearly one million of London's inhabitants dwelt and to offer a model for their rehousing that focused not solely on the provision of accommodation but also on the enhancement and improvement of tenants' lives by the incorporation of social amenities and activities into new estates.[4] In all, five exhibitions were held: the first, in December 1931, at Westminster Central Hall. The other four were held at Olympia as part of the biennial Building Trades Exhibition.

I focus on several issues. First, the development by the voluntary sector of an approach to housing which was determinedly interdisciplinary. This emerged at the same time as various forms of work within the sector were being professionalised and specialised. In housing, for example, this trend led to the appearance of the distinct disciplines of social work, housing management and architecture. Partly in response, the voluntary sector sought to develop mechanisms through which different sorts of expertise could be brought together to work in unity towards the resolution of a great social ill. Interdisciplinarity was seen as crucial to the permanent resolution of, in this case, the housing problem. Second, I signal how reformers identified housing, who and what went into it and the amenities constructed around it as a means of creating better citizens. Finally, I emphasise the significant role played by women in the formulation of this philosophy of housing. Some historians have suggested that as the voluntary sector began to work in collaboration with the state in the inter-war period, women's traditionally strong role within the movement began to decline. It has been argued that whilst the sector was entirely private, women's ideas and influence were central. However, once the shift began to what was labelled the New Philanthropy, although 'women gained the status of paid workers they were no longer positioned in such a way as to exert influence.'[5]

I offer a more nuanced interpretation of this view. Even though it is true that women did not go on in great numbers to assume the parliamentary or civil service roles that might have assured them greater influence over policy after 1945, the fact that they were still active, even central, to the voluntary sector in the inter-war period meant they were ultimately able to influence the form housing policy took in the immediate post-war period, although their influence declined after that. Women (as both paid and unpaid workers) dominated the New Homes for Old Group (NHFO) and the housing associations from which its members were drawn. Elizabeth Denby, a paid housing professional, is a specific example of how central women were in this period in articulating and enacting alternative approaches to (re)housing. I explore her work on Kensal House, a block of flats for the working classes built in Ladbroke Grove, west London, which opened in 1937.

The Voluntary Housing Sector and the New Philanthropy

The activities of the NHFO and the voluntary housing associations from which its members were drawn took place within the context of attempts by successive inter-war governments to resolve housing shortage after the end of war in 1918. The Housing Act of 1919 (and subsequent Acts in 1923 and 1924) laid down, for the first time, the principle of state intervention through subsidy in the production and ownership of rented housing for the working classes, as well as continuing the wartime policy of rent control. These Acts were introduced in the context of high building costs which had stifled the speculative house building market (the traditional supplier of housing for rental), a problem made worse by the decision to continue the control of rents throughout the twenties. This made speculation in building property for rental even more undesirable since landlords would not be able to charge sufficient rents to recover their investment.

Under both Conservative and Labour governments the main type of dwelling constructed under subsidy was the two-storey cottage on estates at the edge of towns or cities. Such housing was aimed deliberately, by the size of the rent, at the better-off section among the working classes in the belief that once their former homes were vacated, the poorer would move in. This policy of 'filtering up' was preferred to the alternative of building for the very poorest because it was believed that the private sector would ultimately resume its traditional role as house provider, once costs came down, and neither party wished to be left with a huge stock of low-rate and unlettable housing on its hands when this happened. For these reasons very little attention was paid to slum clearance by governments in the twenties. Such action was in contrast to pre-war housing policies which had been almost exclusively concerned with slum clearance and the facilitation of philanthropic and, latterly, local authority action to rehouse the poor. Between 1919 and 1930 only about 11,000 dwellings had been pulled down and replaced with blocks of flats and this was under the terms of the 1890 Housing Act.[6]

The policy of governments in the twenties may have had a logical justification but it left an enormous problem unchecked. 'Filtering up' simply did not work in practice, with the result that large sections of the working class remained housed in the most appalling conditions. The existing slums of 1918 were untouched whilst new ones were created as a result of the particular economic and social circumstances faced by the poor. The main problem was that although many of the working classes could afford the rents of houses on cottage estates, their incomes were not sufficient to pay the cost of travel to work as well. Thus they had to stay in accommodation that was close to their place of employment. There remained also the considerable sector of the working class that was refused council housing because of the size of their families and the large number of people who could not afford to rent anything but the most minimal of dwelling space. In inner-city areas, individuals and families were crammed into whatever accommodation was available. The scarcity of rooms exacerbated the problem and created disproportionally high rents for the space inhabited. Multiple occupation of houses, with two or three families per floor in a house originally intended for single occupancy, became common. Any space available was inhabited, including cellars. Since few landlords made adaptations to sanitary facilities, the most horrendous living conditions quickly developed.

It was in this context of lack of action by state and local authorities that a new wave of philanthropic work devoted to housing emerged in the twenties. Across Britain, local groups were formed to campaign that public authorities address the issues of overcrowding and slum housing. Then, in the face of indifference from the authorities, they sought to try and deal with the problem themselves by building new accommodation. These groups perceived the limited action taken by central and local government as a failure of civic duty. They also claimed that the housing which was being constructed, either in cottage estates or in inner-city blocks of flats, was inadequate and failed to enhance the lives of the tenants who would live there. On estates such as that built by the London County Council in Barnes, west London, between 1925 and 1928, 644 cottages were constructed on a site of approximately 50 acres, with no facilities other than a school and one open space. The China Walk estate in Lambeth, central London, a clearance scheme begun in 1928, was similarly ill-equipped. This was an inner-city estate and comprised a series of five-storey blocks around grass courtyards; an asphalt playground was built but no other amenities. So, beyond reminding local authorities that they were acting too slowly against the problem of slum housing, the voluntary sector was also concerned to press for a better model of rehousing. The permanent, and therefore successful, resolution of the slum problem could only be achieved with a housing programme which, to complete Elizabeth Denby's statement, 'wasn't a question of shelter alone, or even firstly, but a question of reclaiming life – of enriching and enlarging the whole sphere of human activities.'[7]

The mixture of propaganda (as it was then called) and action distinguishes such organisations from the philanthropic housing companies of the nineteenth century like the Peabody Trust which, though they benefited from state legislation, did not attempt to influence state policy to any degree. Rather, the groups formed in the twenties were part of a new phase in the history of the voluntary sector as it shifted towards what has been described as a more complementary and supplementary role in welfare provision.[8] This was what the social welfare theorist Elizabeth Macadam defined as the New Philanthropy under which the voluntary sector no longer acted as the main provider of social welfare, a role increasingly taken by the state after 1918, but instead took on a vanguard role, identifying new areas of concern and articulating new responses. She noted that 'private action can push ahead of public opinion.' For Macadam, the primary role of the voluntary sector was now research and experimentation; to build on a foundation of definite facts and seek 'new and practical methods of solving fresh our newly recognised problems as they arise.' Propaganda now took on a central role: it was the 'necessary precursor of all reform.'[9]

The New Philanthropy inaugurated not only a shift towards a different set of activities by the voluntary sector but also a shift in the way groups within it were organised. The adoption of a role as a pioneer investigative body, combined with the fact that the sector now in effect acted as an agency of the state in welfare provision, demanded a more permanent and trained workforce than the traditional unpaid volunteer could supply (although such individuals remained a significant part of the sector). Paid workers, who had taken advantage of the training which had become available for social workers in the early years of the century, were recruited to work alongside volunteers.[10] The new areas of work also tended to precipitate a move towards specialisation within the sector with groups focusing on particular issues, like housing, at a local level but with reference to a coordinating body, such as the National Council of Social Service (NCSS), at borough or national level.[11]

The entry of paid workers into voluntary work, the creation of specific focus groups and large coordinating bodies like the NCSS epitomise the 'modernising' aspect of the sector and its evolution from pre-war models of social welfare. At the same time as it underwent these changes, however, it remained firmly tied to its origins in the ideologies and practices of pre-war social welfare. This was manifest not only in the continued presence of a predominantly female workforce but also in the ways in which voluntary groups acted and in the assumptions which underpinned their campaigns. The people and organisations under discussion here operated within the discourse of citizenship and debates about the purpose of welfare provision that had been instigated in the last quarter of the nineteenth century by the British Idealists. In the context of social distress and fears about national decay, philosophers like T. H. Green and Bernard Bosanquet began to reconceptualise the relationship between the state and the individual, proposing that 'the purpose of the state is to promote the good life of its citizens and to develop the moral nature of man.'[12] The Idealists believed that the only way for society to progress was for all its members to participate fully in its collective life.[13] Their guiding principle was that 'the perfection and moral condition of a state is dependent upon the degree of citizenship in its membership.'[14] This entailed a reworking not just of the role of the state but also that of the individual or citizen in relation to it. One manifestation of this was the concept of active citizenship which envisaged a reciprocal relationship between citizen and state in which in return for certain rights, be they social or political, the citizen would participate in the life of the community, pushing it towards a higher state of existence.

In the context of social work, the influence of Idealism was significant because of its demand for action. It was both a political theory and a practical one. The end was the moral state, the means was to draw out from individuals their potential for citizenship for, as Jose Harris has noted, the Idealists and their heirs believed that 'all human beings, however destitute were fundamentally rational.'[15] Incumbent upon those who were already rational citizens was the duty, on the one hand, to participate in civic life and, on the other, to enable the less fortunate to realise their potential. Such ideas gave rise to two main approaches to social work in the latter decades of the nineteenth century. The first focused on work with the individual. Here the work of the Charity Organisation Society (COS) was most important.[16] Its aim was 'to enable disadvantaged individuals to become more effective citizens' by one-to-one visiting and casework.'[17] The second approach, very much an extension of the COS philosophy, was to work on a community-wide level. This was carried out under the auspices of the Settlement Movement which sought to make of local areas environments where 'individual citizenship could become more effective, and in which a sense of civic idealism could flourish.'[18] Such principles suggest a dynamic relationship between the individual and his or her community which it was the duty of all those who could to further. Whilst debate would rage about the best way to achieve this end, such concepts remained fundamental to the practices of the voluntary sector in the inter-war decades.

Perhaps the only significant change that this philosophy of welfare underwent in the twenties was the increasing emphasis placed on the relationship between the citizen and the community, be that a person's immediate neighbourhood or the nation as a whole. The introduction of universal male suffrage in 1918, followed in 1928 by the extension of the vote to all women, meant that reformers became especially concerned with how best to encourage the newly enfranchised to adopt the duties of full citizenship. Weight and Beach have noted that it was generally accepted that a nation could not survive unless its people adhered to certain codes of conduct and in return received certain rights.[19] In this context it became important to encourage the workers or potential citizens to see themselves not just as individuals but as part of a much larger grouping to which they had responsibilities. This now became a central aim of social reform. Everything should be done to enable the newly enfranchised to act as part of and feel part of society as a whole: 'a healthy group and neighbourhood life is a *sine qua non* of a successful democracy.'[20]

The new emphasis was also reflected in the way voluntary groups argued for reform, especially to those of the middle and upper class who were already seen to have attained citizenship but who had, perhaps, forgotten its duties. Reformers presented the good work carried out by a wealthy citizen with time to spare as something which not only benefited him or her, but society as a whole. The middle class public was reminded of its duty to the community and the nation and constantly exhorted not to stand back and do nothing. As an anonymous author in a housing journal put it: 'Each one of us ... is responsible as a citizen of the greatest city in the world for the public opinion which rules the rulers of the city, and is therefore personally responsible for allowing the continuance of such [housing] conditions ...'[21] The task for middle class citizens was to form a coherent public opinion and to contribute to the work of those who were working to develop models of welfare provision which would enable the working classes to achieve citizenship.

The activities of voluntary social workers in the London Borough of Kensington exemplifies the use of these concepts in practice. The New Philanthropy began there in 1919, when the Kensington

Council of Social Service (KCSS) was formed to coordinate voluntary work within the area. In 1923 it formed a small campaign group to lobby the borough council for action against the severe overcrowding in accommodation in the northern parts of the borough. In order to gain more support, this group was expanded in 1925 to become the Kensington Housing Association (KHA), to which members of the public could subscribe. In the face of continued inaction by the council, in 1926 the KHA formed the Kensington Housing Trust (KHT) to acquire sites and to recondition dwellings and to build new ones. By the early thirties, the Trust had built five blocks of flats in North Kensington. Their tenants were eligible for differential rents and had access to a benevolent fund and a furniture loan fund so that they could buy furniture for their new homes at affordable rates. The KHA/T was also involved in establishing a nursery school in the area for local mothers.[22]

Like most of its contemporaries, the KHA/T's workforce was predominantly female; a combination of the sector's traditionally large number of 'lady volunteers' and paid workers. Although men were active in the sector, they tended be the chairmen, presidents and treasurers of voluntary organisations, with careers outside them. The 'real' work of these organisations, visiting, investigating slum conditions, fund raising, day to day administration was carried out by the women members. This work was their 'career', paid or unpaid. In the case of the KHA/T, although its executive committee included a number of men, most notably the well-known peer and housing campaigner, Lord Balfour of Burleigh, the organisation received much of its funding from the Quaker philanthropist and local resident Rachel Alexander. The organisation and administration of the Trust's work was largely carried out and instigated by Alexander and its (paid) Organising Secretary, Elizabeth Denby, alongside a team of female volunteers. Denby was typical of the new generation of paid workers in the inter-war voluntary sector. She had taken the Certificate in Social Science at the London School of Economics and went to work for the KCSS in 1923. Her role in the organisation was broadly defined, encompassing administration, propaganda and social work and, by all accounts, she was extremely influential. A colleague described her as a driving force within the Trust: 'her office fizzed with energy, new ideas and alarming outburst ... Elizabeth, always two jumps ahead of everyone else, impossible to catch up with, unpredictable, immensely stimulating.'[23]

Similarly, in the north of London, in Somers Town, the St Pancras House Improvement Society (SPHIS), founded in 1924 by the resident mission priest, Father Basil Jellicoe, benefited from the work of Edith Neville (a figure not unlike Rachel Alexander) and Irene Barclay and Eileen Perry. Barclay and Perry were two of the first women to qualify as Chartered Surveyors and acted as surveyors to the Society as well as being responsible for the investigation and documentation of slum conditions both in St Pancras and the rest of London.[24] It was the knowledge gathered by such women from their daily acquaintance with slums and slumdwellers, as well as from specific investigations, which enabled organisations like KHT and SPHIS to produce a model of new housing and to campaign vociferously for action by central and local government.

The Campaign Begins

The formation of voluntary housing groups across London in the early twenties that sought through propaganda and, latterly, building to draw attention to the lack of action in housing policy by the State against the problem of the slums may then be seen as a clear expression of the vanguard role being taken by the voluntary housing sector under the New Philanthropy. In 1928, however, voluntary housing groups were faced with a new challenge when the Conservative government committed itself to a policy of slum clearance in the next parliamentary session. This reflected the party's belief that as a result of the post-war housing acts sufficient cottages had been built to end the shortage and the private sector could now be left to meet demand. State intervention was now to be limited to a resumption of the pre-war sanitary policy of slum clearance. These issues would subsequently form a significant part of the platform of all political parties in the run-up to the 1929 general election and added a renewed impetus to the work of housing societies to keep the slum problem in the public eye and, through their building programmes, to offer a model for the next government to emulate.

The possible resumption of a slum clearance programme coincided with a difficult period for London's voluntary housing groups who were faced with considerable difficulties in raising the necessary funds for construction and they began to explore ways of joining together for more effective action.[25] In March 1928, under the auspices of the Garden City and Town Planning Association (GCTPA), the main central body then working in the interests of public utility housing societies, the first joint meeting of London's housing societies took place at Magdalen College Mission in Somers Town. This discussed the problems facing housing societies and considered the possibility of a collective appeal for funds for building work.[26] At a second meeting in June the decision was taken against making an appeal for funding, instead members elected to examine ways in which the societies and GCTPA might more effectively work together. The ultimate aim was twofold: to improve the organisation of the London societies by sharing knowledge and fund-raising techniques and to campaign for more public awareness of the slums and the work of those groups that were working to improve them. This decision represents the sector's realisation that whilst individual societies could achieve much on a local scale, especially in research and experimentation, a more coordinated and 'national' attack was needed if the government were to be pushed towards more effective action, on the lines promoted by the voluntary sector, and the slums finally destroyed and no more rise in their place.

Between 1928 and the holding of the first NHFO exhibition in December 1931, a series of initiatives were made to draw public attention to the slum problem, as well as facilitate cooperative action amongst societies. These initiatives led to discussions within the sector itself and small-scale displays at the Ideal Home Exhibitions of 1929 and 1930.[27] This activity seemed to have met with almost immediate success with the passing, in 1930, of a Housing Act (the Greenwood Act) by the recently-elected Labour government which focused on tackling the slum problem. It introduced clearance and improvement areas, a subsidy per person rehoused and rent rebates for tenants. Finally, it seemed that the appalling problem of the slums, highlighted by the campaigners, would be tackled by a wholesale clearance programme. It was not to happen: within a year Britain's economy was in a slump and the Labour government replaced by a National Government anxious to limit public expenditure.

If the National Government was prepared to sacrifice housing in its pursuit of economy, then the London housing societies were not prepared to accept this capitulation. The experience already gained in raising awareness of the slum problem now had to be harnessed into a more effective programme if the Government were to be persuaded to spend what money was available on housing for low rental. Galvanised, the sector prepared a new campaign. This would be more direct, more shocking and more organised; not the work of one individual group within the sector, but a group of the sector's best activists working together to ensure the slum problem did not go out of the public's consciousness. The chosen method of attack was the public exhibition and it was to prepare this that the first New Homes for Old committee was convened in March 1931 to organise a display, to be held at Westminster Central Hall, in early December 1931.[28]

The New Homes for Old Exhibitions

In all, five New Homes for Old Exhibitions were held in London between December 1931 and September 1938. Each was organised by an Honorary Chairman who appointed an exhibition committee and formulated the general theme of the display. Committee members were drawn from housing groups across London. They seem to have offered their services for no monetary reward and carried on their usual (paid or unpaid) work in their own organisations at the same time. Funding for the shows came from donations from each society which was represented. Societies also contributed models and related data that the committee then worked into a final display.[29] Here I discuss the first two exhibitions, held in 1931 and 1932, in order to outline the theory of housing on display.[30]

The overall responsibility for the first exhibition rested on 'the dynamic chairmanship of Elizabeth Denby and the exuberant charm of its secretary Elizabeth Alington.'[31] The two epitomise the dual face of the voluntary sector in the inter-war period. Denby may be seen as a representative of its modernising face. Her co-organiser, the Honourable Miss Elizabeth Alington, a reminder of the continued presence of the unpaid volunteer enacting her civic duties. She was the daughter of the headmaster of Eton and later married Alec Douglas Home. The aristocratic connections were further reinforced by the exhibition's president, Lady Cynthia Colville, and committee member Lady Pentland, the daughter of Lord and Lady Aberdeen.[32] Both were members of the royal circle and it was through Marjory Pentland in particular that useful royal contacts were made. The involvement of titled ladies in an exhibition on slum housing may seem ironic, however it is clear from conversations with the 'professionals' who worked on the exhibitions that they were, for the most part, seen as committed co-workers.[33] A contemporary described Lady Pentland as 'far more than just a titled do-gooder, bringing a mind and a personality to housing work which everyone respected.'[34]

Together this diverse band worked on what would become the first 'New Homes for Old' Exhibition. Its objective was to display to the public a graphic and easily absorbed representation of the horrors of London's slums in order to emphasise what remained to be done.[35] The exhibition was preceded by the publication of a book, edited by Kathleen England of the Under Forty Club, called *Housing, a Citizen's Guide to the Problem* (1931). The book featured a series of articles on all aspects of the housing problem and the kinds of solutions proposed by the voluntary sector. It also described the latter's activities. The title is significant, underlining the sector's belief that if citizens could be placed in a position to inform themselves, then action would surely follow. The exhibition, which followed the same line of thought, was opened on 7 December and lasted for four days, attracting around three thousand visitors.[36]

In all, twenty-two housing societies contributed to the display, each being allotted wall space for photographs and charts.[37] The SPHIS, for example, exhibited what it called a 'Chamber of Horrors'. This was a display consisting of large models of the vermin and insects that infested the slums of Somers Town. A model of the Isle of Dogs under flood conditions 'was a grim ... sight, as was the diagram from the same spot of a room in which eight people lived.' The use of the chart with housing and overcrowding statistics would become a mainstay of all subsequent exhibitions. KHT showed a model of a slum site it had acquired, flanked by images of the new flats which would rise in its place. The centrepiece of the display was a full-size model of a typical one-room slum dwelling, nine feet by six feet, and its six inhabitants alongside which stood, in contrast, the living room from a brand-new flat. The displays were not left to speak for themselves. Guides and attendants, drawn from the ranks of the housing societies, were on hand to describe conditions and draw attention to distressing details. Expert guides are also recorded as taking parties around the exhibition.[38]

The Duchess of York opened the exhibition and gained the show several pages of press coverage. It is clear from the tone of these articles that the conditions the exhibition illustrated were a revelation to many. Hugh Redwood expressed the hope that it would lead where others might follow.[39] In *The Spectator*, F. Yeats Brown noted that it would no longer be possible to say 'I never knew that such things existed in the twentieth century' and hoped that the exhibition would mark the beginning 'of a real national awakening as to the work which lies ahead of us.'[40] In the light of such coverage the exhibition was deemed a success. It certainly proved that publicity could be made of an unattractive subject if it was presented in an accessible way. The use of posters and film conveyed the message quickly and easily and the *Architects' Journal* commented that it was 'a bright idea to employ the art of the poster in propaganda to establish the evil of slums'.[41]

There were two immediate outcomes of the exhibition. The first was the offer of a site for a new NHFO exhibition at the September

1932 Building Trades Exhibition at Olympia by its organiser Mr H. G. Montgomery.[42] There is no documentary evidence which records why the offer was made, however various charities had stands at this exhibition and it seems likely that a group which advocated the adoption of a vast housing programme would be considered a worthy occupant of space at a show for builders and related trades. The offer, whatever its origins, assured the venture a wider audience in the future. A further outcome was the onset of formal negotiations to create a central housing organisation. Discussions began in December 1931 and finally reached fruition in 1934, when the Housing Centre was established in central London as a coordinated propaganda and information body. The following year the National Federation of Housing Societies was formed with responsibility for the practical side of voluntary housing work. The Housing Centre became the main arena for housing reform debate from the mid-thirties onwards and was responsible for the organisation of the NHFO exhibitions from 1934.[43]

New Homes for Old, September 1932

While negotiations for a central organisation continued, the momentum and attention gained by the first NHFO exhibition was not allowed to dissipate. The show had been designed to be portable and throughout the Spring and Summer of 1932 it was displayed around England, usually at the request of provincial housing groups. In the meantime, in London, a new exhibition committee, chaired by Elizabeth Denby, was formed to work on the display for the Building Trades Exhibition in September. The second NHFO exhibition opened at Olympia on September 14, 1932, and lasted for two weeks. Denby's intention was to 'reveal to those who visited it not only the essential nature of the need for improvement if any social progress is to be made; but the many valuable ways in which the needed improvement can take place.'[44] The emphasis on the latter may be attributed to the fact that in the months following the exhibition a new housing bill, which would become the 1933 Housing Act, would be going through parliament. Hence the visitor followed a display which began with 'slums' and culminated in a model flat.

As at the first exhibition the display included models, photographs and statistical charts, using the data from the recently completed 1931 census, to underpin the message about the human cost of the slums. A catalogue, produced by Lady Pentland, also provided a longer lasting reminder of the problem. The organising committee benefited from a grant from the Carnegie Trustees that enabled them to produce better visual displays.[45] *The Spectator* observed that it was 'the most impressive, the best arranged and the most comprehensive housing exhibition yet seen in this country'.[46] Each section of the exhibition was curated by a member of the committee chosen for her specific expertise in one aspect of housing. From the voluntary sector Denby drew workers to organise displays on slums, reconditioning, new building and to deal with the catalogue and publicity. For the sections on town planning, the model flat and for technical advice and assistance, she chose architects and town planners who had work experience with the voluntary sector.

The first section of the exhibition was devoted to slum conditions and was curated by Avice Trench, a member of the Manchester & Salford Better Housing Council, probably known to Denby through the public utility society conferences of the GCTPA. Once again SPHIS's 'Chamber of Horrors' was on display. This was complemented by charts and photographs that showed the correlation between bad housing and bad health in several of England's major cities. From here the visitor moved into the first section to proffer a solution, 'Reconditioning', curated by Kathleen England of the Under Forty Club. The display here was mostly of photographs of work carried out and once again included statistical charts. The work of Octavia Hill-trained housing managers was also illustrated in order to remind visitors that 'well-qualified and trained management is a vital factor in the success of any reconditioning or new building scheme'.[47]

The next section, on Town Planning, was the work of Jocelyn Abram. The first woman member of the Royal Town Planning Institute, she had strong connections with the Fulham Housing Association and, later, the Housing Centre.[48] Her exhibit stressed the need for the public to press for the practice of town planning, especially in the wake of the passage of the Town and Country Planning Act in the summer of 1932. Hence the display was essentially educative, outlining the main objects of planning. It also included a history of town planning and examples of contemporary planning schemes. The message was that the public should require that 'the fuller planning powers [now] made available are used to preserve the manifold beauty of the countryside and to increase the amenities and conveniences of the town.'[49]

Having passed through an information and literature stand, the visitor reached the climax of the exhibition, the section on new building and the model flat. The former was curated by Denby and Alexander. It offered a survey and commentary on the type of work being carried out both by local authorities and voluntary groups; a map of London was used to show densities of population and housing provided in each area. The display also contained a series of charts which showed the figures for unemployment in the building trade and the variations in the cost of money since 1928. The main display was devoted to photographs of council cottage estates, the most common type of development outside London. Denby noted in the catalogue that the self-contained cottages with gardens built on such estates 'are undoubtedly most congenial to British taste.' In recognition, however, that it was flats which were most likely to constitute the common form of rehousing in areas like London, where high cost of land made this unavoidable, the two women devoted much of their attention to a consideration of the factors necessary for such flats to succeed. They insisted that care had to be taken in their design and management: 'It is ... vital that the pre-war barrack tradition should be discarded, and that flats should be planned as centres of happy, family life.'⁵⁰ Photographs were shown of the amenities that would facilitate this model of existence: verandahs, playgrounds, gardens, community halls amongst other things. Denby and Alexander also emphasised the importance of economy of design and low running costs and showed examples of the use of space in flats in Germany, Austria and Sweden. Cooking, heating and furniture, especially built-in, were also considered.

The last section of the display featured a model flat 'to show the use that can be made at a reasonable cost of the 760 square feet which is the area recommended by the Ministry of Health for a three-bedroomed non-parlour dwelling.'⁵¹ This type of flat, which had a living room but no parlour, was the most common type of flatted accommodation built by local authorities. The NHFO model flat was designed by two women architects, Janet Fletcher and Alison Shepherd. Fletcher was a member of the KHA/T and had contributed to the 1931 exhibition. She and Shepherd, with whom she had joined forces when they were both studying at the Architectural Association, produced, according to Denby, 'what seemed to be an eye-opening revelation to the thousands of people who came to look[:] ... the enchanting, gay, airy, charmingly proportioned colourful three-bedroomed flat.'⁵² The flat itself was designed for a family of seven and had three bedrooms so that separate sleeping accommodation could be provided for boys, girls and their parents. Most space was given to a large living room with dining recess; the kitchen was well-equipped and designed to a labour-saving layout. It also featured built-in and specially-designed furniture, all within a budget of £30, intended as prototypes for what tenants could make themselves.

According to Denby, the exhibition created a furore.[53] The display clearly pitted the progressive approach of the voluntary sector towards housing design and policy against that of successive central governments which built accommodation and little else. The exhibition also reiterated the sector's criticism of the continued inactivity of local and national government. Charts were displayed showing how different local boroughs spent their rates on housing, or did not.[54] As visitors left the exhibition, a panel reminded them that 'a million new houses are needed to-day to relieve overcrowding, sweep away the slums, give work to the unemployed.'[55]

The greater sophistication of the 1932 show and its location within a major public exhibition was a further step in the anti-slum campaign. It was reported to have attracted 20,000 visitors and gained more press coverage than had the first exhibition, in particular from architectural journals.[56] Its reception is summarised by the comment in the *Architect and Building News*: 'taken as a whole, the exhibit is stimulating and provocative, and should have a useful influence.'[57] The extent to which these two exhibitions were a cause or a symptom of a growth in awareness about the slums and whether they were a stimulus to action is almost impossible to establish, though Elizabeth Macadam noted in her book *The New Philanthropy* that 'a travelling exhibition of models, photographs, and graphic statements and a film did much to educate the public.'[58] Certainly, by 1933 the amount of attention paid to the slum problem was far greater than when the NHFO group first began its work. Ernest Simon commented on a new consciousness amongst the public and of how 'in 1933, we are ... in the midst of the biggest wave of public opinion since 1920.'[59] During the rest of the thirties a stream of books on the slums was published, some documentary, some rather more sensationalist.[60] In addition, newspaper articles and a new means of mass communication, the wireless talk, were used to keep the problem in the public eye. Between January and March 1933, listeners to the BBC heard Howard Marshall's series 'Other People's Homes' in which he visited slum areas across Britain and gave first hand descriptions of what he saw, generating a great deal of comment.[61] This series coincided with the presentation of a smaller version of the NHFO exhibition at 24 Grosvenor Place under the title 'Housing, the Present Opportunity'.[62]

In March 1933, the Minister of Health declared 'a mass attack on the slums' with the introduction of a new Housing Act. This abolished subsidies for all housing except slum clearance schemes and ordered local authorities to produce five-year clearance programmes. On 6 March the Minister also set up a departmental committee (the Moyne Committee) to investigate the possibility of the state working with voluntary housing groups to provide housing.[63] The resulting report, issued in July, which recommended that public utility societies might play a role in reconditioning work, was never implemented but it must have seemed to many in the voluntary sector that government policies were at last starting to move in their favour. Over the next three years the NHFO group, now under the auspices of the Housing Centre, would continue to lobby through the medium of the exhibition for the voluntary sector's model of housing to be more widely emulated. At the same time housing associations, and those who had worked within them, continued to build and develop models of housing practice and it is to the practical expression of the philosophy of housing articulated at the NHFO exhibitions that I now turn.

Kensal House, 1937

At the NHFO exhibitions Elizabeth Denby and her co-workers had conveyed the theory developed by voluntary housing associations that any accommodation built should not just provide tenants with a decent, well-built home but should also enable them to fulfil their potential as citizens and to become useful members of society. Of the many schemes built according to this philosophy in the inter-war period, I examine Kensal House as an exemplar. This small estate of 68 flats was completed in March 1937 and built by the Capitol Housing Association, a subsidiary of the London public utility society, the Gas, Light and Coke Company (GLCc). In all respects it was a piece of New Philanthropy. The project was both an attempt to facilitate citizenship among its tenants and an act of citizenship by the company that commissioned it. It was a collaboration among experts in housing, gas technology and architecture. The result was a remarkable scheme.

The Directors of the GLCc had made the decision to commission a block of working class flats in the wake of the 1933 Housing Act. They were keen to promote the use of their fuel and products in social housing and in November of that year the Company's Director, David Milne Watson, announced the formation of an Architects' Committee 'to advise the Company on architectural and kindred matters of common interest.'⁶⁴ The committee had six members, of whom the only woman, and non-architect, was Elizabeth Denby who had resigned from the KHA/T in October 1933 to pursue a career as a housing expert. While other members were asked to work on the re-design of gas showrooms and products, Denby was appointed with her fellow committee member, the architect Maxwell Fry, to design a block of dwellings for employees of the company and others. This was to be built on part of a gas works site at Kensal Green, the poorest part of Kensington, containing some of the borough's worst slums. To qualify for state subsidy, the GLCc formed the Capitol Housing Association to construct and run the flats which meant that they had to conform to Ministry of Health guidelines. Initially the Company described the scheme as 'primarily to prove the merits of the all-gas flat or house for people of small means', however, it was subsequently decided that the project might also be a means to signify the company's commitment to public service and so it was agreed that 'the estate should be an enlightened contribution to rehousing in a wider sense.'⁶⁵

The decisions about exactly what constituted 'an enlightened contribution' seem to have been left entirely to Denby and Fry. For both, the project offered the opportunity to make a definitive statement about the processes necessary, socially, architecturally and professionally, to best rehouse slumdwellers. Fry's particular concern was to demonstrate that an architect using modernist design principles could produce an efficiently planned and cost-effective block of flats. He and a small group of British architects were working at this time to advance the cause of architectural modernism in Britain. The commission for Kensal House from a large quasi-municipal company offered a particularly public demonstration of a commitment to a new architecture that he and his contemporaries hoped would be emulated widely.⁶⁶

For Denby, Kensal House was an opportunity to demonstrate her expertise. Having resigned from the KHA/T, she decided to use the propaganda skills and knowledge of slums and slumdwellers gathered in her decade with the organisation to create a new type of housing worker, the housing consultant. She won a Leverhulme scholarship to investigate the different types of housing built to replace slums across western Europe; a project which culminated in the publication of her book, *Europe Rehoused* (1938). Denby's figure of the housing consultant who had a detailed knowledge of both the needs of slumdwellers and the types of building solutions available to resolve them was, she said, the person in the best position to advise those involved in the new slum clearance programmes. Denby's attempt to create a figure who in one person blended the interdisciplinarity which characterised the sector seems to have been unique in this period. It was not without success. Kensal House gave her the opportunity to demonstrate what a housing consultant could do. Her role was to decide what should constitute the estate as a whole, the type of flats to be built and the amenities which should be included. Fry would then translate these ideas into architectural form.[67]

The collaboration among the GLCc, Denby and Fry resulted in Kensal House, an estate of 68 flats in three blocks, housing 380 people on a site of one and a third acres. (Fig. 1) As might be expected from someone steeped in the philosophy of the voluntary sector, Denby's scheme was, as Fry noted, 'no ordinary block of flats but a community in action, with social rooms, workshop, a corner shop, with larger flats, better balconies, even a separate drying balcony, and ... a nursery school.'[68] Denby called her scheme 'an urban village'.[69] Here tenants could live close to their place of work yet also enjoy a simulation of the community life of an English village through the surroundings that Denby and Fry created. The notion of an 'urban village' grew out of a cultural heritage that Mike Bartholomew, Anna-K. Mayer and Chris Lawrence discuss in their chapters; a tradition of 'Englishness' that idealized the

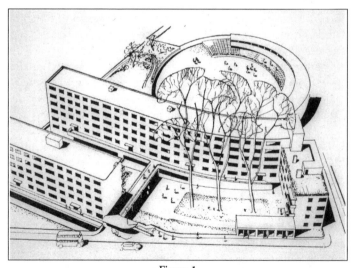

Figure 1
Drawing of Kensal House, from F. R. S. Yorke and F. Gibberd,
The Modern Flat, London, 1937. Courtesy of the Architectural Press.

wholesomeness of country ways, stipulating that village life was the embodiment of all those personal and civic values that secured individual and collective happiness. Kensal House was designed to be a location where the poor could reclaim the life denied them in the slums. It typifies the hope invested by many in architecture during this period, the hope that architecture would solve the social problems of the modern world by transporting traditional values into the modern era. This hope is also apparent in Keith Vernon's chapter on the civic universities. The former slum dwellers of Kensal house were to be transported into a bright, airy home where the opportunity to develop as both a private and public individual would be provided. This meant that Denby and Fry took great care in the planning not just of the tenants' flats but also of the estate's communal areas.

What made Denby's approach different from that of professional architects was that in her view architecture alone could not solve the problems of the modern age: according to the voluntary sector, only by a combination of social provision, management and architecture could society progress. Recalling her exhortation in the NHFO exhibitions for flats to be planned as centres of happy family life, great attention was given to how the inhabitants' new homes might best be planned to secure 'serenity and quietness'.[70] Each family lived in either a two or three bedroom flat which included a fully-equipped kitchen, a large living room (approximately 15 feet by 12 feet), a bathroom and lavatory. Storage space for prams or bicycles was provided at ground floor level. (Fig. 2)

Of the rooms in the flat, Denby and Fry saw the kitchen and living room as the most important. The efficient plan and array of equipment in the kitchen served both as a vivid contrast to the cooking facilities available to tenants in their former homes and as a location within which the woman tenant could develop as a housewife and mother. The GLCc stressed that a well-planned kitchen would alleviate the excessive burden of housework which it thought made the woman 'a worse human being, a worse wife, and a worse mother than she could be'.[71] The kitchen was designed by Denby to be labour-saving, hence its small size (11 feet by 7 feet 5 inches) which allowed every feature to be within reach.[72] (Fig. 3) It was extremely well-equipped with a gas copper, a spontaneous gas water-heater, continuous work-surfaces, cupboards, and gas iron and cooker. Laundry would be done here and Denby included an enclosed drying balcony which led off the kitchen. This meant that washing could be carried out in private and hung up away from

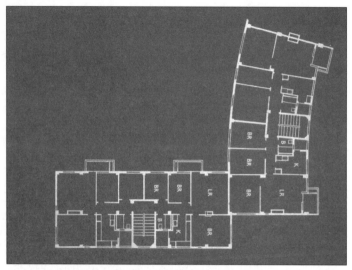

Figure 2
Plan of Kensal House, from Ascot Gas Water Heaters Ltd, *Flats, Municipal
and Private Enterprise,* London, 1938.

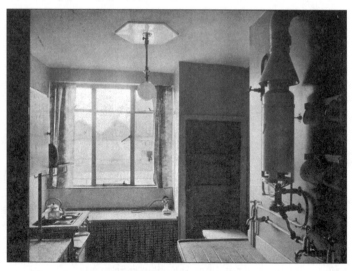

Figure 3
Kitchen at Kensal House, from Ascot Gas Water Heaters Ltd, *Flats,
Municipal and Private Enterprise,* London, 1938.

prying eyes; another way the privacy of the family could be ensured.

The kitchen was, then, the wife's workshop where, as Fry explained, 'the important work of the house [could be] carried on without disturbing the life of the living room and with a lighter mind for that blessing'.[73] A door (and a hatch) led from it into the room to which it was a complement, the living room. This was the space where family life would be lived to the full. The smallness of the kitchen meant that the family meals would have to be eaten here, thereby providing a location for the daily coming together of the family. A coke fire provided the modern equivalent of the family hearth and, since it could not be used for cooking, further reinforced the idea that the living room was just for living. From the living room a door led onto a balcony which Denby believed to be another vital aspect of the design. It compensated for the lack of a garden and provided access to the sun. It was designed to be large enough (8 feet by 5 feet), to hold a table or give sufficient space for children to play within sight of their mother. Window boxes were fixed into the balconies enabling tenants to use them to grow plants or vegetables. (Fig. 4)

If the individual flats of Kensal House were intended to provide privacy and reinforce family life, the areas outside the tenants' front doors provided the location in which they would learn to become part of a larger group within society. Denby and Fry used various techniques to achieve this. As soon as they left their flats, tenants entered the public sphere of Kensal House. Each family belonged to a staircase committee, responsible for looking after the communal areas around their flats, and from which a representative would be selected to serve on the estate's tenants' committee. Inside the blocks, communal life was also enhanced by the provision of two social clubs to which tenants, and others in the surrounding area, could belong. These clubs, one for the adults, the other for the children, were branches of the Feathers Club. The Feathers Club Association was a voluntary organisation that provided community centres for the poor and unemployed near areas of slum housing. It had been formed in 1935 at the instigation of Denby and was funded by the Prince of Wales and his circle of friends. The clubs at Kensal House were the first to be integrated into an estate. They provided not only a space for entertainments, refreshments and meetings but also workshops with sewing machines and boot-mending equipment.

When tenants left their block, they would find a further set of amenities through which communal life would be facilitated. The absence of space and greenery in slum areas was replaced by spacious

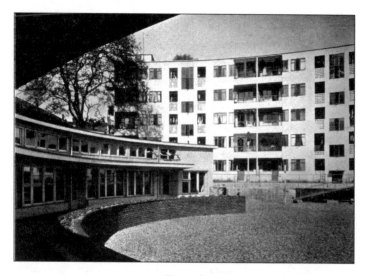

Figure 4
Nursery and rear block of Kensal House, Ascot Gas Water Heaters Ltd,
Flats, Municipal and Private Enterprise, London, 1938.

communal areas. Fry kept as much of the original planting as possible
and the space between the front and rear blocks was grassed over. A
children's playground was placed on the site of the former gas holder.
Allotments were laid out for the male tenants, providing them with
healthy exercise and cheap food. Overlooking the playground was the
estate's nursery school. Mothers from the estate and those who lived
nearby could leave their children at the nursery all day in the care of
a Macmillan-trained nurse. Each child received a daily medical
inspection, a dose of cod liver oil, a healthy dinner, plenty of play and
fresh air and a training in good manners.

The final element of the urban village was its tenants' committee.
This was formed of the tenant representatives from the staircase
committees and was responsible for the day-to-day running of the
estate. It reported to Denby who was appointed as the estate's Housing
Director on the flats' opening. To my knowledge the committee was
unique for its day. It may be understood as one further way in which
tenants were to be educated for citizenship. Denby seems to have held
that Kensal House offered proof that a combination of material and
social provision was the most successful way to rehouse the poor. She
commented that 'the tenants of Kensal House are to my biased mind
a fine example of the latent potentialities in every slum dweller which
only need freeing from weed before they flower.'[74]

Conclusion

In this chapter, I have drawn attention to the distinct approach to rehousing that was developed by the voluntary sector in the inter-war period and was 'theorised' in the exhibitions of the NHFO group and put into practice by Elizabeth Denby in the building of Kensal House. I contend that there is a link between a model of housing that saw as its goal the drawing out of the potential of the nation's citizens and the creation of community life, with the housing built during the first ten years of the Welfare State. Much of post-war housing policy was based on the Central Housing Advisory Committee report, published in 1944, called *Design of Dwellings*, which stressed the need for housing estates to be designed as living communities with extensive amenities. It was also deeply critical of pre-war council housing for both its design and lack of social facilities.[75] Among those who served on the committee were several members of the Housing Centre; it also heard evidence from Elizabeth Denby. The ideas expressed through the various NHFO exhibitions and at Kensal House may then be seen as prototypes for post-war housing development.

It is obvious that women housing workers were central to the development and promotion of this model of housing; an influence which they were able to extend into the post-war period through their presence on wartime committees. I suggest that women did not disappear from influence in the inter-war decades, but remained central to the development of a highly influential housing programme. This is not to say that women workers did not go unaffected by the changing nature of the voluntary sector in the inter-war decades. The transformation of the sector from a substitute for the state to an adjunct of the state gave rise to paid workers with academic qualifications, like Denby. It is, however, important to stress that although figures like her were a new presence in the voluntary sector they were by no means dominant. In fact they were often the only paid workers in voluntary groups. The sector had yet to reach its post-war state, when the treatment of social problems, as Harris has observed 'had become technical, specialised and hived off into discrete areas of expert, professional concern.'[76] This process was underway but in the thirties, just as there was a mixed economy of welfare exemplified by the New Philanthropy, so too existed a mixed economy of labour within the sector. While it remained less formalised than it became after the war, it was possible for women to be active in many of its spheres. Denby stands as a good example of someone who crossed boundaries at this date but who, after the war, was forced to withdraw from housing work because her lack of architectural qualifications made it hard for her to practise the interdisciplinary role she had developed in the thirties.

Professionalisation and specialisation also had the effect of marginalising the lady volunteer. It may be, in fact, that when historians have spoken of the decline of women's influence in the voluntary sector it is to the lady volunteer that they refer, rather than all the women involved in the sector in this period. The demise of the lady volunteer can be traced in the changing composition of the personnel of the NHFO organising committees. After the first exhibition, the lady volunteer became less and less active and was replaced by experts in particular fields. This process, in turn, had a particular impact on the ways women could operate within the voluntary sector. The growth of areas of specialisation within welfare practice led to women becoming particularly associated with the 'caring' aspects of social work, rather than areas associated with decision making and design. This may be explained by the fact that specialisation required academic and professional qualifications and since women tended to have qualifications in social science, they were more likely to end up as social workers or housing managers rather than architects. As the demand for architect-designed social housing rose, especially after the war, this area of work almost inevitably became male dominated since the majority of the architectural profession was male. Again, Kensal House may stand as a symptom of this tendency. Fry's involvement in the project can be interpreted as the first step in a process which led architects to monopolise an emerging area of work and be awarded credit for the design solutions they produced, when, as has been seen, they merely grafted architectural solutions onto concepts generated by women voluntary workers.

In this chapter I have taken steps to revise the history of the origins of Welfare State housing policy and suggested that it is to the voluntary housing sector that more attention needs to be paid. I have also pushed forward the date of the decline in women's influence over social policy to after 1945 and returned to history the work of a remarkable and visionary set of people.

Notes

1 See, for example, the papers in *Charity, Self Interest and Welfare in the English Past*, M. Daunton (ed.), London, 1996.

2 See, *inter alia, ibid.*; also M. J. Moore, 'Social Work and Social Welfare, the Organisation of Philanthropic Resources in Britain, 1900-1914', *Journal of British Studies*, 16 (1977): 85–104; M. Cahill and T. Jowitt, 'The New Philanthropy: the Emergence of the Bradford City Guild of Help', *Journal of Social Policy*, 9 (1980): 359–82.

3 Elizabeth Denby, 'Speech' to Senior Speech Day recorded in *Bradford Girls Grammar School Chronicle*, 1944, 31.

4 F. Yeats Brown, 'New Homes for Old', *The Spectator*, no. 5397 (Dec. 1931): 761.

5 See Elizabeth Macadam, *The New Philanthropy*, London, 1934; J. Lewis, 'Women, Social Work and Social Welfare in Twentieth Century Britain: from (unpaid) Influence to (paid) Oblivion', in *Charity*, Daunton (ed.), pp. 203–23. Helen Meller also makes this point in H. Meller, *Towns, Plans and Society in Modern Britain*, Cambridge, 1997, pp. 44–5.

6 S. Merret, *State Housing in Britain*, London, 1979, 49.

7 Denby, 'Speech'.

8 Lewis, 'Women, Social Work and Social Welfare'.

9 Macadam, *The New Philanthropy*, pp. 31–2.

10 See J. Harris, 'The Webbs, the COS and the Ratan Tata Foundation', in *The Goals of Social Policy*, M. Bulmer *et al.* (eds), London, 1989, for a detailed discussion of the development of training in social welfare during the 1890s and 1900s.

11 There is not space to discuss the history of the NCSS here. It acted as an umbrella group for the coordination of social welfare provision at both voluntary and state level and was founded from the amalgamation of pre-war Guilds of Help, Councils of Social Welfare (both of which had pioneered collaboration with public authorities) and the Charity Organisation Society. See Margaret Brassnett, *Voluntary Social Action, a History of the National Council of Social Service*, London, 1969.

12 A. Vincent and R. Plant, *Philosophy, Politics and Citizenship*, Oxford,1984, 2. See also J. Harris, 'Political Thought and the Welfare State', *Past and Present*, 135 (1992): 116–41.

13 D. Heater, *The Civic Ideal in World History, Politics and Education*, London, 1990, 62.

14 Vincent and Plant, *Philosophy, Politics*, 26.

15 Harris, 'The Webbs', 33.

16 See *ibid.*, and Moore, 'Social Work', *inter alia*, for detailed accounts of the COS' history.

17 Vincent and Plant, *Philosophy, Politics*, 133.

18 *Ibid.*

19 *The Right to Belong, Citizenship and National Identity in Britain, 1930-1960*, R. Weight and A. Beach (eds), London, 1998, 1.

20 J. Pimlott, *Toynbee Hall, Fifty Years of Social Progress, 1884-1934*, London, 1934, 265.

21 Anon, 'untitled', *The Phoenix* (journal of the Fulham Housing Association), 1 (1931): 3.

22 For a survey of the work of the KHT see, KHT Ltd, *1927-1937 The First Ten Years*, London, 1937. This period also saw the founding of similar groups across London such as the Bethnal Green Housing Association, Fulham Housing Association, St Pancras House Improvement Society.

23 E. Pepler, 'Obituary, Elizabeth Denby', *Housing Review*, 15 (1966): 9.

24 See I. Barclay, *People Need Roots*, London, 1976, for a limited autobiography and more thorough account of the work of the SPHIS (now St Pancras Housing Association).

25 Groups like the KHA/T and the SPHIS relied for their funding on gifts and bequests of money, occasionally using these funds to issue shares.

26 See Anon, 'Conference of London Housing Societies', *Garden Cities and Town Planning*, 18 (April 1928): 90-91. This meeting was attended by representatives from societies including the Improved Tenements Association, KHT, SPHIS, the Bethnal Green Housing Association and the Garden Cities and Town Planning Association.

27 The discussions amongst housing societies are discussed in a chapter called 'Housing Discussions', in *Housing, a Citizen's Guide to the Problem*, K. England (ed.), London, 1931, pp. 65–8. The displays at the Ideal Home Exhibitions were organised by the Under Forty Club ('youth's contribution to the fight against the slums'), whose work is described by A. E. Chaplin in England's book.

28 I have not yet located a complete set of documents relating to the activities of the NHFO group, however it has been possible to piece together the exhibitions' history by using minutes from the archives of the KHT, SPHIS and the Housing Centre Trust, as well as catalogues and contemporary press reports. This reference comes from papers in the KHT's archive held in the Royal Borough of Kensington and Chelsea Central Library: KHT archive, document number 17949 'Minutes of the Executive Committee of the KHA'.

29 *Ibid.*, meeting on 13 May 1931, records the decision to contribute to the cost of the 1931 exhibition, as well as to supply photographs and a model.

30 Subsequent exhibitions were held in 1934, 1936 and 1938. I discuss these in my Ph.D. thesis which explores the work and life of Elizabeth Denby.

31 According to E. Pepler, 'The Evolution of the Housing Centre', *Housing Review*, 33 (1984): 158.

32 *Daily Telegraph*, 8 October 1931, cutting in KHT archive.

33 Interviews with women who worked on the exhibitions: Janet Pott (Fletcher), Margaret Baker (Solomon) and Lady Elizabeth Pepler.

34 M. Baker, 'HCT: The Beginnings, Aims and Activities', *Housing Review*, 33 (1984): 160.

35 *The Times*, 20 November 1931, cutting in KHT archive.

36 Pepler, 'The Evolution of the Housing Centre', 158.

37 Anon, 'Westminster Housing Exhibition', *Architects Journal*, 74 (1931): 793.

38 Anon, 'The New Homes for Old Exhibition', *The Phoenix*, 3 (1932): 7.

39 Unsourced press cutting in KHT archive, 8 December 1931.

40 Brown, 'New Homes for Old', 76.

41 Anon, 'Westminster Housing Exhibition', 793.

42 Anon, 'New Homes For Old', *The Phoenix*, (1932): 7.

43 A full discussion of the evolution of what is now the Housing Centre Trust is beyond the scope of this paper.

44 New Homes for Old Group, *New Homes for Old*, London, 1932 (exhibition catalogue), 4.

45 *Ibid.*, 2.

46 B. Townroe, 'The Building Exhibition', *The Spectator*, no.3439 (1932): 384.

47 *New Homes for Old*, 11. See G. Darley, *Octavia Hill, a Life*, London, 1990, for a discussion of the history and practice of Octavia Hill's house management system.

48 Information on Abram, who later changed her surname to Adburgham, from J. Ledeboer, 'J. F. Adburgham, obituary', *Housing Review*, 28 (1979): 92.

49 *New Homes for Old*, 11.

50 *Ibid.*, pp. 14-15.

51 *Ibid.*, 16.

52 Elizabeth Denby, 'Apprenticeship in North Kensington', undated and unpublished autobiographical sketch, which forms part of her papers held at the Building Research Establishment Library,

Watford. Document number 11 67 75 – 11 68 20.

53   *Ibid.*

54   Anon, 'New Homes for Old', *Town and Country Planning*, (1932):
     page 19 gives the statistics. Paddington with a penny rate which
     raised £7505 had built nothing, Woolwich with a rate producing
     £4,264 had built 2586 dwellings.

55   Lady Pentland, 'The New Homes for Old Exhibition', *The Phoenix*,
     no.3 (1932): 11.

56   Kensington Housing Association, *Annual Report*, London, 1932.

57   Anon, 'New Homes for Old', *Architect and Building News*, 131
     (1932): 397.

58   Macadam, *The New Philanthropy*, 147.

59   E. Simon, *The Anti-Slum Campaign*, London, 1933, 4.

60   See, for example, H. Quigley and I. Goldie, *Housing and Slum
     Clearance in London*, London, 1934; Mrs Cecil Chesterton,
     I Lived in a Slum!, London, 1936.

61   *The Listener* published transcripts of all 12 talks, see *The Listener*, 18
     January 1933 to 5 April 1933. For comments, see relevant letters
     pages.

62   NHFO, *Housing, the Present Opportunity*, London, 1933.

63   GB Ministry of Health, *Report of the Departmental Committee on
     Housing*, London, 1933, better known as the Moyne Report.

64   Minutes of the Directors' Court of the Gas, Light and Coke
     Company (GLCc), copies held at the London Metropolitan Archive.
     Meeting held 3 November 1933. B/GLCc/54.

65   Anon, 'Kensal House', *The Times*, 16 March 1937, 13.

66   There is not space here to give a full account of Max Fry and the
     introduction of modernism into Britain. Fry was a key figure in this
     process and had earlier formed the MARS (Modern Architectural
     Research Group) Group to advance the cause. He met Denby in
     1933 and she invited the MARS Group to exhibit at the 1934 and
     1936 NHFO exhibitions. She also collaborated with Fry on the
     design of R. E. Sassoon House in Peckham (1934) which was very
     much a prototype for Kensal House. See L. Campbell, 'The MARS
     Group, 1933–39', *Transactions of the RIBA*, 4 (1985): 68–79.

67   During the thirties and the war years Denby's housing consultancy
     covered a diversity of areas, reflecting her belief in the need for a
     multi-faceted approach to ameliorating the lives of the poor, as well as
     the fact that sufficient employment opportunities existed for at least
     one figure like her to practise. *Inter alia*, her consultancy involved:
     service on the Executive Committee of the Pioneer Health Centre;
     membership of the committee set up by the Council for Art and

Industry to investigate 'the working class flat: its furnishing and equipment'; work with the SPHIS to establish and run a shop called House Furnishing Ltd to sell good quality furniture at hire purchase rates to the society's tenants. She was later appointed to serve on the Utility Scheme Advisory Committee during the war, a period which also saw her involvement with the Women's Group on Public Welfare and the 1941 Committee. Throughout the thirties she also worked as an adviser to to Political and Economic Planning, Paddington Borough Council and the London County Council Housing Committee. Her book *Europe Rehoused* (1938) was her major textual contribution to the housing debates of the thirties.

68 M. Fry, *Autobiographical Sketches*, London, 1975, 143.

69 E. Denby, 'Kensal House, an Urban Village' in *Flats, Municipal and Private Enterprise*. Ascot Gas Water Heaters Ltd, London, 1938, pp. 61–4.

70 Denby, 'Kensal House, an Urban Village', *The Phoenix* (1937): 12.

71 S. C. Leslie, *Kensal House, the Case for Gas is Proved*, London, 1937, 4.

72 GLCc, 'What the Tenants think of Kensal House', unpublished survey carried out by Marjorie Bruce Milne for the Gas, Light and Coke Company Board of Directors, December 1942, 9.

73 M. Fry, 'Kensal House' in *Flats, Municipal and Private Enterprise*, 58.

74 Denby, 'Kensal House, an Urban Village', 64.

75 GB Ministry of Health, Design of Dwellings sub-committee of the Central Housing Advisory Committee, *Design of Dwellings*, London, 1944. See also, Royal Institute of British Architects Housing Group, *Housing*, London, 1944, for a similar argument presented by a group that included Denby and Fry amongst its members.

76 Harris, 'The Webbs', 27.

7

A Healthy Society for Future Intellectuals:
Developing Student Life at Civic Universities

Keith Vernon

Although the independent intellectual was not quite a thing of the past in the early twentieth century, universities were fast becoming the institutional locations for advancing knowledge and expertise and for educating an increasing proportion of the nation's leaders, whether political, professional or technical.[1] The importance of the university-trained expert had been grimly demonstrated during the Great War of inventions, which had required an unprecedented mobilisation of technological capacity.[2] The university sector had grown significantly from the end of the nineteenth century, with the civic colleges in the large industrial cities gradually acquiring the academic level and chartered status of independent universities, but their place had been decisively reaffirmed by the war. A University Grants Committee (UGC) was established in 1919 to enhance and coordinate the essential work of the universities in producing the growing numbers of leaders, experts and intellectuals required by a modern industrial nation.[3]

The technological carnage wrought during the war had raised considerable fears about the place of science and technology in British culture and in its educational systems, and the UGC was keenly aware of the issue.[4] It regarded as one of its central tasks the maintenance of the humanities at the universities, yet the UGC also recognized the national importance of technical graduates. The danger was that there may be too much emphasis on the mere acquisition of expertise, to the detriment of the wider educative functions of the university. If all students, however, of whatever subject, could enjoy the full experience of a proper university education, then the problem would be much diminished. It was a question, then, not simply of maintaining rigorous academic standards but of ensuring that students emerged from their university education as fully rounded and humane men and women, equipped to take their place as leaders in a civilized society. Thus the UGC gave

179

considerable time, thought and government funding to the issue of providing the right kind of society in which students could thrive. To this end, it emphasised the inestimable value of the corporate life, particularly the hall of residence as a place where a community of students could develop which would itself have a crucially educative role. In similar vein, the Student Union or sports field could encourage the meeting of student with student which formed the basis of a healthy student body, while health and welfare facilities could help to promote physical well-being alongside intellectual and moral growth.

In this chapter, I explore the efforts of the UGC and the universities themselves, to foster the corporate ideal among the English urban civic and London universities.[5] A great deal was achieved at all the institutions through the provision of halls of residence, Student Union buildings, health and sporting facilities, with the mobilisation of private donations which helped to attract the funding offered by the UGC. Running through these initiatives was a concern that the increased number of students entering the universities and especially those coming from relatively poorer backgrounds, should have the opportunity of a full university experience, not merely a course of academic instruction. By the early thirties, students themselves expected a range of extra-curricular activities that had to be delivered if universities were not to lose students to rival institutions. Surmounting this, however, was a desire that the technical experts, with which the civics were most closely associated, should not be tainted by the narrowness of outlook which, it was said, corrupted the graduates of German universities. However brilliant the German trained technologist might be, his moral vacuity, demonstrated in the barbarity of the war, was to be avoided at all costs in the English graduate. Rather, the alumnus should combine high levels of proficiency with a humane largeness of view, derived from his years in a disparate, yet cohesive community of fellow scholars.

The Corporate Ideal

The corporate ideal was, of course, by no means a new thing in the inter-war period but arose, essentially, in the medieval idea of the university as a community of scholars and the collegiate systems of Oxford and Cambridge.[6] That a university education comprised more than simply what was learnt in the classroom was reinforced by the mid- and late nineteenth-century reforms at both institutions. John Henry Newman's classic restatement of the nature of liberal education gave renewed emphasis to the university's function in nurturing the whole man, not merely intellectually, but socially, culturally and morally. This ideal was inculcated through the myriad influences of the academic society and environment in which he lived and worked. The collegiate idea of the teaching university, fostered by the cadre of college based dons and Benjamin Jowett's tutorial system at Balliol College, translated Newman's vision into more concrete practice alongside the growing regard for academic excellence. Similarly, the sporting ethos of many colleges diffused the influence of serious academic achievement, while the promotion of the Union as a proving ground for future politicians continued the tradition of student societies, most notably exemplified in the Cambridge Apostles.[7] By the second half of the nineteenth century, the informal educative function of the universities or, more precisely, the colleges, had not only been perpetuated, but had been firmly established as a central component of the English idea of the university.

The civic colleges which had emerged through the second half of the nineteenth century, principally in the large industrial and commercial cities, presented a rather different kind of situation, but one which steadily incorporated the Oxbridge ideal.[8] The civics served a wide variety of educational functions, being centres for technical and vocational education, particularly for those in work seeking to gain or improve their qualifications; offering courses for professional organisations and teacher training; organising services for local authorities, and providing general higher level education for people studying for London external exams. In this mixed economy, the majority of students were part-time, attended occasionally, and often in the evening, for one or more individual courses. The civic colleges subsisted on fees, philanthropy and a variety of grants from central and local government. From the end of the nineteenth century, central government grants from the Treasury and Board of Education became ever more important, and with them came regulations governing how the colleges should develop.[9] Accordingly, they divested themselves of much of their non-degree work and began to focus increasingly on full-time degree students entering from the secondary schools. From the early years of government grants for university work, the quinquennial reviews, invariably conducted by representatives of Oxford and Cambridge, had urged the indefinable spirit of the university proper, to which the civics should aspire.[10] Primarily, this was conceived as infusing the technical subjects with a more liberal outlook, but there was also reference to the corporate life of students, especially halls of residence. One of the key criteria by which the advancement of the civics was measured was the extent to which the pervasive spirit, characteristic of a university, had been created. By 1907, the reviewing panel was pleased to detect that certain spirit beginning to pervade the universities and colleges which was 'influencing the intellectual growth of their students and producing, as we think, results of the highest importance which are not capable of expression in tables of examination successes.'[11] They concluded that '[t]he students recognize in much fuller degree that they are members of a collegiate community.'[12]

The civics clearly recognized the relevance of this matter, not only from a need to engage with the perceptions of those who assessed them for much-needed grants, but also from the very practical demand for common rooms and refectories, especially from full-time students who, if they travelled in from a distance, or had to spend most of the day at the college, needed somewhere to go between lectures or laboratory classes. The shoestrings on which most of the colleges were run, however, meant that such provisions, while desirable, were low priorities, although some of the better endowed ones, such as Manchester, Liverpool and Leeds, did offer limited Student Union rooms and playing fields.[13] Greater attention to social and welfare issues was required with the admission of women students and the colleges began to create some special, if limited, facilities for them.[14] Halls of residence were seen as very important for women students who could not live at home. Informed by traditional notions of propriety, the colleges accepted a sense of some responsibility both for the health and decorum of the female students under their charge, while for the women themselves, it was important to have a room of their own, away from domestic demands.

The significance of halls of residence for women students was confirmed by the Board of Education which introduced regulations requiring trainee teachers to live in an approved hall.[15] Throughout the Edwardian period, the Board had tried to enhance the status of teaching as a profession and improve the quality of candidates who would enter the state schools.[16] All too often, teachers, particularly for the elementary sector, had barely had more than an elementary education themselves, which was little augmented by the traditional training colleges. From the turn of the century, teacher training had been brought into closer association with the civic colleges and from 1911, the possibility of studying for a degree, alongside the teaching certificate, had been introduced. It was hoped that the university spirit and association with straight Arts and Science students would help to elevate the cultural attainments of largely working-class trainees.[17] Halls of residence would further promote their acculturation while freeing women from domestic duties and a lowly domestic environment. Trainee teachers, though, remained distanced from other undergraduates and continued to be looked down upon.[18]

By the outbreak of the First World War then, actual welfare and social amenities for students at the civic universities remained decidedly limited, making for only marginal levels of corporate life. Women students, primarily trainee teachers, perhaps had greater opportunities, although numbers remained small and future elementary school teachers were barely accepted into university society. Yet the ideal of corporate life was firmly entrenched in the English idea of the university and was contributed to, at least in theory, by the civic institutions. Although shaken further by the decline of student numbers during the war, the still uncertain status of the new universities was considerably improved by the growing recognition that graduates were going to have an ever greater role in a modern society and economy, particularly in the scientific and technical subjects which were the civic's chief strength. At the start of the post-war period, the UGC was ready to ensure that expanded university education was maintained at proper levels and in an appropriate environment, throughout the university sector.

The model university experience, however, remained that provided at Oxbridge, and its centrality was highlighted in the Royal Commission on the old universities, appointed in 1919.[19] Oxford and Cambridge had not escaped the financial ravages of the war and were constrained to approach the government for funding. The Royal Commission was set up to report on this unprecedented situation and to make recommendations on what levels of state support, if any, were appropriate. Unsurprisingly, the national importance of Oxbridge and the special value of the tutorial system were decisively confirmed and substantial grants recommended, yet the commissioners were not uncritical, nor did the colleges escape censure. The historically difficult relationships between the universities and their colleges had left a complex political and financial legacy and college life was open to criticism. While the excessively hedonistic lifestyle of undergraduates was deemed largely a thing of the past, living in college remained expensive and possibly deterred poorer students. Several recommendations were put forward to try to address these problems, primarily involving more professional management and more economical catering arrangements. The Commission did not advocate giving public funds to the colleges, as they would not benefit the whole university community and would raise a variety of intractable problems of finance and accountability.

Despite these reservations, the collegiate system was seen as of inestimable value, both central and crucial to the life and work of the universities, especially in developing a sense of community and identity among students and in fostering their wider personal and intellectual development. The colleges were the means by which undergraduates of all types, subjects and social classes could be brought together, thus preventing sectionalism and avoiding narrowness of outlook, perspective or sympathies. Tutors and students could also get to know each other more personally, in a way which was not achieved anywhere else, and which allowed a number of educational functions to be fulfilled. 'The sense of history and tradition in perfect harmony with the sense of progress and free intellectual activity,' gushed the commissioners, 'seems enshrined in the quadrangles, courts and cloisters ...'[20]

This unique educational experience was seen to have some very real benefits in the modern world. The commissioners noted that the business community was increasingly interested in the value of Oxbridge graduates, not only for the practical importance of science subjects or because of the work of the Universities' Appointments Authorities but primarily because 'the intellectual and moral qualities of the University trained man often render him peculiarly capable of dealing with big economic and business problems, and with the social and human factors which they involve.'[21] The contrast was immediately and pointedly drawn between this and apparently similar trends observed in German universities during the nineteenth century. Undoubtedly, Germany's industrial and commercial advancement had been due, in large measure, to the closer connections between the universities and the business world but, in Britain '[we] are not, it is to be hoped, likely to follow Germany into certain paths connected with that development.'[22] The technically proficient scientist might well be economically useful, but if they were trained in too narrow a fashion, they lacked the large view that allowed the social and human aspect to be taken into consideration. Thus, it was earnestly emphasised that the two universities should not be allowed to follow their distinctive trajectories sufficiently far as for Oxford to become, essentially, an Arts university and Cambridge a Science one. The central role played by the college was to create a community of students which would foster that largeness of view. While the future industrialist or businessman would have to receive a specialist training, at the end of the day, he or she could leave the department or laboratory to return to the timeless beauty of their college, there to have their minds enlarged in the elevating atmosphere and broadened by discourse with fellow students of classics or theology. With this rounded perspective, they could go into the world cognizant of the human and social context in which they made their decisions.

Halls of Residence

What the colleges were to Oxford and Cambridge, halls of residence were intended to become for the civics and London. The hall of residence, a version of the community of scholars which had always been the foundation of a true university education, occupied prime position in the plans of the UGC to generate a healthy corporate life for students. These were the locations where students studying various subjects, with different attitudes, perspectives and backgrounds, could meet at leisure to discuss, to all hours, the great questions which had preoccupied humanity from time immemorial, or which were burning issues of the day. '[T]hese are the influences which stimulate thought and enlarge its boundaries, develop the faculty of judgement and arouse in students that energy of the soul in which Aristotle found the essence of true well being.'[23] Foremost in this endeavour was a desire that the wider range of students that were, and had to be, brought into the universities, particularly from poorer backgrounds with more prosaic, and pressing, circumstances, should also be brought under this influence. We see here, as in the chapters by Abigail Beach and Elizabeth Darling, the importance attributed in these years to architectural planning to enhancing the life of relatively small scale communities.

The UGC gave careful consideration to the best means by which a real community could evolve in a hall of residence.[24] There were three main types: the Oxbridge style college where a good deal of teaching took place besides the residential aspects, the simple accommodation hostel or the hall which offered some social and recreational facilities alongside the living quarters. The first was rejected as too difficult and expensive, the second as too minimal and the model adopted was the mix of residence and social life. While converted dwellings could furnish a suitable substitute, the best halls were purpose built with single bed-sitting rooms. To be run economically and efficiently, but also to enable a sense of community to emerge, somewhere between 75 and 80 students, drawn from all faculties of the university, was optimum. A crucial feature of a successful hall was the warden who possessed the right personal, administrative and academic skills, but who was also a respected member of the university, with a place on the Senate. The warden's post, the UGC suggested, should be of equal status to a senior lecturer; a position that would be regarded by a junior lecturer as a promotion. The Committee estimated that, once the building and equipment were supplied, it should be possible to run a hall without loss at a cost of 30 - 40 shillings a week, which compared reasonably favourably with the calculation of 35 - 55 shillings for lodgings. The social facilities offered might differ, but of special importance was a well-chosen library of general interest literature as well as standard academic books, accessible at evenings and weekends, which would help to ease the pressure on university libraries, and also

> accustom students to living with books and turning to them easily and naturally. Students who come from poor homes where they have not been able to enjoy the companionship of a good collection of books, will derive great benefit from the presence in the Hall in which they live of a well chosen library to which they can have ready access.[25]

In the wake of these recommendations, the UGC was soon confronted with a request for help in implementing them. Early in 1922, the University of London applied for grant in aid to erect a hall of residence in Bloomsbury.[26] The Committee decided to postpone consideration of the matter until the end of the year, but to gather together any similar requests, with the possibility of devoting part of the non-recurrent grant to these purposes. The UGC received a block grant from the Treasury each year to distribute among the universities. This was reviewed every five years.[27] The much greater proportion of the funding went to the core academic work at the universities, but a portion of it was retained each year as a non-recurrent grant which could be used to support occasional extra or novel activities. By the end of the year, five similar requests had been received and early in the following year, the UGC decided that the balance of the non-recurrent grant should, in general, be limited to social projects.[28] Relatively small grants would be awarded as supplementary to local contributions for works that were already in train, not as inducements to universities to launch ambitious new schemes. There was a balance of £126,882 in the non-recurrent grant, £100,000 of which was retained against the uncertain circumstances of the early twenties, leaving the remainder to be distributed.

In the first round of grants, two principal beneficiaries were

Birmingham University and King's College, London.[29] Birmingham already had a women's hostel but was planning a hostel for men students. A house and land had been purchased with donations of almost £12,000, including £5,000 from Sir Charles Hyde. The total cost was estimated at £20,000 and it was reported that if Sir Charles knew that the Committee would make up the rest, he was likely to add another £3,000. There was an acknowledged need for more accommodation in Birmingham; the percentage of its students living in hostels was below the national average, and there were 427 students in lodgings in the city. With all the appropriate factors in place, the UGC readily agreed to a grant of £3,000. Similarly, King's College was in the process of fitting out a hostel that had a capacity of 90, but the College only had resources to complete rooms for 50 students. A grant of £5,000 was awarded towards the £8,500 needed to fit out the extra 40 places to make the hostel fully efficient.

In the mid twenties, the UGC identified the social needs of students as one of the four main principles which university authorities should keep in mind for future planning.[30] The first two were to extinguish debts and put existing departments in order; the third was to take all practicable steps to meet the social needs of students, including suitable residential halls, which should take precedence even over the extension of laboratories and lecture rooms. The UGC conceded that '[m]any Universities would be the better for new or larger laboratories, lecture rooms, etc., but in our view the most urgent and widespread need is for more residential Halls or Hostels.'[31] This need would have to be met primarily by private benefactions, although they would be taken into account when calculating the levels of local support which each university received, and which, in turn, contributed to the levels of grant made by the UGC. However the UGC would also support sound projects from the non-recurrent grant. In 1924, about £80,000 was distributed; in 1927 around £90,000 was provided and applications requiring a further £80,000 were still being received.[32]

Through the twenties and thirties, most of the civic universities significantly expanded their residential capacity, notably for men students. As indicated above, halls had been built for women from the turn of the century, while men were expected to shift for themselves. Accommodation for women increased as well, but the greater proportionate increase was for men. At Bristol, a long time supporter of the university, Sir George Wills, helped to pay for a 'particularly fine quadrangular building' for 150 men, in memory of his brother.[33] The UGC, for its part, helped to pay for a new women's

187

hall.[34] Armstrong College was able to provide accommodation for men with an anonymous donation in the early thirties. Leeds embarked on a major rebuilding plan which included a large new men's hall and two women's halls. Extensions were made to men's and women's halls at Liverpool, for women at Manchester and for men at Reading. The university colleges at Exeter and Nottingham enjoyed handsome donations which allowed them to enlarge accommodation for women. UGC grants went towards a new men's hall at East London College, to extend women's halls at Exeter and men's halls at Liverpool, Reading and Southampton.

The most remarkable exponent of halls of residence was Reading University College, which was the only institution to gain a charter between the wars, in part because of its attention to residence.[35] Reading had the highest proportion of its students in residence outside of Oxbridge, and developed it as a distinctive feature from early in the twentieth century. The mastermind of the Reading plan, the dynamic principal H. Childs, recalled the system as originating in Newman's dictum to consult the genius of the place. 'If the College was to be no more than a mechanism to produce teaching and research, it could do without a hall. If it meant to be a real society, an association of comrades, a hall was a necessity.'[36] Rather more prosaically, the issue of providing more facilities for students was brought to his mind when he had occasion to discipline some male students after an unnamed misdemeanour in 1905. The first hall for men was provided for by longstanding patrons of the college, Lord and Lady Wantage. (figs 1 and 2) For a small college, this was something of a novelty, and Childs turned it into a selling point in its campaign for full university status. He reasoned that there would be a niche for a small college, primarily devoted to general arts and science teaching, but with a specialist expertise in agriculture, and a distinctive residential system: a university, as he later put it, 'with a fine quality of life, doing a few things well under agreeable conditions and at a moderate cost to the student.'[37] By the outbreak of war, there were five halls catering for men and women.

Although Reading's first attempt to secure a charter, in 1920, was unsuccessful, the UGC was supportive and a renewed effort won independence in 1925. The UGC was not without reservations; Reading was still considerably smaller than the other universities and colleges on the grants list, it had limited reserves, the work remained academically weak and it relied heavily on government funding.[38] Nevertheless, Reading had in fact fulfilled the requirements imposed in 1920 and it had some important positive features that the Committee set out in its recommendations to the Privy Council:

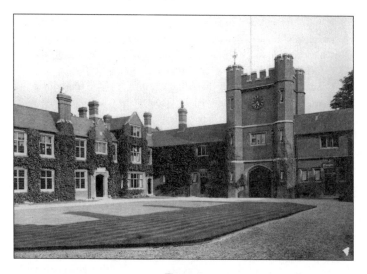

Figure 1
Wantage Hall at the University of Reading, opened in 1908.
Courtesy of the University of Reading.

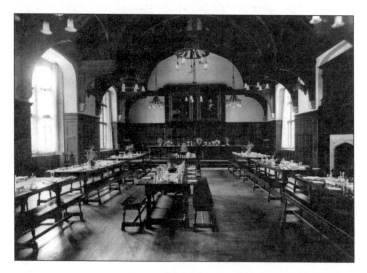

Figure 2
Interior of Wantage Hall.
Courtesy of the University of Reading.

A university which, though small, is yet large enough to ensure the mingling of teachers and students working in a reasonable variety of subjects, and which in addition provides the benefits of the residential system, on a scale unknown except at Oxford and Cambridge, may actually have the advantage as an educational instrument over bigger Universities, where students are so numerous that close personal contact between teachers and taught is impossible and where corporate life is less highly developed.[39]

When the Privy Council communicated its assent to Childs and that the case had been swung, 'mainly owing to the well developed residential system ... and its determination to concentrate its limited resources upon the Faculties of Arts, Pure Science and Agriculture', he concluded that '[t]he human side of our work, then, had carried the day.'[40]

Reading offered a good example of the development of student life that the UGC wanted to see; it was also pleased with a university with modest aspirations. Childs had seen its hall system as an important part of the college's work but also as a marketing strategy which, indeed, paid off. The other university colleges, at Exeter, Nottingham and, to a lesser extent, Southampton (which occupied an ambiguous position in the university sector) also catered disproportionately for student accommodation, perhaps for similar reasons.[41] The UGC was also aware that for some of the colleges in smaller towns, with a shortage of lodgings, halls might help to attract students. Bangor and St. Andrews even had surplus teaching accommodation which might be more efficiently utilised if residences were provided.[42]

Halls soon became an indispensable feature of the urban universities which Sheffield, always one of the poorer relations among the civics, began to notice by the early thirties.[43] Hitherto, the university had not been that much concerned with residences but the new Vice-Chancellor, Pickard-Cambridge, appointed in 1930, made his first priority the erection of a hall for male students. He recognised that there was a financial problem underlying the issue. Inquiries made at local schools as to why relatively few pupils went to the nearest university, compared with Manchester or Leeds suggested:

The answer is always the same – that we have no proper accommodation for men, whereas Manchester has hostel accommodation for about 250 and Leeds for 140. Neither the schoolmasters nor the parents want their boys to be in lodgings in Sheffield, especially in the early years of their University life; and they are undoubtedly right.[44]

To attract even a small number of extra students brought much needed fee income and the grants which went with it.

Pickard-Cambridge was also alive to the educational value of halls of residence. He noted that the one male hall which the university did have, with only 26 members, nevertheless provided 20 of the strength of the Officer Training Corps – a sure sign of the 'spirit of enterprise and public spirit' which hall life encouraged.[45] A hall was subsequently built in two open quadrangles, with a library and staff accommodation, to house 70 students. The builders experimented with corridor and staircase arrangements of rooms and concluded that the Oxbridge style of staircases was superior.

The quinqennial review ending the twenties reiterated the high priority accorded to halls and, again, emphasised the importance for a university education of students learning from each other.[46] Much progress had been made; in the previous five years the number of students living in halls had increased from 1,516 to 2,188 men and from 3,333 to 3,563 women, a noticeably higher proportional increase for men. Since 1921, something over £600,000 had been granted, in relatively modest sums to many institutions, which had helped local contributions to achieve a great deal.[47] There was some recognition, however, that the scale of the task was too great for local philanthropy and occasional government grants to meet.[48] Urban universities could not readily be transformed into Oxbridge or, indeed, Reading style residential institutions, and there would always be a sizable number of students who would stay at home, if for no other reason than economy. Thus, there was something of a shift of emphasis towards other aspects of student life, such as unions and athletic clubs, considered below. Nevertheless, £10,000 was found for a new men's hall at Armstrong College in the early thirties.[49]

The work of the UGC in promoting student life was considerably damaged for the first half of the thirties by the reductions in public spending following the slump of 1931.[50] The austere budget of that year recommended cutting £250,000 per annum from the UGC's budget for the rest of the quinquennium. In the wake of vigorous protests, a compromise was reached in which the Treasury agreed to maintain the level of the annual grant, but would retain the balance of the non-recurrent grant, some £150,000. This, of course, removed the principal source of funding for social facilities, although it meant that the core academic work would not suffer. By the mid thirties the situation had eased, and the grant restored, and the UGC resumed its interest in corporate life and it made 'no apology for putting such essential requirements in the forefront...'[51]

The report published in 1936 did contain the most substantial and thoughtfully argued case for the fundamental significance of the corporate life and it is worth examining in some detail. In practical terms, there were still some 22,000 students living at home and 11,500 in lodgings. Analysing the state of British universities, the UGC posed itself some searching questions. 'How far are the Universities of Great Britain ... in a position to offer their students all that a University education ought to imply?'; 'When the young graduate puts on the gown and hood of his degree, of what inward and spiritual graces are these the outward and visible signs?'[52] The university-trained graduate was expected to have a sound technical training, but had he

> also received that stimulation and enrichment of the whole mind which will enable him to lead a fuller and more interesting human life and to play more adequately his part as a member or leader of the community. In other words, does a University training notably enhance a man's equipment, not only as a skilled worker but as a member of society and a human being?[53]

These questions were of particular relevance to the primarily non-residential universities in the large industrial cities. The civics and the Scottish universities had their own valuable and distinctive traditions, particularly their closeness to their home cities, yet this militated against the traditional idea of university education as forming the whole man and not just the intellect. 'How', the UGC asked, 'is [the traditional belief] to be made effective in a predominantly non-residential University in the heart of a great industrial population?'[54] The UGC's answer was to remove, as far as possible, the student from the industrial populations from which they came, especially the poorer students. These men and women, living at home or in lodgings, could not fully share in the university experience; they may have to travel some distance on overcrowded public transport or contribute to domestic tasks if the family was unfamiliar with the demands of a university course; in poorer homes, there may only be a fire in the one room where the entire family would gather, which could not be conducive to reflective study.[55] The problem was not one which affected the students alone as 'not only is the intellectual training of students apt to be stunted if they remained as isolated units after leaving the classroom; beyond that the training of the students for citizenship is bound to suffer...'[56]

Students' Unions, Playing Fields and Health

The hall of residence remained the ideal means of promoting corporate life, but the UGC acknowledged that few new universities were likely to be able to become even predominantly residential and so encouraged other, less expensive but nevertheless useful, ways of facilitating the meeting of student with student through the development of Student Unions and sporting amenities. Both manifested a growing concern with student health. These areas had also been recognised as important from the end of the nineteenth century and several of the larger civics had made some provision but, reviewing the position just after the war, the UGC found that 'in the majority of cases the provision in both these essential matters is quite insufficient.'[57] The situation improved considerably through the twenties and thirties, primarily through private donations, although the UGC also devoted some of its non-recurrent grant to these purposes. Towards the end of the period, a substantial boost was given to student health services by the national physical training and recreation scheme.

One of the first grants made by the UGC for student welfare was £2,500 towards extending the women's athletic ground and building a pavilion for University College, London.[58] The UGC was wary of making too many grants to the London colleges, which had more opportunities for lobbying, but admitted that, since the potential donors had recently been generous to a similar appeal from the male students, the UCL women needed extra help. For the most part, though, Students' Union buildings and athletic grounds remained the province of individual gifts during the twenties.[59] At Birmingham, the gift from Sir Charles Hyde, which had helped to build the men's hall, also allowed the erection of a 'large and liberally planned Students' Union'. The students at Armstrong College and Medical School obtained a union of 'handsome and commodious design' from an anonymous donor. At Leeds, there had been an athletic union since 1889, and a five acre playing field had been added before the end of the century. In the twenties, though, a new site was acquired which was laid out with labour paid for by the Unemployment Grants Committee. The result was an 'exceedingly fine athletic ground' which was completed with a gift from C. F. Tetley for a new sports pavilion.[60] There was an extension to the union buildings at Liverpool and additional land adjoining the playing fields purchased. Extensions to the men's and women's unions at Manchester allowed for new refectories, senior common rooms and a gymnasium. A gym was built at Nottingham and Southampton University College acquired athletic grounds and built a pavilion in the early thirties.

At Sheffield, a suggestion to provide a substantial Students'

Union building was first raised in 1919, initially to meet the needs of returning ex-servicemen who, following military service, wanted better facilities.[61] Once more, the university felt an unfavourable comparison with Manchester, Newcastle and Nottingham. The same was true of the changing rooms at the playing fields that were too inadequate to permit Sheffield to take its turn in hosting inter-varsity matches. A legacy of £5,000 from a former university official, Sir Albert Hobson, however, allowed a generous new pavilion to be erected in memory of his sons. The building, with dressing rooms, baths and stores, together with a large tea room and maple dance floor, for regular Saturday evening dances, was completed with further support in 1928.

By the late twenties, the UGC was more appreciative of the role union and sporting opportunities could play in fostering corporate life, particularly in view of the expense of residence which, realistically, could only be provided in limited quantity.[62] The virtual moratorium during the slump years made progress difficult, but the new sense of optimism gaining ground by the mid thirties, extended also to health and welfare. Detailed in the minutes for 1936 were plans for two extensive projects at Leeds and Manchester.[63] Leeds University had already laid out athletic grounds and obtained gifts sufficient to build a pavilion. In an ambitious new proposal, the university wanted to develop a social precinct close to the main teaching site by erecting a large new Student Union to go with the pavilion, gym and grounds that were also only a few minutes away from the refectory. They had managed to raise almost £30,000 towards the scheme and sought additional funds to complete the coordinated project. The UGC agreed that this was the most outstanding need of the university and made grants of up to £15,000 to build and fit out the new union.

At Manchester, too, the chance of creating social facilities near the main site was an important consideration.[64] A private donor, McDougall, had bought a drill hall for the university with the intention of converting it into a swimming bath with showers and dressing rooms, plus offices and a drill hall for the Officer Training Corps. He further offered to buy more land adjacent to the first site, which would allow for a more extensive scheme, and it was intimated that if the UGC was prepared to make a substantial grant, the university undertook to raise the rest. The UGC assented and £12,000 was given towards the £19,000 estimated cost. In the same year, the UGC aided the development of the playing fields at Sheffield and paid for squash and fives courts at their new men's hall of residence. Southampton submitted alternative plans for a new refectory, on a larger or smaller scale, and was promised the resources necessary to meet whichever one they implemented.

By the late thirties, most universities had playing fields and pavilions and there was a thriving inter-varsity fixture list, especially in rugby, football and athletics, even rowing at some places. Use of the sporting facilities, however, seems to have been limited and the UGC was surprised that membership of the clubs was rarely more than a third of the student body.[65] Noticeably unpopular was physical training and several universities remarked that the gymnasiums were hardly used. At Sheffield, the brand new gym remained almost empty after the enthusiasm of the first few weeks of term had abated and only a new instructor who emphasised the value of training for games and sports revived it.[66] The UGC's concern was again for the poorer students: 'Zeal for athletics can no doubt be carried too far, but all students would be better for some regular exercise in the open air, more especially those from the poorest homes who are tempted to overwork themselves under the shadow of examinations.'[67] Their fear was that students who were more used to games, primarily those from the public or grammar schools, would monopolise the opportunities available for organised sports. Through the thirties, the UGC registered a growing general concern about the health of students, to which the National Union of Students (NUS) had drawn attention in a report.[68] The NUS rejected any notion of compulsory or elementary health education, but suggested that the rather *ad hoc* arrangements prevailing in Britain had led to average standards of physical well-being falling behind those of other countries. Several Vice-Chancellors voiced their growing awareness of a large number of basically unhealthy looking undergraduates. Some universities began to establish health centres and insurance schemes for their students with local doctors.[69]

The moves to encourage student health and welfare services were considerably boosted by the national plan to promote physical training and recreation launched in 1936. The UGC was advised that grants might be made available to the universities for physical education to the tune of some £200,000.[70] The UGC felt that any university level provision should not merely increase recreational facilities, but that this opportunity should be taken to establish full programmes on a proper scientific basis. This would allow for more extensive study of human physiology and, preferably, be integrated with systematic medical inspection of undergraduates. The UGC was also wary of simply providing more capital projects which would only become a further strain on maintenance budgets. The representative of the National Fitness Council, Pelham, however, was more intent on making access as wide as possible, pointing out that the scheme was designed for the whole population.[71] Thus, he was reluctant to see large portions of the grants going to support a limited number of comprehensive projects with annual costs. Although he acknowledged that, at a university, physical education should be conducted at a higher plane, with the possibility of doing research and certainly with fully qualified instructors. The UGC resolved, therefore, to discuss plans with Vice-Chancellors that would include skilled instruction, medical examination, proper supervision to ensure that a higher level of activity was put in place and lectures to students on health. The UGC also resolved that plans for gyms should include special rooms for medical examination, possibly with apparatus for remedial treatment of students.[72]

Under the recommendations drawn up, virtually every university benefited from the new funding which substantially extended their health facilities.[73] Grants, averaging about £9,000, paid for up to half of the costs of gyms at Exeter, Leeds, Nottingham and Reading, and for swimming baths at Bristol, Leeds, Liverpool, Nottingham, Sheffield and Southampton. Several very large projects were planned, with Oxford and Cambridge to receive £20,000 each and the central scheme for London, £25,000. As Manchester and Birmingham had recently been awarded non-recurrent grants for proposals which would probably have come under the Physical Training grants, they were told that any future applications could be expected to be received sympathetically.[74] The plan from Manchester to build a concert hall and theatre for the students' dramatic society was just the sort of thing the UGC had in mind.

Tempered by Humanity

Establishing social and recreational facilities for students was clearly an important issue between the wars. The UGC accorded it high priority in their views of how universities should develop and the universities themselves regarded them as important areas to expand and improve. Student life had been seen from the early days of the civic universities as a valuable feature which did much to foster the intangible, yet essential, university spirit, constantly sought by the Oxbridge types who reviewed their progress for the Treasury. For non-residential institutions, it was necessary to offer somewhere for students to go when they were not actually in class, and unions with common rooms and refectories were begun quite early on. Halls of residence took on special significance for women students for whom the colleges still regarded themselves as being somewhat in *loco parentis*. For the most part, however, such amenities were secondary to the need to try to put their academic work on a proper level. By the start of the inter-war period, the position of the civic universities was much more secure, with enhanced funding to ensure that they survived and prospered. The UGC, however, was not prepared to see multiple new initiatives springing up and it made a clear commitment to consolidating the academic work at the right level, while improving the quality of university education for the whole, expanding, student body, through the promotion of corporate life. At the same time, there was apparently a vocal demand for such social facilities from returning ex-service men and women who had enjoyed the camaraderie of life in the forces and wanted something like it at the colleges.[75] By the end of the twenties, a university without a reasonable level of provision was going to struggle to attract students with those that did. By the mid thirties, the UGC had identified corporate life as the primary need in university development.

There were two principal issues that the UGC believed could be addressed through a richer student experience. The first involved the requirements of poorer students. Although a university education was still well beyond the reach of practically all the poor, nevertheless, there was a widening of the social spectrum from which university students were drawn, aided by private or state scholarships, which grew significantly after the war.[76] Moreover, the UGC wanted to ensure that this expanded cadre of future leaders enjoyed the benefits of a university education to the full and that meant not merely a formal course of instruction. The poorer students, especially women, might need to be removed from the constraints of a domestic situation. They might also be more worried about career prospects, spend too much time studying and so avoid sports or other exercise, if they were even aware of their benefits, as irrelevant. Such people were in danger of becoming isolated and narrow-minded and missing out on those crucial elements of a proper university experience which were equally important to their future place in society.

The problems were particularly acute at the institutions located in the major industrial centres, but the UGC recognised that its policy posed a dilemma.[77] The civic universities had been established primarily to cater for those of limited means who could not afford to go to the old universities and it remained important that they kept their costs to a minimum. Halls of residence and sports, however, entailed extra expense and also tended to divorce students from the environment from which they came. While the civic ideal had been to reach out to the locality and provide academic service in an accessible form, the UGC was effectively putting up a barrier between the civics and their hinterlands. This model was created as much in the Board of Education's attitude to trainee teachers as in the collegiate system at Oxbridge. While the UGC interpreted the matter as improving the quality of experience for those who managed to gain admittance to a university, the model was based on a suspicion that large industrial cities and poorer homes could not constitute healthy conditions for future intellectuals.

The over-riding point was that the 'mere acquirement of knowledge [was] not enough and, emphatically, that the acquisition of technical knowledge was not enough.'[78] Certainly, it was recognised that universities ought to be centres of technical expertise, and should provide the nation with resources for modern life; a matter clearly demonstrated during the war, but this had its dangers, also amply displayed between 1914 and 1918. The Royal Commission on Oxford and Cambridge noted the important place of the universities in the industrial and commercial development of Germany during the nineteenth century. While not diminishing the importance of technical and other modern subjects, the Commission observed that a narrow focus on the purely technical aspects of training gave rise to the lack of humanity and liberality of the wider view that, to their mind, was characteristic of the German *Kultur* and the barbarity of the First World War. The civics, being more closely modelled on the German professorial type of university and popularly perceived as being dominated by technical and industrial priorities, were obviously regarded as more at risk. It is notewothy that an even stronger reaction took place in America, where the German model had been even more firmly embraced.[79] Many of the major American universities, in the twenties, began to look more to the Oxbridge ideal and to move towards collegiate structures. This too was noted by the Commission: '[s]ince the war there has been an increasing tendency in Universities beyond the ocean to welcome Oxford and Cambridge guests, and to send over here advanced students, who formerly went to Germany to complete their courses.'[80] The anti-German backlash, which had cost R. B. Haldane his position, still reverberated through the university system he had done so much to develop.[81]

By the mid thirties, of course, an even more sinister threat was arising in Germany. The cultured minds of the UGC members could scarcely comprehend the rise of extremism that appeared to threaten with seismic violence the very bases of civilised life and the power of human reason. In such circumstances, they pleaded,

> it is hardly possible to exaggerate the crucial importance of the training to be received by those from whom in the next generation leadership in the various spheres of life may naturally be expected ... To ensure conditions of training which will enable them to go out into the world with minds richly informed, unsleeping in the exercise of a critical intelligence, and imaginatively alive to the human issues underlying the decisions they may be called upon to make, is perhaps the highest form of service.[82]

The humanity of the rounded, university-educated English man and woman, nurtured in the union debates, the athletic club or in the late night discussions in the hall of residence was the bulwark against the rising tide of Fascist illiberality and extremism.

Notes

1 T. W. Heyck, *The Transformation of Intellectual Life in Victorian England*, London, 1982; H. Perkin, *The Rise of Professional Society: England since 1880*, London, 1989.

2 M. Sanderson, *The Universities and British Industry*, London, 1972; K. Vernon, 'Science and Technology', in *The First World War in British History*, S. Constantine *et al.* (eds), London, 1995, pp. 81–105.

3 C. H. Shinn, *Paying the Piper: The Development of the University Grants Committee, 1919-1946*, Lewes, 1986.

4 A-K. Mayer, 'Moralizing Science: The Uses of Science's Past in National Education in the 1920s', *British Journal for the History of Science*, 30 (1997): 51–70; Memo on University Grants etc., 13 March 1918. ED24/1964; Public Record Office.

5 The focus on the major English urban universities is not solely for practical purposes. They were of particular concern to the UGC, although it did encourage similar developments at the Scottish and Welsh universities. The Scottish tradition was quite different although, there too, there were similar trends to those discussed here. See, for example, R. D. Anderson, *The Student Community at Aberdeen, 1860-1939*, Aberdeen, 1988.

6 S. Rothblatt, *The Revolution of the Dons: Cambridge and Society in Victorian England*, London, 1968; S. Rothblatt, *The Modern University and Its Discontents. The Fate of Newman's Legacies in Britain and America*, Cambridge, 1997; N. L. Brooke, *A History of the University of Cambridge*, vol. 4, *1870-1990*, Cambridge, 1993; A.

J. Engel, *From Clergyman to Don: The Rise of the Academic Profession in Nineteenth Century Oxford*, Oxford, 1983; W. R. Ward, *Victorian Oxford*, London, 1965.

7   M. C. Curthoys and H. S. Jones, 'Oxford Athleticism, 1850-1914: A Reappraisal', *History of Education*, 24 (1995): 305–17.

8   Sanderson, *Universities and British Industry*, D. R. Jones, *The Origins of Civic Universities*, London, 1988.

9   K. Vernon, 'Civic Colleges and the Idea of the University', in *Scholarship in Victorian Britain*, M. Hewitt (ed.), Leeds, 1998, pp. 41–52 .

10   *University Colleges (Great Britain) (Grant in Aid)* (245). London, 1897.

11   *University Colleges (Great Britain) (Grant in Aid)* (267). London, 1907, 11.

12   *Ibid.*, 14.

13   H. B. Charlton, *Portrait of a University*, Manchester, 1951; T. Kelly, *For the Advancement of Learning. The University of Liverpool, 1881-1981*, Liverpool, 1981; A. N. Shimmin, *The University of Leeds. The First Half-Century*, Cambridge, 1954.

14   C. Dyhouse, *No Distinction of Sex? Women in British Universities, 1870-1939*, London, 1995; J. S. Gilbert, 'Women Students and Student Life at England's Civic Universities Before the First World War', *History of Education*, 23 (1994): 405–22.

15   Dyhouse, *No Distinction of Sex?*

16   P. H. J. H. Gosden, *The Evolution of a Profession*, Oxford, 1972; A. Tropp, *The School Teachers. The Growth of the Teaching Profession in England and Wales From 1800 to the Present*, London, 1957.

17   *Question of making Building Grants to Hostels*, 18 March 1907. ED 86/63. Public Record Office.

18   Dyhouse, *No Distinction of Sex?*

19   *Royal Commission on Oxford and Cambridge Universities* [Cmd. 1588], London, 1922.

20   *Ibid.*, 15.

21   *Ibid.*, 44.

22   *Ibid.*

23   *University Grants Committee. Report for the Period 1929/30 – 34/35*, London, 1936, 13.

24   *Report of the University Grants Committee* [Cmd. 1163], London, 1921; *UGC Report, 1921*; *UGC Report Including Returns From Universities and University Colleges in Receipt of Treasury Grant. Academic Year 1923-4*, London, 1925.

25   *UGC Report 1923-4*, 25.

26 UGC minutes of meeting, 7 December 1922. UGC 1/1. All UGC files referred to here are held in the Public Record Office.

27 Shinn, *Paying the Piper.*

28 UGC minutes of meeting, 22 March 1923. UGC 1/1.

29 *Ibid.* Appendix III, minutes of meeting, 21 June 1923. UGC 1/1.

30 *UGC Report 1923-4.*

31 UGC minutes of meeting, 5 February 1925. UGC 1/1.

32 UGC minutes of meetings, 10 July 1924, and 3 February 1927. UGC 1/1.

33 Summaries of works which attracted private donations were given in the *Report for 1928/29* and *Report for the Period 1929/30 –1934/35.*

34 A summary of works supported by the UGC is given in Appendix A, minutes of meeting, 2 February 1927. UGC 1/1.

35 W. M. Childs, *Making a University. An Account of the University Movement at Reading,* London, 1933.

36 *Ibid.,* 56.

37 *Ibid.,* 117.

38 Letter from UGC to the Privy Council on Reading's application for a Charter. Reproduced as Appendix B to minutes of meeting, 12 March 1925. UGC 1/1.

39 *Ibid.*

40 As quoted in Childs, *University Movement,* 260.

41 *UGC Report 1923/24.*

42 UGC minutes of meeting, 5 February 1925. UGC 1/1.

43 A. W. Chapman, *The Story of a Modern University. A History of the University of Sheffield,* Oxford, 1955.

44 Quoted in *Ibid.,* 373.

45 *Ibid.*

46 *UGC Report 1928–29.*

47 Totals given in Appendix A to the minutes of meeting 3 July 1935. UGC 1/2.

48 Memorandum by UGC to Treasury, reproduced as Appendix A to the minutes of meeting, 7 November 1929. UGC 1/1.

49 UGC minutes of meeting, 13 February 1930. UGC 1/1.

50 UGC minutes of meeting, 22 October 1931. UGC 1/1.

51 *UGC Report 1929/30–34/35,* 11.

52 *Ibid.*

53 *Ibid.*

54 *Ibid.* 12.

55 These issues were discussed throughout the period and rehearsed more fully in *UGC Report of the Sub-Committee on Halls of Residence,* London, 1957.

56 *UGC Report 1921*, 14.

57 *Ibid.*

58 UGC minutes of meeting, 21 June 1923. UGC 1/1.

59 Summaries are given in *UGC Report 1928/29.*

60 *Ibid.*; Shimmin, *University of Leeds.*

61 Chapman, *Modern University.*

62 Memorandum by UGC to Treasury, reproduced as Appendix A to the minutes of meeting, 7 November 1929. UGC 1/1.

63 Appendix A to minutes of meeting, 2 December 1936. UGC 1/2.

64 *Ibid.*

65 *UGC Report 1923/24.*

66 Chapman, *Modern University*

67 *UGC Report 1923/24*, 24.

68 *UGC Report 1929/30 – 34/35*; E. Ashby and M. Anderson, *The Rise of the Student Estate in Britain*, London, 1970.

69 *UGC Report 1929/30 – 34/35.*

70 UGC minutes of meeting, 16 December 1937. UGC 1/2.

71 UGC minutes of meeting, 4 February 1938. UGC 1/2.

72 *Ibid.*

73 Appendix A to minutes of meeting, 29 March 1938. UGC 1/2.

74 UGC minutes of meeting, 7 October 1938. UGC 1/2.

75 *UGC Report 1921*. Chapman, *Modern University.*

76 There were 200 state scholarships provided for the first time in 1920; by 1936 this had grown to 360. *Education 1900-1950. Report of the Ministry of Education for the year 1950* [Cmd. 8244], London, 1951.

77 *UGC Report 1929/30–34/35.*

78 *UGC Report 1929/30–34/35*, 13.

79 F. Rudolph, *The American College and University*, New York, 1962.

80 *Royal Commission on Oxford and Cambridge*, 46.

81 E. Ashby and M. Anderson, *Portrait of Haldane at Work on Education*, London, 1974.

82 *UGC Report 1929/30–34/35*, pp. 49–50.

8

Potential For Participation:
Health Centres and the
Idea of Citizenship c.1920-1940

Abigail Beach

Positive Health and a Modern Society

The idea of citizenship as an expression of human potentiality gained considerable support during the inter-war period, finding practical manifestation in a range of social policy areas. Medicine and health care provision became particularly fertile arenas for debate.[1] During the inter-war years, with the foundations of the Edwardian world still left unreconstructed, many Britons particularly, though not exclusively, among the intellectual and political élite turned with hope towards science and to 'its humane extension into the lives of working people.'[2] In these years the medical and general press carried a growing number of articles, editorials and letters exploring the meaning of health in a modern society. An interesting feature of these discussions was what Charles Webster has called a 'growing impatience' with the traditional terminology of health care: 'New words were called for to reflect new attitudes towards health and disease.' Amongst them were 'positive health' and 'social medicine': a linguistic development that, arguably, reveals changing attitudes towards people, their needs, rights and the nature of their citizenship.[3] This chapter explores this development, first, by looking at a range of contemporary expositions on the inter-connections between health and citizenship and second, by examining the practical efforts of physicians, politicians and others to foster a more integrated and active citizenry through new approaches to health care delivery.

Examination of articles and correspondence in the *British Medical Journal* during the inter-war years indicates the increasing use of the term 'positive health'. Even before the term itself became common in the later thirties, the concept was attracting the attention of significant figures within and around the medical profession.[4] From a basis that owed much to contemporary understanding of preventive medicine, 'positive health' signified both the need for greater consideration of the 'normal' and attendance to health before the visible onset of disease.[5] From this view, it was insufficient to describe the health of the nation in terms of mortality or morbidity. A much wider definition – one which incorporated signs of 'exhaustion, ill-health, under-nourishment' revealed through 'loss of vitality, deficiencies of growth, in bad nerves, and in bodies which, though whole, are inefficient' – was felt to be necessary.[6]

The appeal of the notion of positive health reflected the strength of a neo-hippocratic holism within some sections of the British medical community. This was a practical philosophy that saw illness not simply 'as the result of discrete biological causes, but rather as a function of a whole life' and health (or the lack of it) as an intrinsic part of 'the complex relations between individual and environment.'[7] In his chapter Chris Lawrence refers to this holism and its origins in so far as it was described by élite clinicians as pertaining to bedside medicine. But the medical planners who were considering the organization of local and national health services also employed it.[8]

The drive towards a positive notion of health also appears to owe much to the 'national efficiency' movement of the early twentieth century.[9] As such, one might question how far contemporaries found it compatible with an interest in the citizenship rights of individuals. Positive health is frequently described in collective terms as a 'material asset' of a nation and thus a prime consideration of the state: the 'cost effectiveness' of taking stock of this 'national asset' regularly appears as a prime reason for the development of positive health policies.[10] However, the call for positive health also entailed a recognition of human potentiality, which for many advocates implied the pursuit of equality of opportunity for health.[11] Health, it was repeatedly argued, meant having all the equipment to fulfil one's potential. It was medicine's role to understand what were the limiting factors, physiological, genetic but also, environmental.[12]

Manifestations of the idea of human potentiality appeared in a wide range of contemporary statements, many of which reveal an awareness of the inter-connections between health and notions of citizenship. In the early twenties, with the memories of the Great War still fresh, *The Spectator* ran a series of reports on the state of the nation's health. Though infused with a concerned tone, the emphasis was firmly on the opportunity for future improvement. A devastating war had been fought and won. But if the nation's resolve had been proved strong, its citizens' flesh was undeniably weak. There was no disguising 'C3 manhood' even if it did contain an A1 spirit.[13] The men in the streets were not shirkers as had often been thought prior to the war but 'lion-hearted youths, with feeble, distorted, ill-developed bodies ... Fine souls in poor bodies.' The implication is clear: the 'lion-hearted youth' was being caged in by inadequate health. The nation and the individual deserved better.[14] Was this a recognition of rights, of the entitlement of each citizen to a standard of health that would enable his (and her) true potential to be unleashed? If this voice was a solitary one in 1919, it certainly became stronger in the following decades. In the inter-war years there were a number of health-related issues that provided a framework for the articulation of the developing ideas of positive health and social medicine. These, arguably, reflect the idea of potentiality in practice.

Throughout the thirties the physical fitness of the nation, or lack of it, was a popular topic for discussion and became a vehicle for the articulation of opinions on the role of the state and the rights and responsibilities of the citizen. This relatively uncontroversial subject thus provided an entry point into the wider issue of responsibility for health care. By the thirties the state's role as provider of some sort of health care service was relatively well established and accepted as necessary and proper. Increasingly, though, emphasis was placed on how far this should extend. In 1933, *The Spectator* noted the emergence of 'a public opinion demanding that the administrator and the scientist ... step in and sweep away the limitations which have kept so much of the population on the C3 level ... opportunities to become physically fit and to have the power of physical self-expression should be denied to none.'[15] However, although there was a general recognition of the state's responsibility to facilitate fitness and healthy living, emphasis was squarely laid upon the co-operative and pluralistic nature of the relationship between the state and the individual.[16] In 1937 the Conservative government initiated a campaign to promote the use of existing health services. Primarily an educational activity, the main object was to teach 'men and women that the maintenance and improvement of standards of health is a co-operative enterprise, to which the private citizen must contribute as much as governments.'[17] The campaign was, undoubtedly, a cosmetic exercise and as such was not without criticism. The medical profession, while giving its support to the campaign, felt it was hugely deficient, if not actually misplaced: *The Spectator* observed that the 'existing health services, which have grown up piecemeal, do not represent a national health policy. The basis of this policy should be the provision for every citizen of a general medical practitioner backed by the necessary specialist, laboratory and institutional services.'[18] But if, in reality, the health campaign was an unsubstantiated verbal statement of the right of equal entitlement to health, the episode was revealing of a changing social and political environment. The initiative indicated the widespread affirmation of the cultural value of the active participation of state and citizen in a common project for health not least since the programme was introduced at a time of stringent Treasury control and general uncertainty as to the desirable limits of state provision. This is particularly clear if the campaign is seen in conjunction with the Physical Training and Recreation Act of the same year, a piece of legislation which sought the development of local health and fitness opportunities through the co-operation of local authorities, the developing community association movement and existing clubs.[19]

Ideological undertones differentiating the ways of Fascism from those of democracy were also influential on the content and format of the fitness and health campaigns of the mid- to later thirties. Although in line with the established publicity policies of the Ministry of Health and Board of Education, the use of voluntary organisations in the campaigns was given philosophical and cultural significance.[20] A mandatory health and fitness scheme was advocated by some, but the prevailing view was that such 'German methods' were incompatible with British traditions.[21] The favoured approach was a combination of voluntary action with state encouragement. The relevance to citizenship was widely noted. Lord Burghley, the Conservative member for Peterborough, echoed the thoughts of many, and not only from his side of the House, when he attested to the value of unforced physical development in the advancement of 'a feeling of the responsibility of citizenship.'[22]

Another issue extremely relevant to the development of ideas on health, potentiality and, by inference, citizenship at this time was nutrition. Awareness of the link between income, diet and nutrition was heightened by John Boyd Orr's study *Food, Health, Income* (1936) which graphically presented the connection between malnutrition and variations in working-class income. A tenth of the population, including a fifth of all children, Boyd Orr concluded, were chronically ill nourished and half of the population suffered from some sort of nutritional deficiency. Poverty was a significant contributory factor.[23] Boyd Orr's work did not escape criticism, not least from officialdom, but it was endorsed by other studies and statements.[24] G. C. M. M'Gonigle, the Medical Officer of Health for

Stockton-on-Tees, for instance, found that the death rate among the poorer section of the population spending only 3 shillings a head on food, was twice that of the most affluent, who allowed 6 shillings a head.[25] Official stubbornness in the face of such findings did soften in the later thirties as the nutrition question was increasingly given prominence in official reports often in conjunction with unemployment. The medical press provided an additional forum, as academic research and government reports relating to the nutrition question were summarised and discussed in editorials and leading articles.[26] Articles in the general press also explored the connection, frequently concluding with an appeal for a better standard of nutrition since however beneficial was physical exercise and training, it could not be 'indulged in upon an empty stomach.'[27] The message from Parliament, particularly though not exclusively from the opposition benches, was similarly blunt.[28] Perhaps the clearest contemporary statement of the need to consider the nation's health within a broad political and economic context, though, came in a survey of health services published by the cross-party research group Political and Economic Planning (PEP) in 1937. If health was to mean 'more than not being ill', as the proponents of positive health and social medicine were advocating, then social policy as a whole needed to be integrated towards this aim. 'The really essential health services of the nation', PEP argued:

> are the making available of ample safe fresh milk to all who need it, the cheapening of other dairy produce, fruit and vegetables, new accommodation to replace the slums and relieve overcrowding, green belt schemes, playing fields, youth hostels and physical education, social insurance which relieve the burden of anxiety on the family and advances in employment policy which improve security of tenure or conditions of work and, finally, education in healthy living through training and propaganda.[29]

These broad discussions on the meaning of health in the inter-war years appear to indicate a changing perception of the social rights of ordinary people: there is a traceable, if imprecise, awareness of the entitlement of all people to health and a broad, if shallow, consensus of the need for some degree of state intervention to achieve this ideal. Yet, here the submerged differences between the various groups and individuals seeking such changes began to impinge upon the debate. The appropriate role of respective statutory and voluntary agencies in shaping health policy and the perceived implications of this interactive relationship to citizenship increasingly became the focus of debates.

Health Centres

Further insights into this limited consensus can be gleaned from practical examples of health care. The health centre, in particular, is a useful reference point for an examination of the relationship between health care provision and citizenship since it is a feature of health debates throughout the inter-war years and directly posed questions of where responsibility and accountability for health care should lie. In 1920, the Dawson report, sponsored by the Ministry of Health, described the health centre as the future direction of primary health care provision. Centres were presented as the means to integrate preventative and curative medicine – a prime consideration of the new Chief Medical Officer, Sir George Newman.[30] They were also presented as a response to the 'increasing conviction that the best means of maintaining health and curing disease should be made available to all citizens.'[31] A conception of the health centre also featured in a Labour Party report of 1919.[32] By the mid thirties the health centre was a major feature in the policy statements of the Socialist Medical Association, Medical Practitioners' Union and the Labour Party.[33] It became a topical phrase in the later thirties, publicised by the Pioneer Health Centre at Peckham and the municipal experiment at Finsbury. The health centre figured prominently in the National Health Service Act of 1946 but this paper prominence was unsupported by concrete initiatives owing largely to the combination of a post-war shortage of building material and, equally important, the marked distrust of centres by medical practitioners.

During the inter-war period a number of widely differing conceptions of the health centre emerged. On one level, the attributes of a centre were generally recognised as including a collaboration of skills and a division of labour among a range of personnel working under one roof and the use of modern therapeutic and diagnostic techniques. There was also a 'diffuse implication that health centres would pay more positive regard to maintenance of health rather than merely react by treating disease.'[34] However, crucial questions of responsibility and administrative structure, questions vital to an understanding of the relationships between the patient, the community, the medical profession and the state were left undefined. For instance, while clearly evolving at similar times, the Labour party's policy on health centres and that of Dawson had one very distinct difference. As Charles Webster has pointed out, 'Dawson's predominant concern was to devise a fully co-ordinated

State Medical Service free from full-time salaried service.' Labour, however, demanded the opposite.[35] Indeed, as late as 1943, A. Robb-Smith, a Reader in Pathology at Oxford, noted that while there was general agreement that groups of general practitioners with secretarial assistance would be a good thing, there was 'considerable disagreement as to who should provide and equip these centres.'[36] Between the twenties and the forties, several different interpretations of the health centre were put forward (many on paper, far fewer in practice) and an examination of these reveals the open-ended and contested nature of the idea of citizenship and the varied definition of the boundaries between the state, both central and local, and civil society.[37] As in the chapters by Elizabeth Darling and Keith Vernon we also see the importance attributed to architectural planning to create harmonically working small-scale communities.

A general feature of contemporary discussions on health centres is how they were to have a particular association with a community of people: they were designed to serve a particular neighbourhood or area and to be the focus of that area's health services.[38] This inherent feature makes the discussions on health centres in this period an important source for understanding conceptions of the relationship between the providers and recipients of care and between the centre and the local community. It is interesting to speculate whether, in a period in which rural life was idealised, images of the village hall as the centre of communal life played any part in conceptions of health centres. Sir Bernard Dawson's view of the health centre was undoubtedly localist: the services of the health centre, he suggested, would be 'established by local enterprise'.[39] However, to Dawson, this meant the centrality of the medical practitioners of the area, rather than the local people themselves.[40] There was little sense of mass active participation in Dawson's idea beyond the Edwardian view that the people themselves should be, in large part, responsible for their own health, with responsibility to be fostered through on-going health education.[41] The profession-dominated model of Dawson can be contrasted with that of Ernest Barker, Professor of Political Science at Cambridge and Chairman of the National Council for Social Service (NCSS), developed over a decade later in the mid thirties. Barker saw health centres as complements to the neighbourhood community centres which the NCSS had advocated.[42] A similar vision was advanced by PEP in a commentary on the 1944 Health Services White Paper. The involvement of local people in the life of the centre, it argued, was fundamental to the effectiveness of the whole project: 'If the people of a neighbourhood regard it as their own institution, established at their wish, they will take full advantage of its services.'[43] To PEP, as to Barker, the health centre could be a socially integrative force. People could 'meet their doctors outside the surgery and the sick-room in the centre's lecture-hall or in the community centre.' By the mid forties, in the midst of war and thoughts of reconstruction, the health centre had become an example of social citizenship in practice. PEP's health centre was to be an 'arena for mutual discussion and questioning' and a means of 'equipping doctors and other health workers with that intimate knowledge of the "consumer" of the health service which they often lack today.' In this modern local facility, 'doctors would learn to treat their patients not as irresponsible children but as adult fellow-citizens.' It was hoped that as the centres' social and educational activities became a powerful instrument for breaking down the barriers of ignorance, misunderstanding and prejudice, on both sides, the 'bottle of medicine' attitude to health would dissipate.[44]

The Dawson model, as noted above, also contrasted with the health centre policy of the Labour party which stressed the importance of community responsibility for the service, operating through democratically-elected, politically-responsive local authorities.[45] The health centre's administrative relationship with the local community became increasingly pertinent in the later thirties as local authorities began to consider the creation of health centres alongside wider plans for the development of the community. In particular, the health centre became administratively associated with housing schemes and estate building. Health Committee minutes and memoranda of the London County Council (LCC) clearly reflect this tandem development. For example, in 1937 the prospective housing development at Bellingham in Lewisham set in motion LCC discussion on the provision of a health centre as part of the new estate.[46] The Council's Medical Officer of Health, Dr Allan Daley, noted that the provision of an estate health centre was likely to be necessary since the expected population would be of the 'clinic class'.[47] The association of health centres with newly developed areas was to strengthen after the passage of the 1946 National Health Service Act but it was a connection that owed little to PEP's or Labour's interest in neighbourhood responsibility for health.[48] It related more to a political desire to avoid problematic clashes between Local Health Authorities and Local Medical Committees. Consequently, 'the few positive moves towards health centre development' that emerged from nearly three decades of debate 'were conducted in the context of new towns and housing estates with more than 2,500 houses.'[49] The ambivalence of the medical profession, and fears about what the health centre meant for professional autonomy, overshadowed and complicated the issue from the start.[50]

Original intentions rarely survive the rigours of practical expression unscathed and certainly in the case of the community health centre this move was an awkward one. In the thirties the Local Authority-run Finsbury Health Centre and the independent Pioneer Health Centre at Peckham received considerable professional and press attention.[51] The following section examines the implications for the idea of citizenship raised by these centres. An evidential point should first be mentioned in this context. Peckham had the advantage of having been established and run by two extremely committed people, eager to use the centre as a vehicle to publicise their own scientific ideas. As a consequence, the Peckham Health Centre's aims were amply recorded. Finsbury, as a local authority centre, has not left such information: the borough council minutes are characteristically brief. However, supplementary information is obtainable from the writings of the architect, Berthold Lubetkin, whose partnership Tecton was commissioned by the council for this project.[52] An examination of Lubetkin's ideas for the health centre reveals an active conception of citizenship less readily apparent from the official records of the centre and its status as a local authority service.

Finsbury

The Finsbury Health Centre opened in 1938 under the auspices of the Labour-controlled metropolitan borough council. It was based on the provisions of the Public Health (London) Act of 1936 that empowered borough councils to provide suitable medical services for their poorer inhabitants. Within this framework, accommodation was found for administrative, sanitary and health visiting staffs, the tuberculosis clinic, public health laboratory, cleansing and disinfecting stations and mortuary. The centre was built beside an existing mother and child welfare clinic and included a dental clinic, foot clinic, women's clinic and a physiotherapy department in addition to the statutory service requirements. Finsbury Borough Council, it appears, attempted to make full use of its rather restricted powers and in doing so, it could be argued, accepted responsibility for the health of its citizens.[53]

The philosophy of local authority public health departments in the middle thirties seems to have been an amalgamation of a collectivism inspired by 'national efficiency' and an individualistic approach. The services offered at Finsbury attest to the preoccupation with the hygiene and treatment of the individual but the basic rationale seems to have been the health interests of the wider community. A pertinent example is the disinfecting station where the family and its possessions 'can be rendered sanitary', for the good of the community as much as for the individual benefits such activity could be expected to bring.[54] There seems to be little immediate evidence that Finsbury utilized an active conception of citizenship in its provision of services apart from the health education approach that had been common in mother and infant welfare centres since the early years of the twentieth century.[55] A Webb-like emphasis on centralized expertise and efficiency seems at first sight to have been the strongest motivation. However, a closer look at the events leading to the building of the Health Centre encourages a modification of this interpretation. Although the health centre is often discussed in terms of 'rationality', of the efficiency of a purpose-built centre housing all the borough's general medical services and public health administration, it seems to have represented much more than this.

There seems little doubt that the motivation for the building of the centre owed much to the political prominence of the Left in Finsbury and also on the LCC. Labour managed to gain control of the LCC and fifteen borough councils in London in 1934. Under the LCC's wing these boroughs began to attempt the implementation of Labour policies. Finsbury undertook this task enthusiastically, motivated by its leader Alderman Riley, a 'devout socialist'.[56] A Labour representative until the end of the war, Riley took a great interest in the conditions of borough residents, regarding health care and housing as the most pressing questions facing the borough.[57] In the area of public health this enthusiasm was bolstered by the presence of Dr C. L. Katial, the chairman of the public health committee and probably the prime motivating force for the creation of a health centre.[58] The Left-wing press repeatedly emphasised the connection between the centre and the ideals of socialism.[59] Its importance to citizenship, particularly in the sense of equal entitlement, was invoked as an example:

> The improvements and facilities that the health centre offers to its patients is in harmony with the whole direction of Socialist control. The patient is no longer to be considered as a charge upon a State machine – an unfortunately necessary charge to be dealt with in the speediest and cheapest manner. It is now being appreciated that a

citizen is entitled to all the advantages of modern science and that he must receive these advantages ungrudgingly as is his right as a citizen.[60]

As the Annual Reports of the Medical Officer of Health, Nicholas Dunscombe, reveal, Finsbury had urgent need of improved medical care.[61] Yet the services offered at the centre went beyond the statutory requirements for borough councils.

The health centre seems to have been conceived with more than functional considerations in mind. According to John Allan, Lubetkin recalled that 'the recurrent analogy in the formative stages of discussion was that of an open-access club, with an atmosphere that would inspire confidence in the public such that they would feel comfortable in calling in at any time – regardless of appointment or even of any desire to see a clinician'. Indeed, it was initially suggested that no reception counter should be located in the foyer 'in order to avoid even the hint of bureaucratic supervision'.[62] This notion of a health centre was also reflected in the choice of furnishings. The original use of loose furniture and standard lamps to be 'informally strewn around the foyer instead of the usual serried rows of benches, was a deliberate attempt to underline this relaxed "drop-in" ambience as opposed to the stereotyped image of interrogation and antiseptic.'[63] Allan suggests this marked a divergence from the Peckham Health Centre's emphasis on clinical observation, yet in fact this was a point of conjunction between the two centres. Both centres wanted to recreate the informality of a 'club' atmosphere and to play down expert control.

This unceremonious approach was combined with a didactic element. As noted, this had always been a marked feature of the mother and child welfare centres of the early twentieth century. In the case of the Finsbury Health Centre, the building was designed to further an instructional relationship. Murals by Gorden Cullen exhorted visitors to spend time outdoors and carried slogans such as 'Chest Diseases are Preventable and Curable'.[64] By turning the venue into a 'sort of teaching vehicle', Allan argues, Lubetkin was echoing the Constructivist ideal of the building as a 'social condenser'.[65] As clinic, club and conveyer of knowledge the centre did indeed go beyond the rather authoritarian approach of the earlier mother and child clinics. A similar awareness of the importance of an interactive relationship between the providers and recipients of health care was evident in Bermondsey Borough Council's experiments in health care provision and publicity. As early as 1924, for example, the Public

Health Committee of Bermondsey Borough Council asserted the need to move beyond a conception of preventive medicine characterised by the making of laws and regulations. It believed such directions to be of limited value without the 'intelligent co-operation on the part of the individuals in the community…'[66]

The Finsbury Health Centre was intended to be part of a much larger strategy of local regeneration and development, an initiative referred to in the press as the 'Finsbury Plan'.[67] Council minutes do not refer to a plan in any specific sense, though it is clear that the health centre was approved in the context of possible housing development.[68] Certainly, by the time the health centre opened in autumn 1938, Lubetkin and Tecton had been re-engaged on housing commissions at Busaco Street and Sadler Street.[69] The Centre itself was intended to sit within an enlarged area of public gardens: this was, in fact, substantially achieved. Other elements were to be new housing schemes on slum-cleared sites, incorporating community centres, laundries and various other tenants' facilities.[70]

The developments at Finsbury in the thirties are examples of contemporary interest in the idea of physical determinism.[71] The health centre and the wider schemes for housing and other environmental improvement were conceived within an ideological framework which stressed the importance of extraneous influences on social life. The contemporary preoccupation with the therapeutic properties of light and air, for instance, is evident at Finsbury where Lubetkin justified the use of glass bricks 'not only from the point of view of hygiene but also as a medium of propaganda of light and air in the homes of the patients, and as a powerfully stimulating psychological factor'.[72] The causal connection between environment and society, indeed, found an effective symbol in the health centre. A phoenix risen from the rubble of the slums, the health centre was a powerful image of progress. It was utilized by Abram Games in his series of wartime posters, 'Your Britain – Fight for it now!', which depicted alternate visions of society before and after the war in the areas of health, housing and education. A controversial poster, it contrasted an image of a rickety slum child with the pristine facade of the Finsbury Health Centre.[73] (Fig. 1.)

Peckham

The experimental health centre set up by George Scott Williamson and Innes Pearse in Peckham, South London, to test their ideas on the nature of health and the conditions necessary for its maintenance also attracted considerable attention during the short and uncertain period

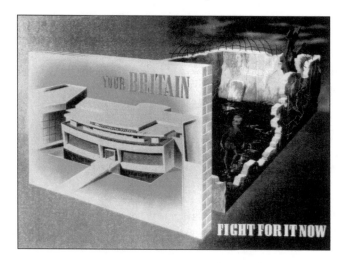

Figure 1
Abram Games, 'Your Britain Fight For It Now' (Finsbury Health Centre)
By permission of *The Imperial War Museum, London* PC 0289
Cat. No. IWM PST 2911.

of its existence. The Pioneer Health Centre, open between 1926–1930, again between 1935–1939 (in new premises specially designed for the purpose) and for a period after the Second World War, was an unusual mixture of health centre and family club, the two facets designed to complement the health development of the members. A fundamental feature of the Peckham experiment was the demand that the members be left to interact freely and spontaneously with the environment provided by the Centre. Williamson attached great importance to the concept of self-responsibility, asserting, in his 1938 publication *Biologists in Search of Material,* that 'health demands that a man shoulder his own burden. It is better that he receive a whole wage and himself take responsibility for his own welfare than he be given what is presumed to be good for him and robbed of responsibility. The one spells health, the other atrophy and degeneration.'[74]

Williamson's exposition of individual responsibility for health carried echoes of the social reform rhetoric of the late nineteenth and early twentieth centuries. Indeed, A. D. Lindsay, idealist philosopher, Master of Balliol College and the author of the preface of the first published report of the Pioneer Health Centre, identified the Centre's aims as 'social self-maintenance' and compared its ideals to those of the late nineteenth-century settlement movement.[75] These

215

principles found ample expression in the organisation of the Pioneer Centre. From the outset, Williamson and Pearse tried to ensure that the decision to join the Centre was freely taken by prospective members. The neighbourhood within half a mile of the Centre was circularized but no other incentives to join were offered.[76] Also, the Pioneer Centre was designed to become self-supporting on the achievement of full membership, on the basis of weekly subscriptions of members (an amount that was felt to be well within the 'capacity and acceptance' of the wage-earners catered for).[77] The benefits of this arrangement were stressed by the founders in the Centre's Annual Reports. Not only did it contribute to the 'inculcation of responsibility' but it was a means of giving power to the members: 'The staff, including the doctors, will then be the paid servants of the members, with no intervening loyalties to undermine mutual confidence.'[78]

Indeed, in their published writings Pearse and Williamson stressed the minimal role accorded to general staff at the centre. The principle of self-service in the family club activities was fundamental to the general organisation of the Centre. 'A healthy individual', Pearse argued, 'does not like to be waited on; he prefers the freedom of independent action which accompanies circumstances so arranged that he can do for himself what he wants to do as and when he wants to do it.' Consequently, the self-service organisation of the Centre had the 'merit of engendering responsibility and of enhancing awareness as well as of increasing freedom of action.' Further:

> As unhampered in the Centre as in their own houses, the members are free to improvise to suit all occasions as they arise ... each new family emboldened to strike out for itself in this living social medium can add its own quota of 'organisation' to the Centre – the outstanding characteristic of which is the abiding fluidity of its constitution, permitting continuous growth and the functional evolution of its society from day to day and year to year.[79]

In practice this meant no attendants, no waitresses, stackable furniture and accessible equipment. The role of the small band of staff was 'to be used by the members as a means of reaching and sustaining their own maximum health.' In summarizing four years of the Peckham experiment, Pearse and Lucy Crocker concluded, that there was 'little to distinguish members from staff in the social interplay of the Centre. The whole medium is social – Science socialised. The Centre has, in fact, shown itself to be a potent mechanism for the "democratisation" of knowledge and of action.'[80]

Nevertheless, Jane Lewis and Barbara Brookes are right to question how far the Peckham regime actually corresponded to the outward face presented by Williamson and Pearse.[81] Peckham's novelty and its modernity were emphasised by the language of its founders in their reports and publicity. The 'democratisation of knowledge' is a pertinent example: in practice, in the consulting rooms of Pearse and Williamson this may have been indistinguishable from 'guidance' or 'influence'. Indeed, many who observed the work of the Centre first-hand attest to the dominant personality of Williamson: to Dr K. E. Barlow, he was the 'ring-master', to Frances Donaldson, he was a 'dictator'.[82] However, most people only saw the outward face of the Centre. As a pioneer health centre the Peckham experiment occasioned much discussion in both the medical and the general press and among politicians and administrators. To Ernest Barker of the NCSS, the Pioneer Centre represented an example of the link he sought between active citizenship, community-feeling and health. Like many of his contemporary social commentators, Barker urged upon society the pursuit of 'national fitness' and questioned the proper framework for this collective effort:

> Not, I should hope, in State-organised institutes or camps. Far better... would be a system under which a natural local community sought to make the best of itself and its members by including fitness among its aims and objects... The Pioneer Health Centre at Peckham is teaching a lesson which deserves general application.[83]

The local, self-propelled responsibility for healthy living and fitness which Peckham typified, was, to Barker, an expression of a vital kind of citizenship.

The other main features of the Peckham experiment were its roles as a family social centre and in aiding the integration of local society. In this respect, the Centre's founders shared the ideals of the Finsbury planners. In the case of Peckham, the aim of social assimilation was publicly stated. Williamson and Pearse repeatedly stressed this aspect of the experiment in their scientific literature and in the Centre's publicity. Again, the language of physical determinism was prominent:

> The whole building is in fact characterised by a design which invites social contact ... It is a field for acquaintanceship and for the development of friendships ... In these times of disintegrated social and family life in our villages, towns, and still worse in cities, there is no longer any place like this ... The Centre is just such a place...

an open forum ... an arena for the unfolding of the consecutive and integrated leisure activity of families.[84]

Peckham was promoted as a model for social planners grappling with the problems of modernity and such inter-war social anxieties as 'urban dislocation, family instability, and the declining birth rate'.[85] 'It is ... a major function of statesmanship to see that there is social opportunity. A nation seeking health cannot leave that to football promoters, dog racers, and the brewers as we do now', Peckham's founders argued.[86] The Pioneer Health Centre was an alternative: a social facility, overseen but not dominated by experts in healthy living, that could provide urban families with much needed companionship and the opportunity 'to cultivate their faculties within a community.'[87] It was, in their view, a bulwark against 'social malnutrition'.

The Pioneer Centre struggled to balance its books throughout its short lifetime. Member's subscriptions and grants from the Halley Stewart Trust proved insufficient to meet its costs. The problem came to a head in 1950 when appeals were made to the LCC to find a niche for the Centre in the National Health Service. Massive stumbling blocks stood in the way of incorporation, however, not least of which was the LCC's requirement that Peckham abandon its restricted catchment area and its member subscription policy.[88] The 1946 commitment to the idea of universality in health care provision meant that the Centre would have to be free and open to the whole borough. This was a different age from that of Peckham's heyday of the mid thirties.

The Centres and Participatory Citizenship

Both health centres, although operating within different circumstances, offer insight into contemporary intellectual and political analyses of the relationship between health and citizenship. Environmental determinism was an important feature of much of this commentary, in line with the broad principles of 'positive health' and social medicine. The move away from a narrow, biologically-determined conception of health and the adoption of the idea of unfulfilled potentiality are also present in the ethos and activities of the two health centres. As such, both centres reflect a growing interest in citizenship characterised by entitlement to a good standard of health. The Finsbury Health Centre and the Peckham Experiment also have implications for a more active and participatory conception of citizenship, one that has much in common with idealist thought and, more particularly, with belief in the organic connection between the individual and the locality. This was expressed in Scott Williamson's descriptions of the Pioneer Health Centre. The plan of Lubetkin, Riley and Katial for Finsbury also contained a participatory element, although this was a far more collective expression of participation, mediated through the democratically-elected borough council rather than through the individual family. The Finsbury Plan was to be a statement of 'civic valour', an exercise in the rebuilding of a community that placed a local centre for health at its core.[89]

In the inter-war years and more so in the forties, health and medicine figured strongly in plans for the reformation of social policy. Much of this was politically driven; for instance in the growing prominence of Labour's health and social policies (particularly after a series of significant gains in local government elections during the mid thirties brought more tangible evidence of Labour's aims and priorities). These policies may well have contributed to the renewed, if still rather subdued, Ministry of Health activity during the mid to late thirties.[90] Plans to reform social policy also reflected the intellectual drift of key elements within the medical profession. On the one hand the need for a new kind of doctor and health service became an increasingly familiar refrain in press and political commentary. On the other the necessity for a more holist approach to health and medicine became a notable strand in the thought of many distinguished clinicians.[91] But while an identifiable consensus had emerged over the value of a positive conception of health, both for the nation and for the individual citizen, the debate had also opened up a series of contentious issues, not least of which was the question of the location of responsibility.

In the inter-war years the health policy documents of the Labour party demonstrated a clear desire to replace the private services of the general practitioner with a salaried medical service. The party had a number of influential allies in this broad aim including Sir Robert Morant, the first Permanent Secretary of the Ministry of Health, and Sir George Newman, the Chief Medical Officer, both of whom wished to see the reorientation of general practice towards preventive medicine. This move, in their view, could best be achieved through the managerial control of the public health authorities.[92] For Labour, though, the prime consideration of this policy was rather different, that is, the institution of a universal and publicly accountable service. During the twenties this concern for accountability pitched the party against the larger 'approved societies' responsible for administering the 1911 National Health Insurance scheme. The hope that the National Insurance Act would produce a democratic scheme 'controlled by the insured for the insured' was deemed by Labour in 1925 to be 'almost a dead letter.'[93] For the Labour party, the best solution for the development of a national health service (at least for the time being) lay in extending the responsibilities of the local authorities.[94] Policy documents of the thirties and early forties continued to accentuate the importance of public accountability in health service provision. In 1942, for instance, the party argued that:

> a medical service provided by the community and paid for to a large extent out of public funds, ought to be controlled and directed by public representatives. A doctor in such a service must have a responsibility to the nation and must understand it. He must be something more than a tradesman whose sole duty it is to please his customers, and whose practice and remuneration depend almost entirely on the way in which he succeeds in this.[95]

The rising inter-war 'frustration at the subversion of the self-governing approved societies' undoubtedly 'led to a greater acceptance of the state providing democratic accountability.' However, this acceptance could not remove the fear of the medical profession that Labour's health service vision would gravely compromise their autonomy and their interests.[96] This fear was particularly marked among the élite who practised in the prestigious London voluntary hospitals, As reconstruction plans took shape during the last years of the Second World War and the first years of the peace, the debate openly centred around the question of control.[97] Issues of local interest and community responsibility, the desirability of democratic control and the elective principle as against expert management and professional autonomy pervaded discussions, and the contested nature of the concept of citizenship were laid bare in the process.

Notes

1 Abigail Beach, 'The Labour Party and the Idea of Citizenship 1931-1951', Ph.D. thesis, University of London, 1996.

2 Gary Werskey, *The Visible College. A Collective Biography of British Scientists and Socialists of the 1930s*, London, 1988, 44; Dorothy Porter, 'Social Medicine and the New Society: Medicine and Scientific Humanism in Mid-Twentieth Century Britain', unpublished paper read at Institute of Historical Research, 16 May 1995.

3 Charles Webster, 'The Origins of Social Medicine', *Bulletin of the Society for the Social History of Medicine*, 38 (1986): 52.

4 In the early 1930s, features in the medical press on broad questions of health are not usually indexed under general terms but are tied to particular problems, for example, 'tuberculosis' and 'maternal mortality'. Where a generic term, is used the favoured term until *c.*1933 seems to be 'public health'.

5 See, for example, J. L. Brownlie, Chief Medical Officer, Department of Health for Scotland, 'National Health Policy: A Critical Survey', *British Medical Journal* (1933): ii, 275–7. The concept was often illustrated by reference to the work of Pearse and Williamson at the Pioneer Health Centre, Peckham. See for example, G. Godwin, 'The Peckham Experiment', *The Fortnightly* (February 1934): 187–92; A. S. Playfair, 'The Health Doctors', *St Bartholomew's Hospital Journal* (November 1938): 38–40; *British Medical Journal* (1938): ii, 131, 1056–7. For the historical strength of the preventive health movement in Britain see Dorothy Porter, '"Enemies of the Race": Biologism, Environmentalism and Public Health in Edwardian England', *Victorian Studies*, 4 (1991): 159–78; and Anne Hardy, *The Epidemic Streets. Infectious Disease and the Rise of Preventive Medicine, 1856-1900*, Oxford, 1993.

6 'A Palace of Health', *The Spectator*, 27 March 1936, pp. 565–6.

7 Steve Sturdy, 'Hipprocrates and State Medicine: George Newman Outlines the Founding Policy of the Ministry of Health' in *Greater than the Parts: Holism in Biomedicine, 1920-1950*, Christopher Lawrence and George Weisz (eds), New York, 1998, pp. 112–34.

8 *Ibid.*

9 Michael Freeden, *The New Liberalism. An Ideology in Social Reform*, Oxford, 1978; Geoffrey Searle, *The Quest for National Efficiency. A Study in British Politics and Political Thought 1899-1914*, Oxford, 1971. There was, indeed, a renewed concern for national efficiency in the 1930s fuelled by anxiety that levels of infant mortality were

still too high, particularly in the light of the falling birth-rate. See for example, Richard Titmuss, *Poverty and Population. A Factual Study of Contemporary Social Waste*, London, 1938.

10 'A National Health Policy', *The Spectator*, 5 December 1931, 759; 'The Nation's Health', *The Spectator*, 22 September 1933, pp. 361–2; 'A Positive Health Policy', *British Medical Journal* (1932): ii, 107–8.

11 Porter, 'Social Medicine and the New Society'.

12 *Ibid.*; J. Huxley, *The Uniqueness of Man*, London, 1941.

13 This phrase, common in press reports at the time is a reference to the lowest category used in army medical examination reports.

14 'National Health', *The Spectator*, 1 March 1919: 256–8.

15 'Health as a Duty', *The Spectator*, 27 October 1933: 565.

16 This was a common theme in the House of Commons Debates on the question of physical fitness. See, for example, *Parliamentary Debates*, 3 November 1936, cols. 18–19.

17 'The Nation's Health', *The Spectator*, 1 October 1937, pp. 537–8.

18 *Ibid.*

19 The co-operative principle was written into the Act; the 22 Local Area Committees established by the Physical Fitness National Advisory Council, were to receive applications for grants from both local authorities and local voluntary organisations. The link between the new Act and the community centre movement was frequently discussed in the pages of *Community*, the journal produced by the Midlands section of the National Council of Social Service. See for example, K. Lindsay, Parliamentary Secretary to the Board of Education, 'Forward to Fitness', *Community*, 1, i (1937); Lord Aberdare, Chairman of the National Fitness Council, 'The National Fitness Campaign', *Community*, 1, iv (1938); also see Beach, 'The Labour Party and the Idea of Citizenship', ch. 2.

20 Mariel Grant, 'The National Health Campaigns of 1937-1938', in *Cities, Class and Communication. Essays in Honour of Asa Briggs*, D. Fraser (ed.), New York, 1990, pp. 216–33.

21 *The Times*, 22 October 1936.

22 *Parliamentary Debates*, vol. 317, cols 175–9. Harold Nicolson, the National Labour M.P. for West Leicester, urged a place in the scheme for existing voluntary clubs and associations on a similar basis.

23 See Virginia Berridge, 'Health and Medicine' in *Cambridge Social History of Britain*, F. M. L. Thompson (ed.), Cambridge, 1990, vol. 3, pp. 231–2.

24 Charles Webster, 'Healthy or Hungry Thirties?', *History Workshop*

Journal, 13 (1982): 112–3.

25 *Ibid.* See also, for example, Sir R. McCarrison, Cantor Lecture on
    'Nutrition and National Health', summary in *British Medical Journal*
    (1936): i, 427–430; the report of the International Labour Office,
    'Workers' Nutrition and Social Policy', summarized in the *British
    Medical Journal* (1936): ii, 75–6. Contrast the optimistic reports of
    the Ministry of Health Annual Reports throughout the 1920s and
    1930s.

26 The medical press often used international or foreign reports and
    surveys as the basis for their articles on nutrition, a tactical
    distancing, perhaps, but nevertheless an indication of the increased
    interest in the subject.

27 'Health as a duty', *The Spectator*; 'To Eliminate the C3s', *The
    Spectator*, 21 June 1935, pp. 1053–4; *The Spectator*, 1 October 1937,
    pp. 537–8.

28 *Parliamentary Debates*, vol. 317, 4 November 1936, cols. 97–8, 104,
    150–1.

29 Political and Economic Planning, *The British Health Services* (1937),
    395. This holistic conception of the health of individuals thus
    connects with the holism of much contemporary town planning and
    housing theory. See Beach, 'The Labour Party and the Idea of
    Citizenship', ch. 2.

30 George Newman, *An Outline of the Practice of Preventive Medicine: A
    Memorandum Addressed to the Minister of Health*, London, 1919.

31 PRO ZHC1/8147/1920. Ministry of Health, Consultative Council
    on Medical and Allied Services, *Interim Report on the Future
    Provision of Medical and Allied Services*, Cmd. 693, 1920, 5. Sir
    Bernard Dawson, the chairman of Consultative Council on Medical
    and Allied Services, had long been interested in the social
    considerations of health. In shaping the notion of the health centre
    Dawson drew heavily on the model of the education service as
    developed by Sir Robert Morant in the early years of the twentieth
    century. It is likely that he took the terms 'primary' and 'secondary',
    which he applied to the local and district health care institutions,
    from this source. In 1919 Morant became permanent secretary at the
    newly established Ministry of Health. In addition, Dawson looked
    to the school medical service, created in the aftermath of the Boer
    War, as exemplifying the interconnectedness of curative and
    preventive medicine. The health centre idea also featured in a book
    of Dawson's *Cavendish Lectures*, 1918. See Charles Webster, 'Conflict
    and Consensus: Explaining the British Health Service', *Twentieth
    Century British History*, 1 (1990): 122–3. See also F. Watson, *Dawson*

of Penn, London, 1950.

32 Labour Party, Advisory Committee on Public Health, *The Organisation of the Preventive and Curative Medical Services and Hospital and Laboratory Systems under a Ministry of Health*, 1919. Reissued as Labour party and TUC, *The Labour Movement and Preventive and Curative Medical Services. A Statement of Policy with Regard to Health*, 1922. In addition, elements of the health centre idea had been present in documents produced by the State Medical Service Association, an organisation established in 1912 and closely aligned with the Labour party.

33 Charles Webster, *The Health Services since the War.* vol. 1: *Problems of Health Care, The National Health Service Before 1957*, London, 1988, pp. 380–1.

34 *Ibid.* The teamwork aspect featured strongly in George Newman's articulation of the health centre. Drawing on his own experiences in developing school clinics and the other public health service initiatives of the pre-war Liberal government, Newman argued that the clinic principle could usefully extend beyond the management of particular health problems to the provision of GP care in general. See Newman, *An Outline of the Practice of Preventive Medicine*, pp. 106–9.

35 Webster. 'Conflict and Consensus', pp. 137–8; see also *idem*, 'The Metamorphosis of Dawson of Penn', in *Doctors, Politics and Society: Historical Essays*, Dorothy Porter and Roy Porter (eds), Amsterdam, 1993, pp. 212–28.

36 A. H. T. Robb-Smith, *The Lancet* (1943): ii, 243–49. Even in 1947 *The Lancet* was asking how, and by whom, would health centres be run.

37 The varying viewpoints developed in the context of health centre policy are reflected in broader health care debates, as noted by Webster in his analysis of the conflict and consensus over the regionalisation of health care debates in 'Conflict and Consensus'.

38 The debate on the community function of the health centre complemented the concurrent discussion of the importance of community centres and other neighbourhood buildings in cementing local relationships.

39 *Interim Report on the Future Provision of Medical and Allied Services*, 7. The locally-organised health centres, however, would be planned and co-ordinated from a regionally-based health authority, which he envisaged would be an *ad hoc* elected body concerned solely with the health services, a mechanism which would be able to protect the autonomy of the medical profession while providing access to public

funds and enabling the distribution of health services to be planned and co-ordinated. The interest in regionalism as an organising concept of local administration, and the contested nature of its contemporary usage, is explored in greater detail in Beach, 'The Labour Party and the Idea of Citizenship', ch. 4.

40 Dawson was echoing the views of his colleagues in the medical profession in his antipathy to local authority control of health centres, seeing this administrative solution as an insuperable challenge to the professional autonomy of medical practitioners.

41 This didactic approach was perhaps typified in the person of Sir George Newman. See Anna Davin, 'Imperialism and Motherhood', *History Workshop Journal*, 5 (1978): 9–60; Carol Dyehouse, 'Working-class Mothers and Infant Mortality in England, 1895-1914', *Journal of Social History*, 12 (1978-9): 248–67, for the development of infant welfare clinics in the Edwardian period.

42 Ernest Barker, Chadwick Public Lecture, 'Community Centres in Relation to Public Health', *British Medical Journal* (1938): i, 1066–7. Barker was particularly impressed with this aspect of the Peckham Pioneer Health Centre.

43 Political and Economic Planning, 'Medical Care for Citizens', *Planning*, 222, (June 1944).

44 *Ibid.*, 33.

45 Webster, *The Health Services since the War*, vol. 1, pp. 380–1. The Dawson approach, as articulated in the Interim Report of the Consultative Council, was also potentially at odds with the Ministry of Health's favoured of control by the public health authorities, a position articulated by Newman. This position also seems to have owed a great deal to Sir Robert Morant whose views on health owed much to his great friends, Sidney and Beatrice Webb. Morant's posthumous influence, however, was countered by the presence of the Permanent Secretary, Sir Arthur Robinson, who, according to Webster, brought 'to his office the parsimonious instincts of the workhouse', 'Conflict and Consensus', pp. 138, 141–2. Labour's commitment to local authority-based health care is replicated in the party's rejection of an extension of medical provision through the National Health Insurance approved societies. Local authorities, they argued, offered greater opportunity for participatory citizenship than did the approved societies which by the 1930s had become dominated by huge insurance companies. See Martin Daunton, 'Payment and Participation: Welfare and State Formation in Britain, 1900-1951', *Past and Present*, 150 (1996): 169–216 at 204.

46 GLRO: LCC/PH/PHS/1/3. Memorandum from the Divisional

Medical Officer of Health to Dr Allen Daley, Medical Officer of
Health, 10 November 1937.

47   GLRO: LCC/PH/PHS/1/3, Memorandum of Dr Allen Daley, 17
November 1937.

48   See, for example, PRO: MH134/48, Health Centre Committee,
minutes of meeting, 9 July 1947; GLRO: LCC/PH/GEN/1/34,
Memorandum, Public Health Department Central Planning
Division, National Health Service Wandsworth Borough Council
Health Centre; A. Talbot Rogers, 'Health Centre Prospects', *The
Spectator*, 17 September 1948, pp. 363–4.

49   Webster, *The Health Services Since the War*, Vol. I, pp. 383.
Somerville Hastings, 'Why no Health Centres?', *The Spectator* (1
June 1951): 713. Soon, however, even this limited application was
overtaken by events. The NHS came under pressure because of the
escalation of costs, with the result that virtually all capital
development was eliminated.

50   Webster, 'Conflict and Consensus', 139; Harry Eckstein, *English Health
Service*, Cambridge, Mass., 1959, pp. 247–52; *Change, Choice and
Conflict in Social Policy*, P. Hall *et al.* (eds), London, 1975, pp.
277–310; M. Ryan, 'Health Centre Policy in England and Wales',
British Journal of Sociology, 19 (1986): 34–46.

51   See, for example, F. Singleton, 'Health Centres: Two Styles', *The
Spectator*, 28 October 1938, pp. 708–9. The health care activities of
Bermondsey Borough Council provide an additional example of
contemporary innovation in the politics of local medical care. See
Elisabeth Lebas, '"When Every Street Became a Cinema". The Film
Work of Bermondsey Borough Council's Public Health Department,
1923-1953', *History Workshop Journal*, 39 (1995): 42–66; Fenner
Brockway, *Bermondsey Story. The Life of Alfred Salter*, London, 1949,
pp. 168–71. The work of the council included the building of a
health centre in 1936.

52   The development of Lubetkin's ideas have been ably demonstrated
elsewhere, most recently in John Allan, *Berthold Lubetkin.
Architecture and the Tradition of Progress*, London, 1992.

53   The health services of metropolitan boroughs were administered
partly by the borough council and partly by the London County
Council.

54   Singleton, 'Health Centres, Two Styles', 708.

55   Davin, 'Imperialism and Motherhood'; Dyehouse, 'Working-class
Mothers and Infant Mortality in England'; Arthur Newsholme, *Fifty
Years in Public Health*, London,1935; see Hardy, *The Epidemic Streets*
for a longer-term view of the role of public health medicine and

Medical Officers of Health since the time of Sir John Simon in the 1850s.

56 A similar motivation is in evidence at Bermondsey which according to Fenner Brockway spread 'the cause of Health with an enthusiasm reminiscent of socialist propaganda', *Bermondsey Story*, 170.

57 P. Coe and M. Reading, *Lubetkin and Tecton. Architecture and Social Commitment: A Critical Study*, London, 1981, 141.

58 Finsbury Borough Council, *Official Minutes*, Public Health Committee, 16 June 1936. See also 'Once a Slum – Now Finsbury's New Health Centre', *Nursing Mirror and Midwives' Journal*, 15 October 1938, pp. 78–79; P. Reilly, 'The Modern Architect is on your side', *The News Chronicle*, 19 October 1938, 10.

59 See for example, 'Labour's Health Centre Example', *The Daily Worker*, 19 October 1938, pp. 2, 5. Of course, much of this was for propaganda purposes, particularly in the build-up to local elections.

60 *Ibid.*

61 See, for example, Finsbury Borough Council, *Annual Report on the Public Health of Finsbury for the Year 1935*, 1936.

62 Allan, *Berthold Lubetkin*, 334.

63 *Ibid.*

64 *Ibid.*, 335.

65 *Ibid.*, 334. The Russian Constructivist movement flourished at the time of the revolution. Their intention was to involve architecture in the integration of society. In many ways this echoes the motivations of the English vernacular architecture and design associated with William Morris and the Arts and Crafts movement.

66 Lebas, 'The Film Work of Bermondsey Council', 49. Bermondsey's use of public relations in the field of health education is particularly interesting.

67 See for example, *Architectural Review* (January 1938): 5–6; 'Finsbury Acts', *Architect and Building News*, 21 October 1938, 58. The programme seems to have covered six areas, housing, open spaces, child welfare services, bath and public wash-houses, air raid precautions and health services.

68 The majority of the Council, it seems, saw the health centre as the 'first step' in an ongoing process. Finsbury Borough Council, *Official Minutes*, Council meeting, 5 March 1936. However, the Finsbury Plan, as far as it existed in any defined sense at all, seems to have a product of informal discussions between Riley, Katial and Lubetkin.

69 Finsbury Borough Council, *Official Minutes*, Housing Committee, 5 April 1937; 13 January 1938; 24 November 1938.

70 Allan, *Berthold Lubetkin*, 349.

71 See Beach, 'The Labour Party and the Idea of Citizenship', chapter 2, for the comparable influence of ideas of physical determinism on town planning. Also, a similar impetus lies behind the work of the Dr Alfred Salter and the Public Health Committee at Bermondsey and with the borough's inner city regeneration and beautification programme. See Brockway, *Bermondsey Story*.

72 Finsbury Borough Council, *Official Minutes*, Public Health Committee, 19 May 1936.

73 Allen notes that Churchill condemned the poster as 'a disgraceful libel on the conditions prevailing in Great Britain before the war...' All distributed copies were recalled and destroyed, though Games saved a few that had not been distributed. Allen, *Berthold Lubetkin*, 442.

74 G. S. Williamson and I. H. Pearse, *Biologists in Search of Material: An Interim Report of the Work of the Pioneer Health Centre, Peckham*, London, 1938, 130. See also PRO MH52/159/718/1037/1, Camberwell Metropolitan Borough Council, Pioneer Health Centre, Peckham, 1933-37, letter from the Centre to the Mayor of Camberwell. Williamson's stress upon the 'whole wage' in some ways echoes J. A. Hobson's belief that a 'living wage' lay at the foundation of less exploitative economic and social organisation. See Neil Thompson, 'Hobson and the Fabians. Two Roads to Socialism in the 1920s', *History of Political Economy*, 26 (1994): 211.

75 Pioneer Health Centre, *First Annual Report*, 1926. A review of Pearse and Williamson's book *A Case for Action*, in the *British Medical Journal* (1931): i, [see fn. 5] 357–8, makes a similar point. Many of the same influences affected other groups urging social reintegration, for example the NCSS's Community Association movement.

76 However, the membership was selected in a broad sense. The first annual report of the Centre in 1926 noted that Peckham was chosen as a suitable site for the Centre because it had a relatively homogeneous and 'moderately good artisan population' which, they argued, was likely to be 'capable of benefiting from educational work', *ibid*. The Peckham founders, it ought to be remembered, deliberately avoided the poor and the social-problem group.

77 The figure varied, starting at 6 pence per family and rising to 2 shillings after the war. I. Pearse and L. Crocker, *The Peckham Experiment, A Study of the Living Structure of Society*, 1943, pp. 73–74.

78 Pioneer Health Centre, *First Annual Report*, 1926, 4; Pioneer Health Centre, *Annual Report*, 1936, 4.

79 Pearse and Crocker, *The Peckham Experiment*, pp. 74–5.

80 *Ibid.*, pp. 77–8.
81 J. Lewis and B. Brookes, 'A Reassessment of the Work of the Peckham Centre, 1936-51', *Milbank Memorial Fund Quarterly*, 61 (1983): 307–50 at 323.
82 *Ibid.*, 323.
83 Ernest Barker, 'Community Centres and Circles', *The Fortnightly* (March 1933): 266.
84 Pearse and Crocker, *The Peckham Experiment*, 69.
85 Lewis and Brookes, 'Reassessment of the Work of the Peckham Health Centre', 309.
86 Pioneer Health Centre, *Annual Report*, 1937, 7.
87 *Ibid.*
88 Williamson was an intransigent negotiator, insisting that the continuation of the Centre's research programme was crucial to any deal. The LCC, however, was not empowered to provide for this work. Between them red tape and stubbornness made any attempt at a satisfactory deal unlikely. GLRO: LCC/PH/PHS/1/7, 'The End of an Experiment – Directors give reasons for closing of Peckham Health Centre', *Manchester Guardian*, 31 July 1951.
89 Interestingly, the contract for the building of the health centre stipulated that at least 90% of the unskilled labour was drawn from Finsbury residents. From March 1938 onwards 100% of the unskilled labour was from Finsbury. FBC, *Official Minutes*, Public Health Committee, 15 February 1938; 22 March 1938. A very similar attitude is evidenced at Bermondsey. See Lebas, 'The Film Work of Bermondsey Council', 60.
90 See, for example, PEP, *Report on the British Health Services; Committee on Scottish Health Services, (Cathcart) Report*, Cmd. 5204, 1936; PRO: MH 80/24, Minutes of Office Conferences, 7 February and 6 April, 1938. Webster, 'Conflict and Consensus', pp. 144–5.
91 Christopher Lawrence, 'Still Incommunicable: Clinical Holists and Medical Knowledge in Inter-war Britain', in *Greater than the Parts*, Lawrence and Weisz (eds), pp. 94–111.
92 Newman and Arthur Newsholme reacted against Lloyd George's decision not to bring health insurance doctors under the control of the public health authorities, believing that it would undermine their hopes for an integrated medical service. See Sturdy, 'George Newman Outlines the Founding Policy of the Ministry of Health', in *Greater than the Parts*, Lawrence and Weisz (eds), pp. 116–7.
93 *The Labour Party: Report of the Twenty-Fifth Annual Conference*, 1925, pp. 289–90; *Report of the Royal Commission on National Health Insurance*, Cmd. 2596, 1926, xiv, pp. 299–304, pp. 306–7,

(minority report), cited in Daunton, 'Payment and Participation', 183, pp. 203–5. The party was not alone in holding this view. Two government committees, the Parmoor Committee of 1920 and the Cohen Committee of 1932, expressed similar unease at the aggressive selling techniques of the major approved societies. See Geoffrey Finlayson, *Citizen, State and Social Welfare in Britain, 1830-1990*, Oxford, 1994, 248.

94 For the Labour Party's move way from a municipally-based to a nationally organised health service during its first year of government see A. Beach, 'The Labour Party and the Idea of Citizenship', chs 3 and 4.

95 Labour Party Archive (LPA): RDR/154, Public Health Sub-Committee, 'Labour's Plan for Health', December 1942, 3; RDR/49, Public Health Sub-Committee, 'First Steps Towards a State Medical Service', December 1941. Two years later, the wartime government's National Health Service White Paper, also drew attention to the importance of accountability asserting that 'If people are to have a right to look to a public service for all their medical needs it must be somebody's duty to see that they do not look in vain'. That duty, it continued, had to be placed with 'an organisation answerable to the public in the democratic way' while enjoying the fullest expert and professional guidance', *A National Health Service*, Cmd. 6502, 1944.

96 Daunton, 'Payment and Participation', 183.

97 Many of the themes which had divided the various interested parties in the 1920s and 1930s resurfaced, for example, the debate over regional or local authority administration.

9

Constituting Citizenship:
Mental Deficiency, Mental Health and
Human Rights in Inter-war Britain

Mathew Thomson

In 1950, T. H. Marshall set out his now famous model for the
development of citizenship rights in Britain: a passage from the
gaining of civil rights in the eighteenth century, to political rights in
the nineteenth century and full citizenship with universalist social
rights under the welfare state by the mid-twentieth century.[1] This
remains a compelling and influential model. However, focusing on
the first half of the twentieth century, especially the inter-war years,
this chapter highlights two of its limitations: first, a history of people
with mental illness and, more particularly, disability points to the
problem of Marshall's model as a universal one and this history also
emphasises the role of difference in constituting the rights of
Marshall's normal citizens. Second, a history of the construction of
'mental health' highlights the role of values and culture in defining
the good citizen. In both cases, the emphasis on a process of
'constitution' indicates the importance of a cultural, rather than
Marshallian 'natural', history of citizenship, a history in which
medicine and, in particular, psychological medicine and policy
played an important role in the first half of the twentieth century.

Histories of mental illness, written from the perspective of late-
modern liberal society, have been dominated by the issue of liberty.
To very different effect, this has been true at both ends of the
ideological spectrum. Writing still in an era of progressive optimism,
the earliest historians of the subject tended to trace a progressive path
from a world of no rights, in which the madman was neglected,
subjected to ridicule and treated like a beast, to one of liberation,
with an unchaining of the insane, a defence of their civil liberties in
asylums, the eventual breakdown of stigma, the opening of asylum
walls and the emergence of a social right to mental welfare. Though
critics of liberal society have subsequently eroded confidence in such
a narrative, they have done so by constructing a mirror image of the

'whig' story which still centres of the relationship between mental order and liberty: the extension of psychiatric welfare is recast as one of the main ways in which the modern state has denied or constricted freedom; and the very construction of the irrational is presented as a tool to police and restrict the freedom of the normal.[2] Despite this focus on liberty, historians have rarely examined in any detail the relationship between the psychiatric domain and broader contemporary theories of citizenship. In inter-war Britain in particular, where a political culture of citizenship was still so prominent and pervasive, such a relationship clearly needs to be addressed.[3] This chapter responds to the challenge. I argue that the emergence to prominence in inter-war Britain of two new psychological concerns, the control of 'mental deficiency' and the promotion of 'mental health', can only be fully understood if we recognise the ways in which these concepts and also their problematisation were framed by contemporary thinking about citizenship.[4] More important still, this framing in turn would help reshape citizenship itself. As such, the chapter will explore the ways in which the psychological played an integral role in the imagining and actively constituting the 'democratic subject'.[5]

Defining Mental Deficiency

The history of mental illness has shown that the notion of temporary mental incompetence was a site of tension and dispute between the medical and legal professions, particularly in relation to crime and punishment.[6] This work, like studies of the controversy surrounding commitment, wrongful confinement and use of mechanical restraints has revealed a profound concern for civil liberties in the nineteenth century. This concern hampered the advance of a rights-threatening psychiatric domain and as such is consistent with a Marshallian model of the era as one of civil-rights citizenship. At first sight, the history of mental deficiency appears to offer fewer prospects for advancing our understanding of rights. For, defined as permanently *non compos mentis*, unlike the temporary and therefore more challengeable condition of insanity, 'mental defectives' seem less likely subjects of legal disputes about the boundaries of mental competence and the defence of individual rights. In fact, this was not the case. For the stretching of mental deficiency to cover moral and social as well as intellectual retardation led to considerable confusion and a certain degree of conflict between legal and medical interpretations of criminal action. Courts and penal authorities, assisted by psychologists, were faced with the difficult task of distinguishing the responsible, and thus immoral, behaviour of criminals from the irresponsibility of the 'weak-minded' criminal (in the second half of the nineteenth century), the moral imbecile (set in legislation from 1913) and the moral defective (from 1927): all of who had an innately defective moral sense but could be of average or even above average intelligence.[7] More generally, the idea that inferior mental ability should be taken into account seemed to open up a potentially even vaster territory of partial responsibility.[8] However, since such medico-legal conflict over the existence of mental competence has already attracted considerable attention in histories of the mentally ill, it will be largely passed over here. Instead, this chapter will concentrate on the idea that the 'mentally defective' were permanently incompetent and thus incapable of ever exercising rights or responsibilities. In this respect, the mentally defective were profoundly 'other' to the rational, autonomous citizens of liberal society in a sense that even the mentally ill were not, and this is crucial in accounting for the intense alarm which surrounded the subject in the late nineteenth and early twentieth century.

The existence of so-called 'idiots' defined by a permanent mental incapacity was well established in law, long before the modern period. The early nineteenth century had already seen the development of special schools and institutions to provide them with care and education, but it was only in the last quarter of the nineteenth century and particularly the first decades of the twentieth century that the question of idiocy was reformulated into a major social problem and that the perceived scale of the problem increased dramatically. Historians have tended to attribute this to a growing anxiety about the eugenic fitness of the population. Equally significant, I argue, was the relationship between the problem of mental deficiency and contemporary concern about producing a citizenship to cope with the process of adjusting to democracy.[9]

Between 1867 and 1918, political citizenship in Britain was radically extended. Before 1867, the ability to vote in national elections had been restricted to men of the upper and middle classes; by 1918, virtually all adult men and many women had been incorporated into local and national franchise. Such a rapid transformation focused attention, and often anxiety, on the question of whether these new voters had the necessary qualities to act as responsible political citizens. In part, this problem was alleviated by continuing limitations of the franchise.[10] Most fundamental, women were excluded or discriminated against (a limited number of propertied and married women were introduced into the franchise for local elections) on the basis that they were not naturally fitted to exercise political responsibility. Despite the fact that the barriers had been lowered to incorporate the urban and rural working classes, there was still a widespread feeling among 'democrats' that the residuum should still be excluded.[11] The maintenance of a householder or ratepayer rather than manhood qualification (perpetuating the plural vote for multiple property holders) ensured that voting remained in principle the right of 'the responsible', rather than a right of manhood. In practice, this was of considerably more than mere symbolic importance: the residency-based registration procedure tended to ensure that a high proportion of the itinerant, lodgers, the young and the single were effectively disenfranchised; early one third of the adult male population at most elections were perceived as lacking the responsibilities and stability of home and family.[12] In the longer term, however, such anomalies were clearly not the answer. The new members of the political nation would need to be moulded, educated and even disciplined into the path of good citizenship.[13] However, whether the culture of active citizenship that was established in the last third of the century would be able to persist as Britain shifted from a limited to a mass democracy was far less clear.[14] In this respect, it is now a commonplace that the introduction of a mass elementary education in 1870 was closely related to the extension of the franchise to the urban working classes in 1867. The emergence and heightening of anxiety about mental defectives and the radical extension of the perceived parameters of mental deficiency beyond idiocy to the so-called 'feeble-minded' who were on the borderlines of normality were also intimately related to this concern about producing good citizens. The category of mental deficiency provided a way to conceptualise a group within the population who were non-citizens, not on grounds of wealth or class but because of an innate incapacity and social inefficiency. This group was also recognised in the new education system to be non-educable as citizens.[15] Of course, the creation of a new, more extensive category of mental deficiency was not a conscious strategy to exclude members of the population from the franchise. However, the removal of older property-based boundaries to citizenship naturally encouraged the conceptualisation of new ones, and the pervasive interest in citizenship shaped the category of mental deficiency as all that the active citizen was not. The authority of science, moreover, gave this new boundary legitimation. Exclusion based on religion was now fast disappearing; exclusion based on the possession of property or wealth would disappear; exclusion based on wilful social inefficiency disappeared with the removal of the exclusion of able-bodied paupers in 1918; in the inter-war period, exclusion based on sex disappeared, leaving only exclusion based on age: the mental defective, as such, was effectively positioned in the inter-war period as the permanent child.

Although early twentieth century liberalism and the ideology of citizenship which it framed opposed policies of state assistance to the fit and able as undermining independence, liberals were more willing than previously to accept the need for intervention in the private lives of the incapable; indeed, this was increasingly regarded as a responsibility of the responsible.[16] Mental defectives, by definition, were unable to help themselves. As such, there was a powerful argument that it was inhumane and unjust to place these 'innocents' in poor law institutions, or at least to stigmatise them as paupers (the same applied, it was believed, to placing them in mental asylums), or to punish them in prisons, when their behaviour and social inefficiency could be no fault of their own. Instead, they needed to be housed in special institutions, with life-time care. Thus, like the insane, like paupers and like children, mental defectives were provided with state-funded welfare well before the independent citizen gained 'social rights'. But in the process, the idea that they were inherently unable to function as independent, responsible citizens was confirmed and subsequently fossilised by institutional stigma within the nation's welfare culture.

An Act of Parliament establishing a national system for the life-time segregation of mental defectives was passed, by overwhelming majority, in 1913. The Mental Deficiency Act put into operation during the inter-war years covered nearly 40,000 in institutions and even more under forms of care and control within the community. This legislation has attracted some notoriety, since it seems to evince a remarkable and exceptional degree of eugenic influence on British social policy. Undoubtedly, eugenic concern about the feeble-minded was a factor behind the Act, but the function of mental deficiency as a biological boundary to rights-bearing citizenship also deserves attention. The contrast in parallel areas of social policy helps to demonstrate this: although there was serious contemporary debate about segregating other problem groups within the population (habitual criminals and inebriates and even the long term unemployed), none of these proposals had ultimately any success. The key objection to them was that permanent segregation would unjustly infringe the civil rights of any able-minded individual, removing the sanction of the just deterrent and leaving them no incentive or opportunity for reform.[17] But if, some said, criminals proved unreformable through the 'rational' deterrence of a prison sentence, if inebriates failed to respond to punishment or cure and if the unemployed really were unemployable, then (it was argued) this could be taken as a sign that the real problem was not the immoral choice of a life of crime, drunkeness or lethargy but an inherent mental deficiency and should be treated as such.[18] Mental defectives could not respond to deterrence or reform, therefore they could not be blamed for their actions. But they also had no meaningful right to personal liberty: as such, their permanent segregation was, uniquely, deemed a just, humane and progressive measure. After 1913 arguments about segregation of those in special problem groups abated as, in practice, they were segregated as defectives.

The Mental Deficiency Act did stimulate a debate about rights, outside Parliament rather more so than inside where radical Liberal MP Josiah Wedgwood was something of a lone figure, protesting against the threat to individual liberties. Moreover, what criticism there was concentrated on the dangers to democracy posed by placing control and authority into the hands of the experts who defined mental deficiency, and the potential dangers of misdiagnosis and abuse of the very loosely defined notion of mental deficiency; but there was little if any substantial rights-based opposition to the idea of segregating those who really were mentally defective.[19] The common refrain was that these individuals had no real liberties to protect and that there was no liberty in the present situation of leaving them defenceless in the community, or unfairly punished in prisons or poor law institutions. As one Liberal MP put it: there was a 'danger of making a fetish of the word "liberty", and of attempting to deprive these children in the name of a useless liberty, of what I believe under the Act will be the care and guardianship of the State, exercised for their interests, and for their interests alone.'[20] Even the Liberal *Westminster Gazette*, after earlier suspicion of the legislation, admitted: 'it would, indeed be the last crime in the name of liberty if we were prevented, by some fanciful or superstitious regard for our own personal freedom, from applying a rational treatment to these unfortunate beings.'[21] It was this line, even more so than that of the 'rights' or interests of the community (eugenic rights and the right to protection from dangerous and socially disruptive individuals) which was crucial in legitimating the Mental Deficiency Act, and this has been underestimated in an historiography rather obsessed by the spectre of eugenics.

The institutions set up to provide care and control for mental defectives were, like those for the mentally ill, strictly regulated by a code of rules and regulations designed to protect the inmates: for instance, outlawing corporal punishment and mechanical restraints, giving residents the right to a reappraisal of their cases at regular intervals and regulating the standards of diets and clothes. In this sense, the rights of the mentally defective inmates were to be protected, even though their position as inmates and their inability to defend and actively exercise these rights gave them little real force. During the inter-war period, there was remarkably little public concern about the fact that many of these rules and regulations were not being strictly followed: perhaps a sign of the increasing confidence in the authority of psychiatry.[22] This showed little sign of changing until the fifties, when the National Council for Civil Liberties mounted a campaign exposing four decades in which mental defectives had effectively been placed 'Outside the Law'. This helped lay the ground for legislative reform in 1959.[23] However, again the limitations of this rights discourse should be noted: there was concern about the rights of the inmate and there was concern about the rights of the wrongly certified but there was no real critique of the fundamental assumption that the mentally handicapped were unable to exercise the basic rights of citizenship.

During the inter-war period, because of the practical limitations of segregation, there was a serious policy debate about using sexual sterilization.[24] The reasons for the defeat of this policy are complex, but significantly the rights and interests of the community (expressed in terms of eugenic rights and savings to the cost of care) were never enough to override concern about protecting the interests of mental defectives and a more general defence of civil liberties.[25] A policy of segregation was still supported on all sides of the political spectrum and deemed to be in the interests of the defective themselves. By contrast, it was very difficult to argue that sterilization, even on a 'voluntary' basis, was in the interest of the defectives. Sterilization could clearly be damaging: it was almost certainly a danger to their bodies and it was likely to lead to them being cast out from institutions that were in search of economies, leaving them unprotected from the threats of the outside world. Moreover, the proposal that they might voluntarily choose such an operation contradicted the doctrine of permanent mental incompetence that had been so fundamental in constructing the 'defective' in the first place. On the other hand, if such an operation was to be performed on a compulsory basis it would symbolise a break with a putative British tradition of defending individual rights and could have serious broader implications for civil liberties if this precedent was extended. Significantly, even supporters of sterilization turned towards a civil liberties argument: the Eugenics Society claiming, rather lamely, that it was an infringement of rights to deny an operation to the poor and mentally defective when, as a form of birth control, it was already available to the rich via private clinics.[26] In sum, the same set of contemporary ideas about rights and citizenship could lend support to lifetime segregation of mental defectives, yet undermine a policy of sterilization.[27]

Defining Citizenship

Clearly, our understanding of the way mental deficiency was defined as a problem and then tackled is given a new dimension once we appreciate the powerful guiding influence of contemporary ideas about rights and citizenship. In what sense, however, did medical and social policy contribute, in return, to the shaping of the political culture and, in particular, to the meaning of what is was to be a citizen in inter-war Britain? I address this question by returning to the extension of political citizenship through franchise reform and, in particular, to the Representation of the People Act (1918). As noted earlier, by admitting women, the itinerant and paupers, this legislation was seen to erode the principle that the right to vote was gained only in return for the exercise of social responsibility. Fear of erosion of this principle, however, was alleviated by the decision to limit the female franchise to the more mature woman, setting the voting age at thirty compared to the male entry at twenty one and then also to restrict it to ratepayers or the wives of ratepayers. The passage and implementation of the Mental Deficiency Act may also have acted as a brake on anxieties. For in effect it would establish a new, biological (and thus still defensible) boundary line to political citizenship. Speaking in 1912, at least one politician was conscious of the relationship between the two issues, warning: 'as to the Franchise Bill, I confess that I view it as not an altogether unmixed benefit if the extended franchise which the Government propose is to be shared by a very large and increasing number of mentally deficient persons.'[28] His fears were allayed, as just a year later the amorphous legal category of mental deficiency extended the state's power to redefine inadequate citizenship as a mental problem. An inadequacy of will, persistent and unreformable irresponsibility, a lack of moral sense and social inefficiency manifest in an inability to support oneself or one's dependents in the community could all lead to a diagnosis of mental deficiency. Pressure to extend the reach of the Act even further into the territory of social and moral inefficiency continued in the inter-war period. 'Upon whose character does happiness of our country depend to-day?', asked one Conservative MP when discussing an amendment to extend the scope of the Act in 1927:

> It depends upon the character of every man and woman who has a vote, and that is why it is so important to lead public opinion to tighten-up the possibility of people who are fit for it bearing the responsibilites of citizenship through their votes, and by measures such as this restricting the possibility of mentally-deficient people being produced by mentally deficient parents.[29]

Those mental defectives segregated in institutions, nearly 40,000 by the end of the inter-war period, would certainly have been excluded from political rights; whether the same was the case for the larger number under community care is far more difficult to say. Whatever the case, we are talking about a relatively small number of individuals: a maximum of 100,000, almost certainly far fewer. More important, however, was the broader symbolic function of mental deficiency. By emphasising the otherness of individuals who lacked intelligence, will, a sense of responsibility, morality and social efficiency, the concept of mental deficiency helped to construct or at least reinforce cultural understanding of the qualities which constituted, by contrast, the good citizen. Moreover, within institutional settings such as the penal and educational systems, the influence on behaviour of the threat of diagnosis as a mental defective extended well beyond those so diagnosed.[30] Over the inter-war period, there were constant attempts to stretch the parameters of mental deficiency even further. Although there was no extension in law, the high profile of this discourse acted to reinforce common assumptions about a relationship between social failure and mental inefficiency, while new labels could facilitate a shift in the practical interpretation of the law. For instance, it was argued that mental deficiency was the root cause of the existence of a 'social problem group', making up some 10% of the population.[31] New categories such as the 'dull' and the 'backward' emerged to diagnose and mark out those not certifiably mentally defective yet still mentally and thus socially inefficient and in need of some kind of educational segregation. Evelyn Fox, a leading advocate of pushing the reach of mental welfare further into the population, believed that the conditions of modern society had fundamentally raised the mental qualification for competent citizenship:

The competitive conditions between modern states makes fitness of their citizens a matter of supreme importance and at the same time these very conditions render the socialization of the unfit peculiarly difficult. The modern state demands from its citizens a high degree of social adaptation; it enforces these demands through a complex system of laws and regulations. Even within the home and family, the individual's social relations are subject, not only to the traditions and conventions of his class and country, but to the requirements of the country or city in which he dwells. The state of cleanliness of his home and person, the infectious illnesses that he may contract, may at times call for social intervention. His methods of work, his rate of remuneration, his relations to fellow workmen, are regulated by organizations whose aims may appear inimical to his individual well being. Should he, owing to the untoward circumstances or to his peculiarities and idiosyncracies of his temperament or character, come into conflict with this weight of written and unwritten laws, all his powers of social adaptation, with their implications of intelligence and self-control, will be needed to bring his life into harmonious working relations with his fellows.[32]

With segregation limited by resources and law from reaching the whole of this expanding population, new forms of community care and social work emerged to guide mental defectives, borderline mental defectives, the dull and the backward, as well as their families, in the paths of good citizenship.[33] In sum, the category of mental deficiency could have both a direct and indirect influence which reached well beyond its own boundaries, playing an unrecognised role in the management and shaping of citizenship in the inter-war period. In the long term, perhaps equally important was its contribution to the opening up of a borderline territory within the population of individuals with partial responsibility and competence where interference in individual rights was considered justifiable both in their own interests and in the interests of the community. In this respect, as the legal expert A. V. Dicey pointed out, with some foreboding, the Mental Deficiency Act seemed to herald a significant broader shift in relations between the citizen and the state: it was 'the first stage along a path on which no man can decline to enter, but which if too far pursued, will bring statesmen across difficulties hard to meet without considerable interference from individual liberty.'[34] Indeed, the acceptance that citizens were only partially responsible for their own problems, broached in part by the inter-war recognition that mental and social inefficiency extended beyond the strict boundaries of mental deficiency, helped pave the way for the emergence of a universalist yet still peculiarly paternalist welfare culture.[35]

Mental Health and Citizenship

From early in the twentieth century, a discourse about the right to mental as well as physical health, mental as well as physical hygiene, had begun to emerge. However, in terms of state policy, this vague rhetoric had little practical impact apart from boosting general programmes of public health and preventative medicine, particularly those aimed at children.[36] The lunacy services remained primarily custodial and had little to do with mental health. Concern about civil liberties had led to a system in which patients had to be certifiably mentally ill before treatment was possible. The 'shell-shock' episode of the First World War can be seen as the turning point at which the right to freedom from certification began to recede in the face of the right for early treatment. The war had shown that even the nation's fittest and bravest citizens could succumb to mental breakdown and, as such, that a temporary mental disorder might visit any citizen and this was in no sense a sign of innate, shameful mental debility.[37] Shell-shocked troops, as a mark of respect, were treated away from public asylums, however, shell-shock did less than often assumed for the civilian insane. On a voluntary basis, outpatient clinics and child guidance clinics slowly emerged and in 1930 the Mental Treatment Act introduced voluntary treatment in public mental hospitals. In line with this trend towards open access to treatment, mental hospitals were placed under the Ministry of Health in 1918, rather than the Home Office, and under the NHS in 1946. In sum, there was a slow movement towards more easily available mental treatment, as in general medical care, as a social right of citizenship.[38]

For all the rhetoric about mental health, state services of this name remained directed towards 'mental illness'. The widespread popular interest in promoting mental health was largely pursued through voluntary, private or popular medicine, outside of the state's orbit. Here, considerable energy was expended in promoting individual self-development and in furthering progress towards ever greater, or 'higher', mental health. Mental health, like physical health, was conceptualised as more than the mere opposite of illness. An older discourse about the development of 'character' was given a psychological twist, 'personality' becoming the new ideal. (On the importance of 'personality' for the sound social body see also Anna-K. Mayer's contribution to this volume.) With recognition of

241

the power of the unconscious mind there was a shift from thinking about personal development in terms of good conduct, to thinking about it in terms of managing an internal psychological economy and tapping into the hitherto hidden depths of the mind. There was a shift from emphasis on self-control and will-power, to an acceptance that becoming a whole person entailed an end to mere repression of instincts and drives.[39] Inevitably, this was to have some impact on a notion of citizenship that had been founded on ideas about 'character'. Psychology, in this case, provided not a tool for the control of citizenship and the restriction of rights, but a model for the reconstruction and potential liberation of forms of behaviour. The new psychology, for instance, suggested that there should be a right to greater sexual freedom; that sexual drives were natural, and that it was unnatural and unhealthy to repress them. These visions of ideal psychological development which emerged continued to draw on existing models of citizenship and character: they did not promote a purely individualist model of the citizen, rather, they still emphasised the importance of service. On the other hand, they provided a new alternative: a less public, less political vision of ideal personal development. This reflected a broader shift in social life: economic growth and increased leisure time providing greater opportunity for privatisation, consumption and investment in personal growth.[40] For some, pursuing the psychology of personal development may also have tapped into an energy which was no longer devoted to the struggle for civil or political rights, such battles largely won by this date.

From the start of the century, there had also been calls for an understanding of the new psychology to be taken up by the state as a new tool for analyzing and managing society.[41] But it was not until the inter-war period that this new broader conceptualisation of mental health began to enter the public sphere of governance to a significant degree. The experience of mass society manifested in crowd politics and popular crazes, the mobilisation of public aggression in the mass warfare of 1914-18 and then the rise of extremist politics, the attraction of anti-semitism, the appeal of dictators and the willingness of civilized humans to agitate for another world war all precipitated enquiry into the mental health of the seemingly normal citizen. The irrational, impulsive 'other' was increasingly recognised as an inherent part, rather than an antithesis, of the normal self. There was also a growing awareness that individuals were psychodynamically tied to the collective. This had significant implications for thinking about citizenship, for it implied that citizenship and rights could no longer be conceptualised in purely individualist terms.

Psychologists and the increasing number of intellectuals and politicians who were alert to this reconceptualisation argued that society would have to take into consideration this new vision of mental health: first, because mental health was necessary for a successful society; second, because it was increasingly apparent that the whole organisation of society had a bearing on mental health. As such, mental health became positioned as a key mediator between the health of the individual citizen and that of the community. Mental health was no longer simply a question of the right to mental treatment or preventive services; it was an issue of the right to the good society and it was also a measure of that good society. In the inter-war years, such concerns were articulated within a discourse of 'mental hygiene', where the collapse of the healthy independent citizen – manifest in anything from the declining birth rate, the anomie of suburban life, rising levels of psychosomatic sickness and the appeal of totalitarianism – were attributed to the difficulties of maintaining mental health when faced by the pressures of modern life. The end product of mental hygiene, as such, was not higher intelligence or a higher mental health, but as the physician Lord Horder said, the 'Quiet Mind ... a means to right conduct. Not only conduct in relation to individual life, but to family life, to community life, to national life and to the whole brotherhood of man.'[42] Various psychological strategies were set in place to address the threat of the collapse of the nation's mental health. For instance, education was to be reformed to suit the developmental needs of the child's mind: play and the release of aggressive instinct were essential, for otherwise drives would remain repressed, leaving a future citizenry fragile to the temptations of violence and intolerance.[43] Indeed, in this period there was much debate about aggressive instincts and their impact on the progress of civilization, as Hayward and Mayer show in their chapters.

Delinquency was reframed as a problem of mental health, with the child guidance clinic to adjust the young back onto the path of good citizenship. The workplace and industrial relations were to be redesigned to take into account the 'human factor' and thus turn workers into integrated rather than alienated citizens.[44] Recognising the powerful influence of press control and propaganda in totalitarian regimes, freedom of information was positioned as not simply a prerequisite for active citizenship but also for mental health.[45] Such thinking about the relationship between the healthy mind and the healthy (that is democratic and peaceable) society was already well developed by 1939, and it would prove influential in shaping the 'British way' in propaganda when war came.[46] Although the expansion of preventative and curative mental health services in the post-war welfare state would be disappointingly limited, at a much more diffuse level the idea of a right to mental health and the desire to avoid the mental pathology which seemed to have beset German political development, would influence the whole ideological climate of post-war reconstruction.[47]

Conclusion

In certain respects Marshall's model of the development of citizenship remains useful in understanding the changing ideological environment within which policy for mental defectives was developed. For instance, his era of civil rights can be seen as precipitating the recognition of the 'idiot' as a category of person in need of asylum; the era of political rights coincided with a search for new forms of difference, the formulation of new boundaries to full citizenship and a heightened anxiety in particular about the mental efficiency of citizens. Last, the era of social rights led, by contrast, to relative neglect of those who could not actively or equally exercise such rights, mental defectives, now that the state's resources were stretched by the demands of a universalist welfare system. However, in other ways Marshall's assumptions about citizenship sit uncomfortably with a history of mental deficiency. Most obviously, such a history highlights inequality between citizens. Moreover, it points to the way that the normal citizen was in part constituted in relation to the deviant and pathological: in particular, acting as a biological boundary to citizenship, mental deficiency offered one way to help police the qualities of the good citizen in an era of democracy. The history of deficiency also demonstrates that civil, political and social rights were not necessarily absolute: the category of mental deficiency opened up and highlighted a hazy area of partial responsibility and partial rights. For instance, civil rights were no barrier to liftetime segregation or strict supervision in the community, but they were a concern when protecting the rights of defectives in institutions. Political rights could not be exercised by mental defectives in institutions, but for the greater number in the community or for those on the borderline the practical impact of this biological boundary to the franchise was far less clear. In terms of social rights, mental defectives were among the first groups to attract state welfare, but this 'social right' was merely a passive entitlement, resting on the responsibility of citizenship to provide for those incapable of providing for themselves, and as such confirmed the exclusion of mental defectives from a normal rights-bearing status.

The concept and practices of mental health also played a role in reconstituting citizenship in the inter-war period. Citizenship was now conceptualised within an intellectual environment in which human nature was being reinterpreted by psychology and in which mental health provided an increasingly powerful secular ideal for self-development. This new vision built on rather than rejected the values of citizenship: indeed, the life of the good citizen was regarded as just as essential for mental healthiness as mental healthiness was essential to the good citizen. But psychological theory also contributed to a reinterpretation of the nature and potential of citizenship. If all psychology was social psychology, as now seemed indubitably the case, then the individual was also a social citizen: one whose mind was shaped by membership of the group and whose rights and responsibilities were inseparable from this social identity. If human nature was as potentially irrational, instinctually impulsive and dangerous as psychology claimed and, as the experience of this era of mass warfare and conflictual, often demagogic politics seemed to confirm, then the persistence of democratic, tolerant citizenship would demand a much more interventionist nurture, management and control of mental health. In these circumstances, the liberal model of the autonomous, rational, self-independent citizen was increasingly difficult to sustain.

The history of inter-war citizenship, in sum, is not simply a narrative of the winning of new rights. It is also a history of how a more diffuse set of values and attitudes – like the negative image of the mental defective and the positive ideal of mental health – constituted the cultural meaning of citizenship. As such, the history of two constitutions, the constitution of mental health and normality, on the one hand, and the unwritten, citizen-centred British constitution, on the other, had far more in common than might at first be recognised and were to a degree mutually constitutive: two sides of a single process of redefining the good self in the first half of the twentieth century.

Notes

1 T. H. Marshall, *Citizenship and Social Class and Other Essays*, Cambridge, 1950.

2 For Britain, the 'Whig' position is represented by the rather 'Marshallian' work of K. Jones. For instance, Jones, *A History of the*

Mental Health Services, London, 1972. The leading critic of nineteenth century confinement has been A. Scull, for instance Scull, *Museums of Madness: The Social Organisation of Insanity in Nineteenth Century England,* London, 1979. On the extension of psychological control in the twentieth century, see N. Rose, *The Psychological Complex: Psychology, Politics and Society in England 1869-1939,* London, 1985. The idea that the construction of the irrational was intimately related to the emergence of modern ideas about freedom and liberty was of course opened up in the work of Michel Foucault, particularly his *Madness and Civilization* (1961), which was translated into English in 1967. Foucault's ideas have been pursued in Nikolas Rose's work on twentieth century psychology; Rose, *Governing the Soul: The Shaping of the Private Self,* London, 1989.

3   Particularly important was the influence of the British Idealists. See A. Vincent and R. Plant, *Philosophy, Politics and Citizenship: The Life and Thought of the British Idealists,* Oxford, 1984. For a contemporary expression of the centrality of citizenship to British political and civic culture, see W. H. Hadow, *Citizenship,* Oxford, 1923. For accounts of welfare, citizenship and voluntarism during this period, see for instance G. Finlayson, *Citizen, State and Social Welfare in Britain, 1830-1990,* Oxford, 1990.

4   The history of people with learning difficulties has a longer history, particularly care of 'idiots'. See *From Idiocy to Mental Deficiency: Historical Perspectives on People with Learning Difficulties,* D. Wright and A. Digby (eds), London, 1996. However, the language of 'mental deficiency' and the emergence of this problem to the forefront of national concern took place in the first half of the twentieth century. See M. Thomson, *The Problem of Mental Deficiency: Eugenics, Democracy and Social Policy in Britain, 1870-1959,* Oxford, 1998. For the escalation of a language and concern about mental 'health', 'hygiene', and 'welfare', see Rose, *The Psychological Complex.*

5   For an opening up of this territory, though paying little attention to the psychological, see P. Joyce, *Democratic Subjects: The Self and the Social in Nineteenth-Century England,* Cambridge, 1994; *Re-reading the Constitution: New Narratives in the Political History of England's Long Nineteenth Century,* J. Vernon (ed.), Cambridge, 1996.

6   On law and insanity see Roger Smith, *Trial by Medicine: Insanity and Responsibility in Victorian Trials,* Edinburgh, 1981.

7   J. Saunders, 'Quarantining the Weak-Minded: Psychiatric Definitions of Degeneracy and the Late-Victorian Asylum', in *The*

Anatomy of Madness vol. 3, W. Bynum, R. Porter and M. Shepherd (eds), London, 1988, pp. 273–96; S. Watson, 'Malingerers, the "weak-minded" Criminal and the "moral imbecile": How the Prison Medical Officer became an Expert in Mental Deficiency, 1890-1930', in *Legal Medicine in History*, M. Clark and C. Crawford (eds), Cambridge, 1994, pp. 223–41; *idem*, 'The Moral Imbecile: A Study of the Relations between Penal Practice and Psychiatric Knowledge of the Habitual Offender', Ph.D. thesis, University of Lancaster, 1988.

8 For a contemporary discussion of the history of these disputes, see R. Jones, 'Responsibility – in Regard to Certain Forms of Unsoundness of Mind', *Transactions of the Medico-Legal Society*, 13 (1912-13): 70–95. Similarly, G. H. Cook, 'The Liability of the Insane in Respect of Civil Wrongs', *Transactions of the Medico-Legal Society*, 15 (1921-2): 108–25.

9 For a fuller account, see Thomson, *The Problem of Mental Deficiency*.

10 This situation and tension was pithily summed up by M. Bentley, a leading historian of the politics of this era: 'At no time during the period discussed in this book did Britain experience democracy. At no time, equally, were politicians unconscious of its existence as an inspiration, a dismal inevitability, or a remote and controllable tendency.' See Bentley, *Politics without Democracy, 1815-1914*, London, 1984, 1.

11 J. Harris, *Private Lives, Public Spirit: A Social History of Britain, 1870-1914*, Oxford, 1993, 180.

12 C. Matthew, J. Kay and R. McKibbin, 'The Franchise Factor in the Rise of Labour', *English Historical Review*, 91 (1976): 723–52.

13 On the importance of education for citizenship: Harris, *Private Lives*, pp. 191–3. This remained a powerful concern in the inter-war period. For instance, 1934 saw the launching of the Association for Education in Citizenship: B. Harrison, *The Transformation of British Politics*, Oxford, 1996, pp. 417–19. For a series of essays emphasising the disciplinary nature of the emerging relationship between state education and welfare and the citizen, see *Crises in the British State, 1880-1930*, M. Langan and B. Schwartz (eds), London, 1985.

14 Harris, *Private Lives*, 255.

15 G. Sutherland, *Ability, Merit and Measurement: Mental Testing and English Education, 1880-1940*, Oxford, 1984.

16 M. Freeden, *The New Liberalism: An Ideology of Social Reform*, Oxford, 1978.

17 L. Radzinowicz and R. Hood, *The Emergence of Penal Policy in*

Victorian and Edwardian England, Oxford, 1990.

18 On the transition from regarding the criminal as the subject for penality and short-term punishment, to one of welfare and long-term custody and often towards a rediagnosis as mentally defective, see D. Garland, *Punishment and Welfare: A History of Penal Strategies* Aldershot, 1985; M. Wiener, *Reconstructing the Criminal: Culture, Law, and Policy in England, 1830-1914,* Cambridge, 1990; L. Zedner, *Women, Crime and Custody in Victorian England,* Oxford, 1991.

19 E. Larson, 'The Rhetoric of Eugenics: Expert Authority and the Mental Deficiency Bill', *British Journal of the History of Science,* 24 (1991): 45–60.

20 House of Commons Debates, 3 June 1913, volume 38, col. 835.

21 Quoted in Freeden, *The New Liberalism,* 192.

22 For the suggestion that the growing authority of medicine in this area was taking such questions outside of politics, see S. Ramon, *Psychiatry in Britain: Meaning and Policy* London, 1985, pp. 97–126.

23 National Council for Civil Liberties, *50,000 Outside the Law,* London, 1950; M. Lilly, *The National Council for Civil Liberties: The First Fifty Years,* London, 1984, 74.

24 J. Macnicol, 'Eugenics and the Campaign for Voluntary Sterilization in Britain between the Wars', *Social History of Medicine,* 2 (1989): 147–70.

25 For longer term histories of this policy and its relation to rights, see P. Reilly, *The Surgical Solution: A History of Involuntary Sterilization in the United States,* Baltimore, 1991; P. Reilly and S. Trombley, *The Right to Reproduce: A History of Coercive Sterilization,* London, 1988.

26 Thomson, *Problem of Mental Deficiency,* chapter 5.

27 M. Thomson, 'Sterilisation, Segregation and Community Care: Ideology and the Problem of Mental Deficiency in Inter-War Britain', *History of Psychiatry,* 3 (1992): 473–98.

28 House of Lords Debates, 5 December 1912, volume 13, col. 62.

29 House of Commons Debates, 202 1927: 2364–5.

30 See for instance P. Cox, 'Girls, Deficiency and Delinquency' in *From Idiocy,* Wright and Digby (eds), pp. 184–206.

31 J. Macnicol, 'In Pursuit of the Underclass', *Journal of Social Policy,* 16 (1987): 293–318.

32 E. Fox, 'Modern Developments in Mental Welfare Work', *Eugenics Review,* 30 (1938): 165.

33 M. Thomson, 'Community Care and the Control of Mental Defectives in Inter-war Britain', in *The Locus of Care. Families,*

Communities, Institutions and the Provision of Welfare since Antiquity,
P. Horden and R. Smith (eds), London, 1998, pp. 198–216.

34 A. V. Dicey, *Law and Opinion in England*, 2nd edn, London, 1914,
pp. l–li.

35 J. Harris, 'Enterprise and Welfare States: A Comparative Perspective',
Transactions of the Royal Historical Society, 11 (1990); M. Ignatieff,
'Citizenship and Moral Narcissism', *Political Quarterly*, 60 (1989):
63–74.

36 A major impact not discussed here was the introduction of mental
testing, special schools for mentally defective children, special classes
for the dull and backward, and streaming and child-centred
education to fit the learning process to the mental needs of the child,
see A. Wooldridge, *Measuring the Mind: Education and Psychology in
England, c.1860-1990*, Cambridge, 1994. In terms of the arguments
pursued in this paper, such a system supports the idea that liberal
rights shaped the care provided within institutional systems: in
particular, the ideal of equality of opportunity according to ability.
But it again shows that the pursuit of mental health was closely tied
to a recognition and exclusion of the mentally unfit, here through
testing and special education.

37 M. Stone, 'Shellshock and the Psychiatrists', in *Anatomy of Madness*,
Bynum, Porter and Shepherd (eds), pp. 242–71.

38 Though, it was not until the legislative reforms of the 1959 Mental
Health Act that the welfare state settlement came to embrace mental
as well as physical health. See C. Unsworth, *The Politics of Mental
Health Legislation*, Oxford, 1986.

39 M. Thomson, 'Psychology and the Consciousness of Modernity in
Early Twentieth-Century Britain', in *The Consciousness of Modernity*,
M. Daunton and B. Rieger (eds), (forthcoming).

40 T. J. Jackson Lears, *No Place of Grace: Antimodernism and the
Transformation of American Culture, 1880-1920*, New York, 1981;
T. Richards, *The Commodity Culture of Victorian England: Advertising
and Spectacle, 1851-1914*, London and New York, 1990.

41 R. Soffer, 'New Elitism: Social Psychology in Pre-War Britain',
Journal of British Studies, 8 (1969): 111–40.

42 Horder, 'The Hygiene of a Quiet Mind', *The Lancet* (1938): i, 764.

43 S. Isaacs, *Social Development in Young Children*, London, 1933;
Selected Papers of Margaret Lowenfeld, C. Unwin and J. Hood-
Williams (eds), London, 1988, pp. 12–33, 100–7.

44 Rose, *Governing the Soul*, pp. 55–79.

45 Horder, 'Hygiene', 763.

46 E. Glover, *War, Sadism and Pacificism*, London, 1933; E. Glover and

M. Ginsberg, 'A Symposium on the Psychology of Peace and War', *British Journal of Medical Psychology*, 14 (1934): 274–93; E. Durbin and J. Bowlby, 'Personal Aggressiveness and War', in *War and Democracy: Essays on the Causes and Prevention of War*, J. Bowlby, G. Catlin, R. Crossman *et al.* (eds), London, 1938, pp. 3–150; W. Brown, *War and Peace: Essays in Psychological Analysis*, London, 1939.

47   Thomson, *Problem of Mental Deficiency*, chapter 8; *idem*, 'Before Anti-Psychiatry: "Mental Health" in Wartime Britain', in *Cultures of Psychiatry and Mental Health Care in Postwar Britain and the Netherlands*, M. Gijswijt-Hofstra and R. Porter (eds), Amsterdam, 1998, pp. 43–59.

10

The Biopolitics of Arthur Keith and Morley Roberts

Rhodri Hayward

Morley Roberts: The Intellectual as Outsider

In an interview with the *Evening News* in 1935, the novelist and painter Morley Roberts (1857–1942) explained the basis of his pioneering medical research.[1] His discoveries had not emerged in laboratory experimentation or formal study, rather, they had been won through a rugged engagement with life. As Roberts made clear, 'the author gets ideas which are denied to the specialist.' His own major scientific discoveries had been formed during episodes of shark killing, sheep dismemberment and social unrest.

As a young man, Roberts had been forced by a family argument to seek his fortunes in Australia and the South Seas. Whilst working as a sailor on the SS. Corona, Roberts had removed the living heart from a freshly caught shark, holding the beating organ for twenty minutes in his hands. During this time he had formulated a series of ideas and observations on cardiac anatomy and action, which he later communicated to Arthur Keith, then lecturer in anatomy at the London Hospital. Roberts claimed that these observations had formed the basis of a whole series of papers, from Keith's 1903 article on the anatomy of the valves in the heart, to his own contribution to the *British Medical Journal* on the inhibition of the cardiac vagus.[2]

Roberts' second major discovery had not met with such widespread scientific acceptance. In 1884, Roberts had again been forced to leave Britain after assaulting a pedestrian.[3] Working in Texas as a ranchman, he was called upon to cull a rogue sheep.[4] After dismembering the beast, he realised that it possessed only the tiniest fragment of liver. This discovery provoked a new series of anatomical and physiological ideas. Roberts hypothesised that the liver was an unnecessary or rudimentary organ in herbivores: in its current form, it represented a tumourous outgrowth, providing little evolutionary advantage save the ability to digest a diet of meat.[5]

It was Roberts' experience of social unrest, however, which

provided him with his most enduring medical theory. After a passing involvement in labour demonstrations and anarchist outrages which permeated the closing decades of the nineteenth century, Roberts began to explore the parallels between cancerous growths in the human body and malignant developments in the body politic.[6] Although the metaphorical equation of cancer with social unrest was a commonplace in both political and medical discourse, Roberts developed the analogy far further than most other commentators.[7] Indeed, he used the analogy between social and somatic pathology as a point of departure for a theory which would lead him to a fundamental redescription of the human body and human society as a whole. In his four major biological works, *Warfare in the Human body* (1920); *Malignancy and Evolution* (1926); *Biopolitics* (1938) and the *Behaviour of Nations* (1941), Roberts pursued the organic analogy, developing a monadological model of the caste system which he believed was reflected in every layer of natural organisation, from the individual protozoa through the animal and the human to the modern nation state.[8]

The brutal episodes in which Roberts attained his scientific insights appear as fairly typical elements in his biography. Before his career as a novelist and painter, Roberts had led a passionate life of travel and adventure. His eighty five years seemed to encompass all the classic elements of nineteenth-century melodrama: he had experienced exile, poverty and disappointed love. His biographer, the poet Storm Jameson, considered him the last of the great Victorians.[9] Likewise his close friend, Sir Arthur Keith, waxed lyrical on the romance of Roberts' life:

> a career so crowded in adventure and so varied in experience it is scarcely possible to find a parallel in biography, ancient or modern. Tall, athletically built, he combined great strength with fierce pride and mental ability of high order. While still an undergraduate at Owens College, Manchester, a quarrel with his father sent him out as a wanderer on the face of the earth, for a period of 11 years during which time he earned his livelihood, as a sailor, navvy and ranchman. Then becoming a denizen of London's Bohemia, he succeeded in earning a scanty income by the sale of his experiences in the form of fiction.[10]

With his unconventional biography, penchant for global theory, bizarre claims for priority and outlandish methodology, Roberts seems to stand as a classic example of the outsider intellectual.[11] He had lived a life of exile and economic insecurity, surviving on the sale of popular novels and reviews in the penny magazines.[12] In an era when science and medicine were stressing the importance of specialisation and teamwork, Roberts appeared as a figure from an earlier age: a Victorian autodidact constructing systems and theories piecemeal from chance encounters and random readings in the medical press. Such a pedigree would seem to militate against the author's easy acceptance into the world of science and medicine, yet Roberts won the support and friendship of some of the most significant figures in British physiology and anatomy. In 1935, Sir Walter Langdon-Brown, then Regius professor of physic at Cambridge, could claim that Roberts had influenced his work for the previous fifteen years.[13] Likewise in 1950, Keith confessed that their lives' projects had been thoroughly entangled: 'In writing our books we were in agreement about many things; it is hard to say how much I borrowed from him and how much he borrowed from me.'[14]

The strength of Roberts' support from the medical establishment becomes apparent when one compares the reception of his work in literary periodicals and the medical press. Whereas papers such as the *Times Literary Supplement* consistently denigrated Roberts' biological theories, scientific publications maintained a far more enthusiastic response.[15] The *British Medical Journal* under Dawson Williams published many of Roberts' early articles and supplied extensive and favourable reviews for his longer works.[16] Within these pieces, Roberts was celebrated because of his outsider status. He was depicted as a thinker of ability and a writer of genius, whose distance from the pressures of laboratory research granted him a global and synthesising perspective on current advances in medicine. Thus an anonymous reviewer of *Warfare in the Human Body* noted:

> there was never a time when arm-chair philosophers were more at a discount than they are now, and we dare to believe that never at any period were thinkers more needed than they are today. We have become worshippers of new facts and sceptics as regards the new ideas and principles; our bookshelves groan with files of new observations piled on them year by year. We need in all branches of medicine – indeed in all branches of biology – that form of synthetic imagination which brooding over our harvest of facts will bring order out of chaos. It is a task which men in our modern departmental scientific laboratories do not dare to embark upon; yet it is one which has been essayed with success by a professed writer of fiction – Mr Morley Roberts.[17]

Six years later this same position was iterated in an review of

Malignancy and Evolution. This piece depicted Roberts as a kind of Renaissance man or polymath who reconciled the different forms of fiction and science into a seamless organic whole:

> Without laboratory training and dependent for his facts on others, he nevertheless handles his tools as if he had been accustomed to them from youth upwards. In his dexterity Mr Roberts stands almost alone among 'outsiders'. There are numerous examples of medical men and of biologists who have turned from medicine and from science to fiction and to letters, but in turning form fiction, letters, poetry and painting to sound the depths of modern biology, Mr Roberts has broken all precedent. If we follow him through his later work, we see him becoming more involved in the deeper problems of life, and it becomes plain that he is really a man of science who sought for the expression through the medium of fiction and of narrative.[18]

There is a twofold process operating within these repeated and insistent appreciations of Roberts' work. Alongside the obvious excitement engendered by the author's synthetic theories, the reviewers' attitudes to Roberts were part of a wider agenda surrounding the definition of medicine and its relationship with society as a whole. The acceptance of Roberts' ideas despite his lack of laboratory training militated for a particular view of the life sciences that stressed the importance of holistic integration over and above the reductionist calculation of modern bio-medicine.[19] In the twenties, this view was promoted by a conservative élite which included Roberts' most prominent supporters, Keith and Langdon-Brown. For these authors, the doctrine of holism served a particular social and political purpose: it argued for the necessary autonomy of the individual clinician against the increasing specialisation demanded by biomedical research. Thus, this conservative élite worked hard to promote Roberts' work in both the medical and the popular press. In a letter to *The Times*, written conjointly with Sampson Handley, Arthur Hurst and G. W. Nicholson, Keith and Langdon-Brown celebrated the literary approach which Roberts had been able to bring to the problem of cancer:

> How has it been possible, it may be asked, for one who has been known in the last four decades as a writer of fiction, to say anything original regarding the mysteries of life and disease? As a writer of fiction, it was Mr Roberts' business to study human nature and human action, and to grasp the conditions under which millions of

individuals might be massed in regulated communities and yet remain healthy and orderly. In the body of a living animal, such as the human body, where billions of vital units are massed together in ordered harmony, Nature has accomplished this miracle.[20]

In his elision of the differences between the population of cells in a body and the population of individuals in society, Roberts demonstrated the need for an integrated approach which would combine the rigour of the biological sciences with the manifold insights contained in literature and sociology. Roberts coined his own neologism for this integrated approach: he termed it the science of 'biopolitics'.

The Genealogy of Biopolitics

The metaphorical conflation of the body and society has a long history.[21] In his letters to the Corinthians, St. Paul had drawn from the corporeal analogies of Plato, Seneca and Menenius Agrippa to develop the eucharistic idea of the Church and its members as the continuation of the body of Christ.[22] In the seventeenth century, this imagery was transformed from the universal Church to nation state. The frontispiece and opening pages of Thomas Hobbes' *Leviathan* suggested that the population joined in an organic relationship around the king as head; however, the actual system articulated within the work remained far more mechanical.[23] Alongside this political tradition, there was also a series of psychological explorations which suggested that the personality could be interpreted as a semi-integrated society. Beginning with the spirit-seer, Emanuel Swedenborg's idea of the 'man monster', this philosophy had been refined in the nineteenth century to suggest that the organisation of the personality was analogous to the social structure achieved in animal colonies of polyps or insects.[24]

Keith claimed that this speculative tradition had little connection with the new philosophy of the social organism which had re-emerged in the nineteenth century. In his attempt to trace a genealogy for biopolitics, Keith insisted that the notion of a social organism had first been placed upon a true footing by the work of Herbert Spencer.[25] Spencer's investigations emerged at the nexus of two important nineteenth-century innovations: the growing faith in an evolutionary model of society and increasing knowledge of the composite structure of plant and animal bodies revealed through innovations in microscopy. In a tentative addendum to his work, *Social Statics* (1868), Spencer drew attention to the apparent analogy

255

between the organisation of society and the cellular organisation of the body revealed in works such as W. B. Carpenter's *Principles of Mental Physiology* (1874).[26] Spencer suggested that the body could be interpreted as a 'commonwealth of monads' in which each cell was allotted a particular social role. This cautious analogy was given a firmer exposition in Spencer's essay of 1860, 'The Social Organism'.[27] Written in the knowledge of K. E. von Baer's work on embryology, cell division and differentiation, this essay provided a model of social evolution as a process whereby the roles of individuals would become more fixed and specialised. Human society was depicted as an imperfect approximation to the biological co-ordination achieved in the animal body.

By the end of the nineteenth century, the theory of the social organism had largely fallen into disrepute. Spencer himself had abandoned the analogy in the face of stinging criticisms from T. H. Huxley. Writing in the *Fortnightly Review* in 1871, Huxley highlighted the tensions between Spencer's faith in *laissez faire* individualism and his concept of the social organism. As Huxley argued, 'if the resemblances between the body physiological and the body politic are any indication, not only of what the latter is, and how it has become what it is, but of what it ought to be and what it is tending to become, ... the real force of the analogy is totally opposed to the negative view of state function.'[28] Faced by this choice between political principle and explanatory metaphor, Spencer had quietly dropped his theory of the social organism.[29]

Keith interpreted this rejection of social organicism as an act of intellectual cowardice. He claimed that Spencer had sacrificed his scientific insights in favour of his political beliefs. The theory of the social organism had not been disproved by contrary evidence or superseded by superior explanations, rather, it had been rejected because its idea of a natural caste system was incompatible with the civic vision of Victorian Britain.[30] Keith's conceptual history thus provided a justificatory myth of origins for the notion of the social organism. In his attribution of its nineteenth-century rejection to a series of external and often unworthy influences, Keith reasserted the theory's inherent viability and integrity.[31] It was this fertile and untarnished notion which Keith claimed has been resurrected in the work of Morley Roberts.

Roberts himself claimed a quite different genealogy for his work. In his prefaces and interviews, he repeatedly insisted upon his ignorance of Spencer's theorising in this area. Instead he traced his theory's genesis to two more eclectic sources. Alongside the influence of his anarchist experiences, Roberts claimed to have been directly inspired by his discovery in 1889, of Henry Gawen Sutton's *Lectures on Pathology* (1886).[32] Gawen Sutton, a pathologist at the London Hospital, had maintained that diseases could be caused by both internal and environmental factors: he claimed that the stresses of city hygiene and modern living could disrupt the harmonious coordination of the cells in the body.[33] For Roberts this movement between biological and sociological models of pathogenesis was a revelation. It held out the prospect that biological and social life were interrelated as parts of one overarching system.

Roberts' repeated protestations in favour of his work's eclectic genealogy would thus seem quite convincing were it not for a striking analogy between his own situation and that of a fictional character in George Gissing's novel, *Our Friend the Charlatan* (1901). Gissing was a close friend and colleague of Roberts, they had studied together at Owens College and their friendship had been resumed as they pursued new careers as hack writers in London.[34] They each made allusion to the other in their fictional works: Roberts' *The Private Life of Henry Maitland* (1912) is now widely regarded as one of the best biographies of Gissing, whilst Storm Jameson claimed that Gissing's characters of Malkin, from *Born in Exile* (1893), and Whelpdale, from *New Grub Street* (1891), were thinly veiled portraits of Roberts.[35] However, it is in *Our Friend the Charlatan,* one of Gissing's lesser known novels, that Roberts seems to have received his most accurate portrayal.

Our Friend the Charlatan concerns the career of one Dyce Lashmar, a penurious intellectual who claims to have invented a new philosophical system called 'biosociology'. Biosociology is a prescriptive and anti-democratic programme based upon the natural order of the human body. It suggests that the intellectuals are examples of 'nature's aristocracy', a race of biological superiors who are the only group fitted for government. As such, they are urged to seize the bases of political control from the idiot mass of society, just as the brain and nerves have seized control of the dumb animal body. Lashmar's exposition of his system can be read as a very prescient anticipation of Roberts' theory of biopolitics.

> Here's the central idea. No true sociology could be established before
> the facts of biology were known, as the one results from the other. In
> both the ruling principle is that of association with the evolution of
> a directing power. An animal is an association of cells. Every
> association implies division of labour. Now progress in organic

development means the slow constitution of an organ, the brain – which shall direct the body. So in society – an association of individuals with a slow constitution of a directing organ, called the Government. The problem of civilisation is to establish government on scientific principles – to pick out the fit for rule – to distinguish between the Multitude and the Select ... It is nonsense to talk about equality. Evolution is engaged in cephalizing the political aggregate, as it did the aggregate of cells in the animal organism.[36]

Gissing's novel ends with Lashmar's humiliation and exposure. He is forced from his intellectual sinecure into paid employment with the rest of the mass. Moreover, biosociology, the personal philosophy upon which he had based his intellectual credentials, was revealed as a piece of plagiarism copied from Jean Izoulet's *La Cité Moderne* (1891), a work which had developed the idea of the body politic, insisting that both animal and national coordination emerged from the surrender of an aggregate of cells or individuals to their nervous superiors.[37] In comparison, Roberts seems to have fared far more successfully than his fictional counterpart. Few critics questioned the originality of his work, even if they did draw attention to its structural similarities with the earlier work of Herbert Spencer.[38] Likewise, no Gissing scholars have acknowledged the obvious comparison between Morley Roberts and *Our Friend the Charlatan*.[39] This evasion can be attributed to two causes. First, as we saw in the previous section, Roberts had earned the support and protection of a powerful coterie of practitioners in medicine and the life sciences. Second, and more important, the complexity and turgidity of Roberts' writings militated against their easy assimilation to previous theories or contemporary movements. As we shall see in the subsequent sections, their unorthodox mixture of Lamarckism, endocrinology, crowd psychology and Spinozist ethics placed Roberts' work in a position which few would ever want to completely adopt or follow.[40]

Biopolitics as a Conservative Ideology

Biopolitics initially appears as a deeply reactionary ideology. In its language and argument it fulfills all of Karl Mannheim's criteria for a conservative style of thought, which Mannheim had identified in the literary and philosophical responses to the radical enlightenment of the late eighteenth century. Against the language of atomism, individualism and natural rights contained in the work of the *philosophes*, conservative thought stressed the complexity of lived relations. It located the fundamental aspects of reason and humanity within a seamless web of history, authority and religion.[41]

For Keith and Roberts this conservative vision of the organic community was encoded in the human body. In their writings they had repeatedly argued that the dynamic of evolution consists in a movement towards specialisation and differentiation. This was a process in which the individual cells gave up their potential freedom in favour of a fixed mission which entailed new relationships of dependence upon others. As Keith wrote:

> With each stage onwards in the progress of development, just as in each step upwards in the evolution of human culture, appears a greater and greater restriction of independence or of freedom of the individuals and an ever increasing degree of specialisation in the kind of work they have to do.[42]

This perspective allowed Keith and Roberts to rank the individual cells of the body upon an evolutionary scale. Those cells which achieved a degree of mobility such as the osteoblasts or phagocytes were depicted as protozoan creatures, retaining their 'primitive independence'. This association between freedom and atavism was repeated throughout their work. Thus Keith wrote:

> White blood corpuscles move in the blood and in the tissues with the same facility as does the ancient amoeba. Many kinds of cell can under certain conditions, cease to be "fixed" and again become wanderers just as staid town-dwellers may become the inhabitants of traveling caravans. The male sperm still retains a method of movement which was practiced by simple organisms in the earliest unicellular times.[43]

Within Roberts' work this imperative towards stability and differentiation maps onto a general model of health and illness. For Roberts, sickness is intimately connected with mobility, either through the invasive action of foreign bodies or the inner irruption of restless cells within the individual. This second movement provides Roberts with his model of cancer. Cancer is seen as a form of social breakdown, brought about when cells refuse their proper station in life. He defined malignancy as: 'the diversion of energy from high differentiation into the proliferation of hardy low grade epithelia.'[44] From this situation, in which cells refuse their predefined tasks in the body politic, cancer emerges. The disease is seen as part of a general war in which the cells become toughened and irritated by the body's continuing attempts to police them. Roberts likened the situation to that of revolutionary Russia in which state repression generated sympathy for the insurgent groups, precipitating a general social breakdown.[45] Within such episodes, new forms of destructiveness emerged. Cut off from their relationship with the remainder of the body, Roberts believed that the cancer cells would exhibit famine behaviour. Like the peasant communities of Siberia during the Bolshevik Revolution, they would develop pathological appetites. Just as Siberians had burnt down their barns and houses for firewood and turned to murder and cannibalism for sustenance, so would the cancerous tumour devour its own environment in the body.[46]

From the perspective of biopolitics the animal body thus provided a naturalistic justification for the conservative vision of *Gemeinschaft*. In its organisation and pathology it demonstrated the need for social stability and differentiation. The implication of this system went much further, however, when it was combined with the data of embryology and heredity. These sciences depicted the development of the embryo as following a preordained pattern. Within this pattern, the future role and destiny of the individual cell was fixed, just as in highly stratified societies the future profession of an individual was fixed by his or her ancestors. Thus, the form of society realised in animal flesh was not simply a nostalgic reflection of liberal England. Rather, the organisation revealed was something more alien – the caste system or slave societies of Ancient Mexico or India. As Keith wrote:

> The immense society which we find built up in man's body is based on a system of hereditary trade castes. Nature has worked out her marvelous results on a caste basis. Every step in the development of the foetus has this end in view ... each unit has to be born into an appointed place and each unit has to become a serf or slave to all the other members of the State. A successful society, as seen in Nature's kingdom, is based on each individual sacrificing its liberty of action for the benefit of the whole. The society represented by the animal body is in reality a slave State.[47]

This hereditarian language, with its implication that individuals were destined to take up roles of government or servitude, returns us to Lashmar's ideal of a natural aristocracy of the intellectuals. Certainly Roberts does seem to echo this rhetoric in his own writings. In *Biopolitics* the human nervous system is repeatedly represented as a privileged caste of aristocratic government:

while the untold masses of working cells in the body do their work and perish, the highly endowed brain and nerve cells ... are lapped in lecithin and luxury and live forever, or at least for the life of the body which they help to rule ... For what is the brain which the overlogical are ready to obey like slaves, but a somatic assembly of would-be dominating aristocrats, a cerebral senate or House of Lords.[48]

As the quotation should make clear, there is a central tension in Roberts' attitude to the aristocratic government of the brain. Although the implication of his argument suggests that aristocratic government is the natural telos of social evolution, Roberts' language conveys a much more suspicious attitude. His denigration of the 'overlogical' who submit to the 'would-be aristocrats' of the nervous system seems more redolent of his original anarchist sympathies. Against the conservative imagery with which Keith had approached the social organism, Roberts deployed a more subtle and pessimistic analysis. Despite his equations of evolution with hierarchy and unrest with malignancy, it is possible to read Roberts' biological writings as a hermetic manifesto for the anarchist visions he had pursued in *fin-de-siècle* England.

Biopolitics as an Anarchist Ideology

Roberts' mistrust of the human nervous system extended from his working philosophy into his waking life. In his writings on malignancy and cancer, he argued that the brain could be seen as a tumorous outgrowth. It marked the decadent expansion of this aristocratic caste of intellectuals at the expense of the labouring population of the body. As Roberts noted in an address to the Hunterian Society:

The history of man has been the rise of brain to power. Is it not possible that these domineering cells, the conquering cortex, may in some sense become malignant and destructive? They may learn to want everything their own way, for power possessed is rarely not abused, either in human societies or the marvelous cellular society of the human body. If this is so, we can so overbalance due order that the brain may destroy life and itself.[49]

This apprehension of nervous tyranny haunted Roberts. In 1937, he complained to his biographer, Jameson, that: 'My friend, my brain, is a curse. It's a devil possessing an otherwise healthy man.'[50] This imagery of the brain as an alien invader had its basis in certain extrapolations which Roberts had made from the neurological researches of W. H. Gaskell and the endocrine investigations of Langdon-Brown. Gaskell had argued that the nervous system had originated in an invasion of alien tissues, which had constructed a mesh of supporting cells.[51] Roberts drew upon this theory, depicting the brain and nerves as part of a system of colonial or imperial government:

> Swarms of neuroblasts migrate: they build ganglia and entrench themselves in masses; they burrow as Trotter thinks, against the hostility of the other tissues and subdue them. We may even imagine ... that they make slaves of the muscles ... The migrations of the prevertebral sympathetic ganglia resemble the formation of the early Roman colonies in yet unconquered Italy. The parts they rule are subdued to the commonweal and put in communication by the *rami communicantes* with the central nervous system which was itself invasive to begin with ... Langdon Brown says: "It is not too fanciful to compare the origin of the nervous system to a group of settlers on the coast who gradually invade the interior, first singly and then in an organised army ... Once stabilised the invader assumes control over the indigenous inhabitants, fortifying itself as it goes."[52]

Concomitant with this imagery of the nervous system as an alien invader or imperial forces, lies the suggestion of an older, indigenous pattern of government. Roberts and Keith both identified the endocrine system as the basis for this primitive form of integration. The mechanism of communication achieved through the hormones carried with it suggestions of the primal and the prehistoric. Against the nervous system with its associations of electricity and telegraphy, the hormones in Keith's analogy were depicted as an ancient postal service.[53] Thus Keith argued that the hormones 'are really errand boys on their way to deliver messages, or parcels, and that the gland masses which are built up around the lymph channels serve both as nurseries for the upbringing of such messengers and also as offices from which they are dispatched on their errands.'[54]

The contrast between the modern nervous system and primitive endocrine system developed by authors such as Keith and Langdon-Brown played onto historical and anthropological divisions between Romans and Britons or colonials and natives. It also echoed more contemporary concerns. The struggle between the rational brain and the impulsive hormones reflected modern fears over the relationship between the intellectuals and the masses. Keith and Roberts made this connection when they contrasted the methods of control and social cohesion deployed by the two alternative forms of somatic government. Whilst the brain operated through the dictates of reason, the hormones achieved integration through more irrational means, namely the unconscious drives of the herd-instinct, as conceptualised by Wilfred Trotter and Sigmund Freud.[55]

This idea of the body divided between two antagonistic forms of government provided the basis for Roberts' somatic anarchism. The social organism was not seen as a peaceable kingdom but rather as a Hobbesian state of nature in which each of the cells were constantly engaged in a war of 'all against all'. Alongside the struggle between the nervous and endocrine systems, Roberts envisaged smaller conflicts between groups or individual cells over oxygen or nutrition. His conception drew upon the earlier work of Wilhelm Roux who had suggested, in *Der Kampf der Teile in Organismus* (1881), that natural selection operated right down at the level of individual cells in the internal environment of the organism.[56] Thus, Roberts imagined that the social organism remained in a state of 'hostile symbiosis' in which each of the cells reluctantly co-operated out of fear of punishment or the dangers of social unrest.[57] This state was well described by the protagonist in his novel of 1914, *Time and Thomas Waring*:

> Men fought against each other and fought against themselves; the essence of the body and the mind was but a strange conflict. He had heard some of his doctor friends declare that the republic of the body was a difficult balance of opposing forces; of stimuli, of inhibitions, of desires that drew on and fears that repelled. Each organ would be dominant, and others again denied it dominance. Every gland did its own work and again inhibited or controlled the work of the other glands. At the best of times in health all the body's organs were in a state of armed neutrality. It was the same in life and in an organised society.[58]

This holographic image of conflict extending from nations through individuals via organs down to cells provided Roberts with a mechanism for social progress and organic evolution. In his own peculiar variant of Lamarckian theory, Roberts suggested that the organism's responses to episodes of infection or stress would be reproduced throughout its succeeding generations.[59] This association of evolution with stress and repair transforms the normative value of sickness and war. Illnesses such as cancer or the outbreak of tribal conflicts were not seen as pathological episodes from which the body, natural or political, would recover its equilibrium. Rather, these the events were seen as necessary parts of the flux of life: they were the cornerstones of future evolution.

Against Keith's conservative view of the social organism, Roberts' work can be seen as a kind of medical Trojan horse. Although his arguments are framed in the reactionary language of social malignancy and organic integration, we can recognise a revolutionary intention in his work. It is a celebration of the primitive flux of life, of the ceaseless struggle of the organism and its endless transformation. This dynamic vision only becomes apparent when one joins Roberts' theories of social disease to his eclectic belief in a pathologically driven Lamarckism. Such is the covert nature of Roberts' radicalism, it could perhaps be argued that this anarchist reading rests upon a perverse misinterpretation or a willful act of partial deconstruction. These accusations would be convincing, were it not for the one small area in which Roberts makes explicit his anarchist ideals: his discussions of the work of Sutton.

Sutton makes an unlikely touchstone for syndicalist belief: a deaf pathologist at the London Hospital, he had a fairly typical if energetic career ministering to the needs of the East End poor.[60] Yet, for Roberts he provided a benchmark in anarchist theory. In 1903, Roberts declared himself 'philosophically as much of an Anarchist as the late H. G. Sutton who would have no doubt been astounded to learn that he belonged to the brotherhood.'[61] Twenty two years later in a tribute to Sutton delivered before the Hunterian Society, Roberts would celebrate the pathologist as a 'natural disciple of philosophic anarchism.' His case seems fairly persuasive. He reveals in Sutton's lectures certain unacknowledged borrowings from Proudhon ('society prepares the crime and creates the criminal') and Spinoza ('every year I am more and more impressed with what the human body can do'). It is this second source which provides the key to Sutton's thought and perhaps to the theory of biopolitics as a whole. Spinoza had developed a radical theory of the body and power which stressed their unlimited or unbounded nature. In his *Ethics* of 1677, the body was presented as part of a general extension of the spirit of God. Likewise, power was seen as force which could not be contained in kings or contracts but which lay in the massing of the multitude.[62] The pantheistic implication of both these arguments fitted in well with Roberts' own programme. If the body was part of the general extension of God then each of its states obtained an equal validity.

Health and disease, as both Roberts and Sutton suggested, were both equivalent parts of a universal cosmic process. Likewise if power rested in the multitude rather than the head of state, Roberts' mistrust of the nervous system would seem justified. Against the idea that the social body should be led by the aristocracy of the intellect, this philosophy asserted its faith in the labouring masses within the body politic. It was in these silent crowds of cells and individuals that true power lay. Against the reactionary modernism of inter-war Britain which had argued for salvation through the leadership of the intelligentsia, Roberts proclaimed his faith in the historic wisdom of the ordinary people.

> [Sutton] taught how wrong it was for the mind to rule the body like a tyrant, and to scorn the accumulated wisdom of the ages, solidly founded in the instincts ... [He] therefore asked all, even the encroaching cortex, to consider the body and the instincts. He knew, as many of you know, that the forebrain can be a tyrant ... For this as I believe is the very essence of the doctrine of pure anarchism of which he was the more or less unconscious prophet.[63]

Roberts thus eschewed a naturalistic fallacy associated with the social organism. The body provided neither a model of good health nor good government. It simply offered a tangible map of the struggles which persisted amongst cells, individuals and nations.[64]

Englishness and the Armed Neutrality of the Organism

In the anxious years of the inter-war period the theory of biopolitics began to take a on a renewed significance. In the rich associations it established between the life and health of the individual and the history of the state, biopolitics provided both a language and an objective legitimacy to such vague notions as citizenship, patriotism and national identity. Both Keith and Roberts contributed to the ongoing attempt to define a distinctively English culture and character, reaching conclusions which radically opposed the pastoral vision of the English then being articulated by their humanist contemporaries.[65]

As Anna-K. Mayer demonstrates in her chapter, Arthur Keith drew heavily upon the patrician language of Englishness. His Second World War essays on evolutionary theory open with a patriotic self portrait of the aged anthropologist returning to work the land as part of his contribution to the nation's war effort.[66] He depicts himself as a kind of Arcadian eugenist: 'digging out the weeds and encouraging our native grasses.'[67] Yet, as Keith makes clear, this pastoral scene is not something which stands opposed to or removed from contemporary science. He works in the shadow of the Buckston Browne Institute for Surgical Research, hoeing the fields that made up Darwin's estate at Downe in Kent.

In contrast to the Christian or liberal-humanistic vision which had identified Englishness with the civilised values of freedom, tolerance and fair play, Keith, as Mayer shows, insisted that the notion possessed a darker side – a vicious evolutionary inheritance which persisted beneath the thin veneer of civilisation. In his popular work, *Ethnos, or the Future of Race* (1931), Keith spoke warmly of this hidden aspect of Englishness:

> I would say after a deliberate study extending over many years that in no people are race instincts, race prejudices, race determination, so strongly entrenched as in the hearts of the natives of England ... But then in no people are these instincts so disciplined and controlled by reason. In the Englishman such feelings are difficult to rouse – but once aroused the effect can be truly cyclonic.[68]

Likewise, in his *Essays on Human Evolution* (1946), Keith noted how 'still after all these centuries of civilisation, the Englishman had much of the old Adam in him', going on to quote the historian H. A. L. Fisher's verdict that '[i]n moments of excitement the English are capable of great savagery.'[69]

This image of the Englishman as a bifurcated individual torn between civil and animal impulses derived from T. H. Huxley's Romanes Lecture of 1893.[70] Huxley had argued that the imperatives of man's evolutionary nature – his instincts for struggle and survival – conflicted with the ethical demands of modern civilisation. The individual was thus torn between two codes: the 'cosmic code' of his primitive impulses and the ethical code of Christian and humanist philosophy. Keith's development of this notion in his definition of Englishness served a twofold purpose. At one level, it provided a normative model of conduct through which Keith could foster his obsessions with racial purity and survival.[71] True Englishness could not be achieved through the Christian ideals of justice and tolerance, rather, its success and survival depended upon that primitive cyclonic ferocity that patrician culture had worked so hard to erase. On another level, Keith's model of English nature could be seen as exposing or undermining the moral authority of the church. In its insistent identification of Englishness with Christian virtues of peace and forgiveness, the church demonstrated, for Keith, its fatal ignorance of national character and its strategy for survival. The church ministered to a one-dimensional model of man, a man deprived of the ability to protect his future or his nation.[72]

Keith's vision of a divided and ambivalent Englishness torn between ethical and cosmic impulses was shared by Roberts. Like

Keith, Roberts recognised how English behaviour, at the level of both the individual and the nation, had been characterised by 'an amusing lack of seriousness'. However, he also insisted that such flippancy had a darker side for it imperiled the future survival of the national organism. As Roberts wrote:

> Their passion for sport, their patience in quarrel, their cynical humour, their inevitable jesting in disaster, and their remarkable use of irony in common speech and their readiness to forgive and forget have led their more serious and solemn enemies to think the British fundamentally weak. In this last respect they are the kindest and most foolish people in Europe. This quality, amongst others has far too greatly influenced their European conduct, and exposed to great and unnecessary dangers their actual survival.[73]

This vulnerability, that had been cultivated in the ethical codes of England's intellectual aristocrats, was countered, however, by the primitive temperament of the British masses.[74] Writing in the wake of Dunkirk, Roberts looked forward to a time when the British peoples, pushed to extremity, would reveal a 'Dionysian' anger beneath the cowering policies of their 'milder-mannered' rulers.[75] Roberts thus shared with Keith an ironic understanding of Englishness. They both recognised that the future survival of national civilization had been safeguarded by the primeval ruthlessness it had once worked so hard to destroy.

However, Roberts went much further than Keith in his redefinition of Englishness. Whereas Keith had deployed a fairly static model of national character, seeing ancient traits preserved through racial prejudice and isolation, Roberts had been led through his Spinozist philosophy to a more dynamic interpretation. Against the familiar synecdoche which reduced Britishness to Englishness and Englishness to an Arcadian vision of the home counties, Roberts argued that the vital essence of Britain lay in its young colonies. He argued that the British commonwealth was a 'multi-nucleate organism' which had escaped central direction and control.[76] As he noted:

> a national organism buds and makes a ring of young organisms about the mother country, the whole centripetal group is fuller of vigour and enterprise than it was and is more moved by the native pull of the young protoplasm than the central originating organism and nucleus which continues to hold the main tools, weapons, catalysts and organising enzymes, with the powerful secretion glands

and the great real but intangible catalyst experience. The young and vigorous family is itself a new kind of colonial catalyst urging the mother organism to new efforts, forcing it to free itself from the kind of elderly and obstinate delusion which lost England North America.[77]

For Roberts, the Second World War was not simply the struggle of the English people to maintain their evolutionary identity, rather, it was part of an inevitable and ongoing conflict between national organisms as they fought for nutrition in the form of land and trade.[78] Against the patrician rhetoric that had cast the war as defence of culture and civilisation, Roberts envisaged a more animal explanation, as the massed mind of the primitive British organism surrendered to the promptings of its own cosmic code.

Conclusion

From the perspective of Keith and Roberts, the escape of biopolitics from its obvious associations with conservatism, organicism and tradition could be see as an apparent confirmation of their world view. It was a reminder of the plasticity of language, suggesting that meaning is not sustained through an easy correspondence with the world, but rather it obtained its significance through its position in a web of words. Similarly Roberts' work undid the liberal ideal of society, in which the individual received their definition through their personal talents of unique history. Within biopolitics, the intellectual and the citizen are each sustained through their position in a shifting mesh of social relationships. Likewise the character of a country was not a product of its culture and history, rather it was defined though its shifting position in a web of international relations. For Roberts and Keith, order and identity were not natural or inevitable, rather they were transient stages in the ongoing struggle of the organism.

Acknowledgement

This article was produced as part of the Wellcome Trust sponsored project, 'The Brain and the Self: Popular Understanding of the Neurosciences in Twentieth-Century Britain'. The generous support of the Trust in the research and writing of this project is gratefully acknowledged.

Notes

1   'They Gave a Dinner to Him', *Evening News*, 8 October 1935.
    Loose cutting in Royal College of Surgeons, Arthur Keith MSS,
    Filebox KL2 (Folder R). On Roberts, see, Storm Jameson, *Morley
    Roberts: The Last Eminent Victorian*, London, [1961]; Morchard
    Bishop, 'Introduction', in Morley Roberts, *The Private Life of Henry
    Maitland*, London, 1958.

2   Arthur Keith, 'The Anatomy of the Valvular Mechanisms of the
    Venous Orifices of the Auricles', *Journal of Anatomy*, 37 (1903): 18;
    Morley Roberts, 'The Function of the Cardiac Vagus', *British
    Medical Journal* (1918): ii, 302; *ibid.*, 201; 'Inhibition and the
    Cardiac Vagus', in *idem, Warfare in the Human Body* , London,
    1920, ch. 4. On the general background see *The Emergence of
    Modern Cardiology*, W. F. Bynum, Christopher Lawrence and Vivian
    Nutton (eds), London: *Medical History* Supplement no. 5, 1985.

3   Roberts, *Private Life of Henry Maitland*, pp. 80–81.

4   Roberts' Texan experiences are recounted in *The Western Avernus*,
    London, 1887.

5   Morley Roberts, *Malignancy and Evolution: A Biological Inquiry into
    the Nature and Causes of Cancer*, London, 1926, pp.108–9. Roberts
    repeatedly claimed to have published his findings in the *British
    Medical Journal*, 22 January 1921, but no such reference exists.

6   Robert's claimed involvement in the London anarchist movement is
    dubious and needs further investigation. In a preface to Isobel
    Meredith's *A Girl among the Anarchists*, London, 1903, Roberts
    claimed that he knew Meredith and had been a contributor to her
    revolutionary paper, *The Tocsin*. However historians of anarchism
    have shown that Meredith's work is semi-fictional account co-
    authored by the Rosetti sisters, Olivia, Helen and Mary. These sisters
    had in fact been responsible for the production of *The Torch*, another
    anarchist paper which ran between 1894–96. See Oliver Hermia,
    The Anarchist Movement in London, London, 1983.

7   For a recent discussion of this slippage, see the papers of Paolo
    Palladino on the work of the cancer surgeon, Lockhart-Mummery:
    '"Icarus" Flight: The Surgeon, the Historians and the Contradictions
    of Modernity' (unpublished, 1997); 'On the Contradictions of
    Humanism: The Medical and Other Writings of Percy Lockhart
    Mummery' (unpublished, 1996).

8   Roberts, *Warfare in the Human Body, Malignancy. Biopolitics: An
    Essay in the Physiology of the Pathology & Politics of the Social &
    Somatic Organism*, London, 1938; *The Behaviour of Nations*,

London, 1941.

9   On Storm Jameson (1891–1986), see *The Oxford Companion to English Literature*, Margaret Drabble (ed.), Oxford, 1995, 511–12.

10 'Obituary notice: Morley Roberts' *British Medical Journal* (1942): i, 775. For Keith, see W. E. Le Gros Clark, 'Arthur Keith, 1866-1955' in *Biographical Memoirs of Fellows of the Royal Society*, 1 (1955): 145–61.

11 On this literary role, see Jacob Korg, 'George Gissing's Outcast Intellectuals', *American Scholar* 19 (1950): 194–202.

12 This part of Roberts' life was caricatured in Gissing's novel, *New Grub Street*, Harmondsworth, 1968 [1861].

13 *Evening News*, 8 October 1935. On Walter Langdon-Brown (1870-1946), see *Munks Roll*, vol. 4, 491. For the organicist aspect of his thought, see Christopher Lawrence, 'Still incommunicable: Clinical Holists and Medical Knowledge in Interwar Britain' in *Greater than the Parts: Holism in Biomedicine 1920-1950*, Christopher Lawrence and George Weisz (eds), New York, 1998, pp. 94–111.

14 Arthur Keith, *An Autobiography*, London, 1950, 425.

15 'Warfare in the Human Body' *Times Literary Supplement*, 1920, 723; 'Malignancy & Evolution', *Times Literary Supplement*, 29 July 1926, 514; 'Biology and Politics', *Times Literary Supplement*, 22 January 1938, 53; 'Struggle in the Nutritional Field', *Times Literary Supplement*, 10 June 1942, 224.

16 'Imagination in Medicine', *British Medical Journal* (1920): ii, 632–33; 'Malignancy & Evolution', *British Medical Journal* (1926): ii, 15; Walter Langdon Brown, 'The Mechanism of Evolution', *British Medical Journal* (1930): ii, 519; [Anon], 'Biology and the Body Politic' *British Medical Journal* (1938): i, 622–23. For more tempered reviews see: *Lancet* (1926): i, 443–4; *Lancet* (1938): i, 1427. For Roberts' debt to Dawson Williams see 'The Study of Malignancy', *British Medical Journal* (1935): i, 279.

17 'Imagination in Medicine', *British Medical Journal* (1920): ii, 632.

18 'Malignancy and Evolution', *British Medical Journal* (1926): ii, 15. The language is almost identical to that given in later reviews by Keith, 'Politics and Biology: The Harvest of Literature', *The Observer*, 16 January 1938; 'Nations on the Table', *The Observer*, 20 April 1941.

19 For the general background, see Christopher Lawrence and George Weisz, 'Medical Holism: The Context' in *Greater than the Parts*, Lawrence and Weisz (eds), pp. 1-22.

20 'Malignancy and Cancer', *The Times*, 21 November 1934, 10. The original impetus for the letter seems to have come from Sir Basil

Clarke, emeritus director of information at the Ministry of Health, see, Keith, *Autobiography*, 615; MS letter, Morley Roberts to Arthur Keith,19 November 1934, Royal College of Surgeons, Arthur Keith MSS, Filebox KL2 (Folder R). *The Times* letter directly transcribes part of Keith's preface to Roberts, *Warfare in the Human Body*, vi.

21 H. E. Barnes, 'Representative Biological Theories of Society', *The Sociological Review*, 17 (1925): 120–30, 182–94, 294–300. For an analysis, see Roger Cooter, 'The Power of the Body' in *Natural Order: Historical Studies of Scientific Culture*, B. Barnes and S. Shapin (eds), Beverly Hills, 1979, pp. 73–92.

22 1 *Corinthians* 12, 8–31.

23 For early conceptions of the body politic, see Peter Brown, *The Body and Society. Men, Women and Sexual Renunciation in Early Christianity*, London, 1988; M. Gosbee, 'Body Politic', in *Oxford Companion to the Body* (in press).

24 Alfred Binet, *Alterations of Personality* [1892], London, 1896, pp. 348–9; John H. King, *Man an Organic Community*, London, 1893; Theodule Ribot, *The Diseases of Personality* [1887], Chicago, 1906, pp. 140–7. For a criticism of this idea of multiple monadism and the idea that it originated in the Swedenborgian concept of the 'man monster': Edward Montgomery, 'The Unity of the Organic Individual', *Mind*, 5 (1880): 318–36, 465–89.

25 Arthur Keith, 'Does Man's Body Represent a Commonwealth', *Rationalist Press Association Annual*, 1924, 4; *idem, The Engines of the Human Body*, London, 1925, appendix M, 'The Human Body as a Society of Microscopic Units', pp. 326–9.

26 Herbert Spencer, *Social Statics*, London, 1851. For critical introductions to this idea, see Walter H. Simon, 'Herbert Spencer and the "Social Organism"', *Journal of the History of Ideas*, 21(1960): 294–99; David Wiltshire, *The Social and Political Thought of Herbert Spencer*, Oxford, 1978, ch. 9.

27 Herbert Spencer, 'The Social Organism', reprinted in *Essays, Scientific, Political and Speculative*, London, 1891.

28 T. H. Huxley, 'Administrative Nihilism', *Fortnightly Review* (1871): 534, reprinted in *Collected Essays*, vol. 1, London, 1896.

29 Simon, 'Herbert Spencer', pp. 298–9.

30 Keith, 'Commonwealth', pp. 4–6. Compare with Roberts, *Biopolitics*, 12.

31 Keith, 'Commonwealth', pp. 5–6.

32 Henry Gawen Sutton, *Lectures on Medical Pathology*, London, 1886, x.

33 On Gawen Sutton, see his obituary, *Lancet* (1891): i, 1408–10.

34 On the friendship of Gissing and Roberts, see John Halperin,

Gissing: A Life in Books, Oxford, 1982, 41f.

35 'Writer & Friend', *Times Literary Supplement*, 27 October 1961, 767.

36 George Gissing, *Our Friend, the Charlatan*, London, 1901, 23.

37 Jean Izoulet, *La Cité Moderne et la Métaphysique de la Sociologie*, Paris, 1891.

38 'Malignancy and Evolution', 15; 'Biology and the Body Politic', 623. Havelock Ellis argued that Roberts' theories derived from the work of the German biologist Hermann Renheimer and the British cancer specialist John Bland Sutton, 'The Novelist turned Biologist', *The Nation*, 20 November 1920, reprinted in *Views and Reviews* 2nd series, London, 1932, pp. 33–44.

39 Jacob Korg has suggested that the character of Dyce Lashmar may be an unhappy self portrait by Gissing, calling *Our Friend the Charlatan*: 'an exercise in self-criticism of a particularly masochistic kind.' Jacob Korg, *George Gissing: A Critical Biography*, Seattle, 1963, 295.

40 See however, Matthew Fuller, 'Metastases: Genetics or Ideology', in *Mind Invaders*, Stewart Home (ed.), London, 1997, pp. 175–8. For Roberts' Spinozism, see below.

41 Karl Mannheim, 'Conservative Thought' in *Essays on Sociology and Social Psychology*, London, 1953, ch. 2.

42 Keith, 'Commonwealth', 9

43 Keith, *Engines,* pp. 328–9.

44 Roberts, *Malignancy*, 204.

45 *Ibid.*, 204.

46 Roberts, *Biopolitics*, 202.

47 Keith, 'Commonwealth', pp. 10–12.

48 Roberts, *Biopolitics*, pp. 25, 56.

49 Morley Roberts, *H. Gawen Sutton: An Appreciation*, London, 1925, 18.

50 Letter to Storm Jameson, 3 March 1937, in Jameson, *Morley Roberts*, 50.

51 W. H. Gaskell, 'On the Relation between the Structure, Function, Distribution and Origin of the Cranial Nerves; together with a the Theory of the Origin of the Nervous System of Vertebrata', *Journal of Physiology*, 10 (1889):153. On Gaskell, see W. Langdon Brown, 'W. H. Gaskell and the Cambridge Medical School', *Proceedings of the Royal Society of Medicine*, 33 (1939-40): 1-12; Gerald Gieson 'Gaskell, Walter Holbrook', *Dictionary of Scientific Biography* vol. 5, pp. 279–84.

52 Roberts, *Malignancy*, 157. The internal references are to W. Trotter,

'The Physiology of Pain', *Medical Science Abstracts* (April, 1921); W. Langdon Brown, 'The Influence of the Endocrines in Psychoneuroses', *British Journal of Psychology*, 2 (1921): 1–12, reprinted in *idem, The Endocrines in General Medicine*, London, 1927, ch. 10.

53 Keith, *Engines*, ch. 21, 'A Postal System of a Peculiar Kind'; *idem, Concerning Man's Origin.*

54 *Ibid.*, 230.

55 J. van Ginneken, *Crowds, Psychology and Politics, 1871-1899*, Cambridge, 1992; H. Greisman, 'Herd Instinct and the Foundation of Bio-sociology', *Journal of the History of the Behavioral Sciences*, 15 (1979): 357–69.

56 For Roux, see his entry in the *Dictionary of Scientific Biography*, vol. 11, pp. 570–5.

57 Roberts defined 'hostile symbiosis' as the idea 'that there is latent in all tissues a deep and fundamental hostility at any time liable to resurgence; and that the cell nucleus is not living matter but what may be called a tool-chest, containing the acquired hormones and catalysts necessary for offence and defence, construction and repair.' Roberts, *Malignancy*, pp. 30–1; *idem, Biopolitics*, ch. 8; *idem, The Behaviour of Nations*, ch. 2.

58 Morley Roberts, *Time and Thomas Waring*, London, 1914, 102.

59 His Lamarckian theory is too complex to be fully explored in this short paper. For Roberts' main exploration of the doctrine, see, 'The Function of Pathological States in Evolution', *Zoological Society Proceedings* (1918): 237–54; *idem, Warfare in the Human Body*, ch. 3; *idem, The Serpent's Fang*, London, 1930, esp. chs. 1, 3, 4. On the resurgence of Lamarckism in early twentieth century Britain, see, Peter Bowler, *The Eclipse of Darwinism: Anti-Darwinian Evolutionary Theories in the Decades around 1900*, Baltimore, 1983, pp. 98–106.

60 See above fn. 33.

61 Meredith, *Girl among the Anarchists*, vi.

62 For current readings of Spinoza which stress the radical implications of his theory, see Antonio Negri, *The Savage Anomaly: The Power of Spinoza's Metaphysics and Politics*, Minneapolis, 1991; G. Deleuze and F. Guattari, 'Becoming Intense, Becoming Animal', in *A Thousand Plateaus*, London, 1991, esp. pp. 253–60.

63 Roberts, *Gawen Sutton*, pp. 15, 18.

64 Roberts, *Biopolitics*, 27.

65 There is now a rich literature on the notion of Englishness in twentieth-century Britain, see *Englishness: Politics and Culture 1880–1920*, R. Colls and P. Dodd (eds), London, 1986; *Myths of the*

English, Roy Porter (ed.), London, 1992; Stefan Collini, *Public Moralists: Political Thought and Intellectual Life in Britain, 1850-1930*, Oxford, 1991, pt. 4.

66 Keith, *Essays on Human Evolution*, London, 1946. This essay had originally appeared in *The Literary Guide* (January, 1943).

67 *Ibid.*, 2.

68 Arthur Keith, *Ethnos*, London, 1931, 38.

69 Keith, *Essays*, 76. For a justification of Keith' attempt to conflate races and nations, see his *A New Theory of Evolution*, London, 1948, ch. 32.

70 T. H. Huxley, *Evolution and Ethics*, London, 1893, reprinted in *Collected Essays*, vol. 9, 60.

71 For an overview of Keith's theories on race struggle and purity, see Nancy Leys Stepan, 'Nature's Pruning Hook: War, Race and Evolution, 1914-18', in *The Political Culture of Modern Britain*, J. M. W. Bean (ed.), London, 1987, pp. 129–48.

72 Keith, *Essays*, pp. 123–8, 195.

73 Roberts, *Behaviour of Nations*, 153.

74 *Ibid.*, ch. 14.

75 *Ibid.*, 23. Storm Jameson has written of the 'astonishing exhilaration' she felt, reading Roberts' manuscript in the wake of Dunkirk and the threat of invasion, *Journey from the North*, [1970], London, 1984, vol. 2, pp. 68–9.

76 Roberts, *Behaviour of Nations*, 94. This model had been anticipated in H. G. Wells, *The New Machiavelli*, London, 1911, which had compared the British Empire to an 'early vertebrated monster', Book III, pt. 2, ch. 5. Roberts wrote to Wells acknowledging the deep impact the book had made on his philosophy. David Smith, *H. G. Wells: Desperately Mortal*, New Haven, 1986, 114.

77 Roberts, *Behaviour of Nations*, 94.

78 Roberts, *Biopolitics*, pp. 83–4.

11

'Not a domestic utensil but a woman and a citizen': Stella Browne on Women, Health and Society

Lesley A. Hall

Old and New Feminism

Women and citizenship and women's relation to the state have been abiding concerns of the movement for female political emancipation since its first stirrings. While it has been argued that there was a transition, subsequent to the achievement of the (limited) suffrage in Britain in 1918, from an 'Old' feminism of equality to a 'New' feminism of difference, these far from clear-cut monolithic camps represented two strands which had been present in the movement for women's emancipation for much longer. There were pre-existing tensions between the 'humanist' case for feminism derived from Enlightenment political philosophy and nineteenth-century liberal thought, most notably expressed in Mary Wollstonecraft's *Vindication of the Rights of Women* (1792) and John Stuart Mill's *The Subjection of Women* (1869) and a more biologically based 'essentialist' case conflating sex and gender. While there were differing interpretations of liberalism, its implicitly gender-neutral concept of citizenship could seem wanting when addressing issues involving specifically sexual abuse and exploitation of women. These were the focus of several campaigns from the mid-nineteenth century, including attempts to improve the position of woman within marriage (e.g. the struggles for the Married Women's Property Act, or greater rights of mothers to custody of their children) or to abolish the Contagious Diseases Acts which gave the force of law to the Double Standard of sexual morality by penalising prostitutes in port and garrison towns but not their male partners.

There was also a strategic use of the doctrine of innate difference to claim that men could not legitimately represent women and moreover that women would, because of their specific womanly attributes, bring something new to the political process and state-creation. This did not include acceptance of the existing hierarchical valuing of gender difference or even the idea of separate spheres of activity. Suffragists challenged the existing delineation of the private and public spheres by envisaging taking the values of the home out into the world, rather than the home providing a haven from a cruel (masculine) public domain.

The idea of motherhood and maternal nurturance was central to this vision. Indeed, the feminists of the late nineteenth and early twentieth century often wholeheartedly accepted stereotypes of gender that defined women as caring, nurturant, altruistic and above all, *motherly*. Even if not personally and physically mothers, women could position themselves as taking on a maternal role towards the larger community or specific groups within it. This view of woman's role and the claims to political representation it implied was seldom distinctly differentiated from the discourse of rights and many advocates of women's suffrage moved between the two as specific situations and campaigns required.[1]

From the beginning of the twentieth century, concerns over national fitness and population issues focussed increasing attention on actual motherhood. Women who were already mothers were, in the lower classes, subjected to various interventions aimed at improving the ways in which they brought up their children and cared for their health, while those in higher classes were the audience for growing numbers of books on the right methods of child-rearing. There was pressure to ensure the competence of future mothers by incorporating suitable lessons into the education of girls. Many of the strategies that were aimed at elevating the quality of mothering focussed on the failings of the individual mother rather than the social factors (poverty, inadequate housing, lack of access to health care, etc) which rendered child-raising a constant struggle against adverse conditions.[2]

Some women, it was conceded, would not marry. Therefore they might need remunerative occupations although of course they could seldom expect to be paid as much as a man, since they did not have to support a family (that they might be supporting aged parents or dependent relatives was usually ignored). Martha Vicinus has suggested that in Britain (and some other countries) there emerged during the nineteenth century a class of women who constituted a third term to the usual dichotomous representation of women as either married mothers or whores. The social and economic circumstances of the time admitted of the possibility of the existence of unmarried women living independently, on their own earnings, outside both heterosexual domesticity (either as mothers themselves or as subordinate helpers of their married relatives) and religious governance. However, this freedom was won at the cost of an adherence to celibacy (at least its appearance): as Vicinus points out, 'the spinster had purity thrust upon her.' These women also often had a self-sacrificing dedication to working for others, engaging in various political, educational and moral campaigns aiming at elevating women's position in society (at least for future generations) and applying themselves to the emerging 'caring professions'.[3] Unmarried women were ideally expected to work for others rather than their own direct gratification (except for a sense of duty well done) and fulfil, as already suggested, the task of 'social motherhood' as recompense for failing to achieve the physical actuality. Women who had succeeded, as they were increasingly doing in the early years of the twentieth century, in gaining professional qualifications or entry to relatively secure and well-rewarded jobs in the civil service, local government or business, could only pursue these if they were committed to celibacy, since formal and informal marriage bars operated.

There was thus a definite but rarely explicitly articulated division of respectable female citizens (as opposed to various categories of 'outcast') into married mothers who did not engage in paid work and unmarried women who might undertake remunerative labour but who had to lead a chaste and respectable life. This was contradicted on all sides by social actualities: married but childless women, women with children but invalid, absent or dead husbands, and the many women who combined some form of paid work with the duties of marriage and motherhood. Nonetheless law, convention and the general social culture of Britain in the early twentieth century decreed this dichotomy.

The camps of 'Old' and 'New' feminism have been characterized as on the one hand representing unmarried career women demanding workplace equality and, on the other, married women (or their champions: Eleanor Rathbone, campaigner for family allowances, was herself unmarried) concerned with the more traditionally womanly areas of mother and child welfare. This dichotomy is, however, false, as can be seen not only in the feminist concern over issues of marriage and maternity well before the winning of the suffrage (and indeed, as central reasons for demanding the vote), but by mapping the involvement of specific women with specific causes. Cicely Hamilton, for example, is sometimes seen as an 'Old', equal-rights, feminist because of her involvement with the Open Door League which campaigned against restrictions on women's employment but she was also active in the 'New' feminist struggles for birth control and legalized abortion.[4]

Stella Browne

A very radical direction in which debates on women's citizenship could be turned can be seen in the writings of Frances Worsley Stella Browne (1880–1955) (always known as 'Stella'), socialist and radical feminist, probably best remembered as a vigorous campaigner for birth control throughout the twenties and for abortion law reform during the thirties, when she became one of the founders of the Abortion Law Reform Association. However, she has perhaps been too narrowly seen by historians as a campaigner for women's rights to reproductive control: for her, these particular issues were located in a context of a much wider concern for women's health and their place within society.

Browne was born in Halifax, Nova Scotia, the daughter of Daniel Marshall Browne, a former officer in the Royal Navy who had transferred to the Canadian Marine Service and his second wife, Anna Dulcibella Mary Dodwell, the daughter of a clergyman, in 1880. She was brought up within what was effectively a single parent family following her father's death in a maritime accident when she was three. Her mother kept a genteel boarding house in Halifax until Stella herself was around thirteen.[5] The family then, it seems probable, moved to Germany: Browne's maternal aunt had married Sir Alexander Siemens, of the distinguished Anglo-German engineering dynasty. After some years in Germany she was sent to the pioneering girls' school, St Felix Southwold, and thence to Somerville College, Oxford.[6] She never returned to Canada and indeed seems to have defined herself as British, alluding to herself as a '(female) Briton'.[7]

Browne's writings are fragmentary and scattered but are copious enough and consistent enough in their arguments for it to be possible to deduce the kind of thinking which underlay her career of activism. While she fits into a British tradition of utopian thinking on health and social issues, she brought to this tradition a worked-out gender analysis which drew attention to the particular plight and needs of women and to the necessity of women being given the knowledge and means to manage their own health. By 1911 (she later wrote) she reached the position to which she adhered for the rest of her life and never retreated from, as a 'Socialist and "extreme" Left-Wing feminist'.[8] While she responded to various specific issues and campaigns, the underlying logic of her agenda never faltered.

Her views, especially on abortion and women's rights to sexual pleasure, were extreme for the period. They were nonetheless put forward to a wide variety of audiences, although their actual influence is not easily calculable. She was an early member of the British Communist Party, from which she resigned in 1923 over its refusal to consider contraception a proletarian question. She continued to be active in the Labour Party, supporting the Workers' Birth Control Group set up by Labour women determined to change the party's policy on the subject and harrying the party leadership for its pusillanimity during the twenties campaign for the right for birth control advice to be given in publicly-funded welfare clinics. A leading figure in the Chelsea Labour Party during the twenties, she was actively involved with the Fabian Society from 1924 to 1946.

She was a vigorous and articulate member of the Malthusian League, probably because it was the only British body, at the time she joined it around 1912, explicitly committed to advocating the artificial limitation of births and providing information on the subject. *The Malthusian,* renamed *The New Generation* in 1922, was a major forum for her views that were anathema to an older generation of Malthusians. The leaders of the League at the time Browne joined were the second generation of Drysdales, Charles Vickery ('C. V.') Drysdale and his wife Bessie, who generally preferred to confine their arguments to the economic advisability of family limitation and in particular were anti-socialist in their views.

However, a distinct feminist strand is discernable within the British Malthusian movement: a tradition going back at least to Francis Place and Richard Carlile suggested that preventive checks would benefit women's health not merely by limiting pregnancies but by permitting regular and unworried sexual intercourse. Later in the nineteenth century, relatively well-known figures such as Annie Besant (prior to her conversion to theosophy), Alice Vickery, Lady Florence Dixie, Jane Clapperton and less prominent female League members, gave a specifically female slant to the sometimes rather austere economic arguments of contemporary male Malthusians for the employment of contraceptives, publicly arguing that contraception was vital to women's health and well-being and should be made more widely available, especially to less fortunate women. Some of their writings and contributions to debates hint at the employment of contraception outside strictly marital sex, although the rhetoric tended to be about protection of vulnerable women rather than erotic empowerment.[9] The suffrage movement at large tended to ignore birth control, given the continuing stigma of the practice, as politically contentious (and still repugnant to many in the movement). However, some committed suffrage campaigners (e.g. Edith How-Martyn, Eva Hubback and Cicely Hamilton), as well as other progressive pre-First World War thinkers, such as H. G. Wells, who had no particular sympathy for its political agenda, were involved with the Malthusian League.[10] Browne's continued involvement with the League, even after other more overtly feminist birth control organisations began to spring up during the twenties, was therefore not incongruous with her passionate feminism, as it might superficially seem, but relates her to a long and somewhat occluded tradition of female sexual radicalism which can be traced back at least as far as the Chartists and Owenites.[11]

In 1916, Browne wrote that she had 'observed the Suffrage movement in England, from within and without, for some years'.[12] Assuming that the Miss S. Browne, Mrs Stella Browne, Miss Stella Browne and Miss Browne who thus variously appear in the Annual Reports of the Women's Social and Political Union (WSPU), 1907 to 1913, were all the same woman and that this was the same Stella Browne who was a vociferous participant in debates in the correspondence columns of *The Freewoman* in 1912, she was a veteran of the militant suffrage campaign.[13] She seems to have resigned as a result of the increasing Pankhurst autocracy: like a number of other activists, somewhat disenchanted with the 'towering spiritual arrogance' she had perceived in the WSPU leadership and the 'dogmatic and tyrannical' bureaucracy within the movement as a whole.[14] From personal experience, therefore, she criticized in 1915 the 'self-advertising *arrivisme* and snobbery' of 'arrant humbug[s]', whose behaviour towards other women and men in a 'less advantageous social position' formed an 'illuminating commentary on [their] incessant protestations of feminism and democracy'.[15] Browne was strongly influenced by the German feminist movement, in particular the radical wing associated with Dr Helene Stöcker, which concentrated less on specifically political rights and more on issues of reproduction and maternity. Browne nonetheless did not decry the importance of the struggle for political enfranchisement, arguing in 1912 on behalf of 'the moral value of this active and articulate revolt against *tradition as well as present conditions*' embodied in the militant suffrage movement, and the claim it advanced for women's right 'to full expression and experience'.[16] Her personal style was powerfully shaped by the movement: in later years she was recalled by colleagues in abortion law reform during the thirties as 'what we used to call a war-horse, a sort of militant suffrage type, rather untidy, careless about her looks and appearance. Quite irrepressible at getting up and interrupting a meeting or asking questions.'[17]

Around 1913 she was trying to initiate a movement for the alteration of the laws on illegitimacy, along the lines of Stöcker's 'Bund für Mutterschutz' (the German Association for the Protection of Mothers), and the plight of the illegitimate child and the single mother continued to be a cause of concern to her.[18] She joined the British Society for the Study of Sex Psychology (BSSSP) soon after its inception in 1914 and gave her perhaps best known paper, 'On the Sexual Variety and Variability of Woman, and its Relation to Social Reconstruction' in the course of the following year. In 1916, she was invited to join the executive committee. Browne was a perennial and lively contributor to its debates and although she resigned from the committee in 1923, she continued to speak at and participate in its meetings well into the thirties.[19] At this time, she was also active in the Federation of Progressive Societies and Individuals (FPSI) and co-chair of its Sex Reform Group.[20]

It might be supposed that Stella Browne had nothing like the influence which Marie Stopes, for example, enjoyed between the wars. She never attained the kind of public media guru status that Stopes did but she was rather more than a lone voice somewhere out on the wilder fringes of sexual radicalism with an audience restricted to tiny vanguard bodies. Browne was involved in other organisations of a left-liberal progressive consensus sympathetic to an agenda of sexual liberation besides the BSSSP: she was active in the Promethean Society, Cosmopolis and the FPSI, and a patron of the post-Second World War Society for Sex Education and Guidance. Throughout the twenties and thirties, Browne was addressing numerous and often large meetings of local Labour Parties (both women's groups and mixed), Women's Cooperative Guilds and secular and ethical societies, as well as making her voice felt within the birth control movement. She spoke on a range of topics, including giving lecture series on health issues in general – as well as practical birth control instruction – for women. She also wrote articles, reviewed books and contributed letters to editors across a wide range of publications. One reason for her relative neglect may be that her thinking was complex and did not lend itself to being summed up in a few simple sentences. She did not posit any single cause or remedy for the ills of women and society.

Reorganizing Society

What women's place was in society, how society needed to be reorganized for women's benefit, were abiding concerns of Browne's writings and, we may hypothesise, of her talks as well. In her earliest known public statements in the correspondence columns of the short-lived feminist periodical *The Freewoman* during 1912, Browne was already dealing with the subjects that would concern her for the rest of her life. Her debate with Kathlyn Oliver on whether women were naturally more chaste than men and her pleas for the female right to sexual experimentation have been much discussed by feminist historians.[21] However, she voiced a range of other concerns in her contributions to this vanguard publication that were repeatedly addressed by her in subsequent years.[22]

Birth control was of course a constant concern and always seen in the context of a woman's right to self-determination. Browne argued in 1917 that the advent of the socialist millennium (the Russian Revolution which took place in the very same year must have made this appear more than a utopian dream) would not render the question of women's reproductive choice redundant, but that women would always 'prefer to experience maternity at their own choice of times, circumstances, and father of their child.' She foresaw that 'in the finer social order for which some of us are working (in however insignificant and piecemeal a fashion), abortion will be very rare. But it will be recognised, and respected as an individual right.'[23] She 'never held that family limitation would *alone* abolish poverty' but argued in 1925 that 'No state which had socialised production and distribution ... would be able to cope with an unrestricted and indiscriminate growth of population.' On a more individual level, 'conscious control of parenthood' was 'absolutely necessary, if equal relationships are to be responsible and selective, and to achieve the dignity and beauty to which they can attain; and if the child-bearing half of humanity is ever to be on anything like an equality with man.'[24] Browne's commitment to women's interest and what she perceived as their truly equal status made her a thorn in the side of the Labour Party throughout the twenties, harassing a leadership which persistently ignored overwhelming majorities within the Women's Section for resolutions demanding birth control advice in maternal welfare clinics. Among those who felt the lash of her contempt were women such as Ethel Bentham and Marion Phillips (personally named and shamed in the pages of *The New Generation* in 1924) who had achieved power within the Labour Party but obsequiously followed the Ramsay Macdonald line and ignored or rebuked the agitators for birth control.[25]

Browne also castigated leaders of feminist organisations. They were, she said in 1927, 'women of the most expensively educated and publicly active type, whose initiative and independence on the private side of their lives as well as on Committees could be in no manner of doubt', who ignored the pressing needs of working women.[26] In the previous year she had suggested that feminist bodies apparently considered 'Lady Rhondda's right to sit and vote in the Upper House more urgent than working women's right to refuse to bear children they do not desire and cannot support.'[27] She condemned the feminist periodical *Time and Tide* during the same year for concentrating on political equality, defining its hostile attitude towards the birth control campaign as 'sexphobia' and 'hardly honest' for women 'themselves exceptionally energetic, articulate [and] fortunate.'[28] However, she did pay tribute to the 'persistent agitation' by the National Union of Societies for Equal Citizenship (NUSEC) and the Six Point Group which by 1927 had obtained the 'tardy and grudging concession' by the Government of franchise on the same terms to women as men.[29] While referring in 1928 to the franchise (which had finally been granted on equal terms) as an 'overrated but often helpful weapon', she paid homage to predecessors who 'believing that we were really human beings, worked and suffered in that cause'.[30]

When the NUSEC finally swung over to support birth control in 1927 Browne commended their 'logical and effective synthesis of the demand for birth control knowledge with that advocacy of Family Endowment which Councillor Eleanor Rathbone has made her life work'.[31] However, her general approval of Rathbone's fight for family allowances was by no means uncritical. In particular Browne protested about the central place Rathbone accorded to married women in her formulation of endowment of motherhood. Condemning Rathbone's 1925 suggestion that the children of unmarried mothers should be handed over to the Poor Law unless their parents were willing to 'stabilise their union', Browne expressed her profound hope that maternity endowment would 'never be used to bolster up stereotyped and outworn forms of marriage' by turning 'a brief – though possibly worthwhile – illusion into a permanent incompatibility'.[32]

Although often characterized as a sex reformer above all, Browne did not believe that sex could be reformed in isolation from other social ills, nor that getting sex right would solve all the problems of individuals and society. All sorts of social pressures, she argued, militated against individuals feeling comfortable with their sexuality and being capable of having rewarding erotic lives. In her well-known study on *Sexual Variety and Variability Among Women* (1917) she began by asserting that 'I do not think that any intelligent, humane and self-respecting attitude towards sex is generally possible, without great economic changes; and a responsible education in the laws of sex'.[33] As she saw it, existing 'sexual institutions [were] founded on the needs and preferences of a primitive type of man alone ... creditable and satisfactory to neither sex.'[34]

While praising 'the admirable advice and badly needed instruction, gracefully and happily expressed' in Marie Stopes's *Married Love* (1918), Browne had two insistent criticisms. The book was quite frankly addressed to 'the educated, prosperous and privileged classes', and Stopes 'does not seem to admit that immense industrial, social and legislative changes are necessary, before the majority of her fellow citizens are able even approximately to develop and refine their erotic nature, sufficiently to follow her suggestions.' Stopes's ideal of life-long monogamy, furthermore, overlooked 'the fact that the present legally sanctioned patriarchal monogamy rests on the subjection of women' and implied prostitution as a male 'safety-valve'. A 'tragic amount of misery and misunderstanding' grew out of the ignorance associated with women's economic dependence.[35]

Browne had a solid feminist objection to the regulation of prostitution and the ways in which prostitutes were pervasively deprived of civil rights as well as being stigmatized. Josephine Butler was one of her heroines for her 'proclamation of individuality and individual worth and choice' and 'enormous courage against odds'. Browne claimed that there was not 'so much steadfast courage or so much honest sex pride or solidarity among women, that we can afford to forget Mrs Butler's work', even if the '"Equal Moral Standard" is not being worked out along the lines many of her colleagues and followers anticipated.' But those (like Browne herself) who believed that 'no sexual acts should take place which are not desired and enjoyed by both partners' were, she felt, surely among those who owed Butler a tribute in her centenary year of 1928.[36]

Browne was a passionate critic of the contemporary sexual system which divided women into 'two arbitrary classes, corresponding to no psychological or ethical differences: as a) The prospective or actual private sex property of one man. b) The public sex property of all and sundry.'[37] As she pointed out in 1917 in *The Sexual Variety and Variability of Woman*, 'the promiscuously polyandrous class of women ... are the necessary concomitants of a system of patriarchal marriage – especially monogamous marriage; and of compulsory chastity for most women before marriage.'[38] But in her view, '[t]he existence of prostitution is a great wrong to women and love, in subtle as well as in obvious ways: it not only debases the whole view of sex, but ... it favours a mechanical facility of the sexual process in men.'[39]

Browne never took the existing state of knowledge about sexual matters as given but always considered this as provisional and likely to be revised in the light of ongoing study. She was interested in the investigation of the problem of prostitution and its causes and possible remedies: in *The Malthusian* of July 1916 she heartily recommended the volume *Downward Paths. An Inquiry into the Causes which Contribute to the Making of the Prostitute* (1916) as 'an exceedingly sound and careful piece of work, avoiding all slapdash generalisations' with 'a real wish to *understand,* instead of the usual cheap cant.'[40] She praised the American volume *The Unadjusted Girl* (1924), especially its conclusions that the social system, as well as the delinquent girl, was in need of adjustment. Browne suggested that too often '[i]nvestigation and "preventive" work among prostitutes and criminals may so easily become a wholesale interference on lines of condemnation, a secret flattery of the "investigator's" own sanctity, a salve to her own repressions.'[41]

She was less impressed by the report of the League of Nations Commission on the Traffic in Women and Children which appeared in 1927. She considered that the members' report, possibly bowing to political pressures, only referred

> very briefly and casually to the economic causation of the facts they recount, and the whole vast network of psychological and physiological motives, the effects of ignorance, of the hideous boredom of much modern work, of the increased mechanisation of much modern leisure, of the inadequacy and disharmony of most modern marriage, of the vast individual range of sexual tastes and 'twists', of the fear of the unwanted child

and instead demanded simply 'still more regulation and control – police control'. In addition she linked the ongoing demand for prostitution and in particular *maisons tolérées* to militarism and 'the system of huge military establishments' which the League's constituents were unlikely to abandon or even reduce.[42] In commending the major recommendation of the report of the British Government's Street Offences Committee in 1928, Browne remarked that 'A modern community cannot with any logic, decency or comfort accept the theory of a rightless class or a rightless sex.' But she believed, perhaps optimistically, that 'the two stereotyped feminine patterns of the sheltered wife and the chivvied outlaw are merging into a more various and spontaneous humanity', although adding acerbically 'the woman of the transition so often wants to have it both ways – to enjoy the privileges of subjection and the rights of freedom!'[43]

Browne did not overlook the problem of venereal diseases which she saw as very largely the outcome of a social system orientated towards the needs of a 'primitive type of male', profoundly resistant to sexual enlightenment.[44] She considered various ways in which this peril could be handled which were equitable to all concerned. In 1915, 'A Warning to Women: The Venereal Diseases Peril in Everyday Life' appeared in *Beauty and Health*, a popular women's magazine published by American physical culturist Bernarr MacFadden. This dealt predominantly with the perils of innocent infection rather than sexual transmission: she argued that '[t]he most chaste life will not always safeguard a woman who is ignorant or careless, or unable – as is the case with so many under present social conditions – to observe scrupulous personal cleanliness.' However, Browne did emphasize the importance of knowledge. She pointed out that both syphilis and gonorrhoea were amenable to treatment, but that there was 'need for legislation, for proper facilities for treatment, and for education on sound scientific lines and the utilisation of scientific knowledge.'[45] In her 1917 paper in *Socialist Review*, 'Women and the Race', in response to an anti-feminist article by the socialist S. H. Halford, Browne made a more forthrightly feminist statement: 'a large percentage of sterility in women is due to venereal infection by their husbands ... a tremendous indictment of men's government of society.'[46]

She was even more outspoken about the whole problem in a 1920 private letter to Janet Carson, the paid secretary of the BSSSP. Commenting on literature of the recently formed Society for the Prevention of Venereal Disease (SPVD) which Carson had sent her, Browne wrote:

> It is perfectly free from the hideous barefaced sex-injustice involved in 'regulation', – though I fear for unavoidable reasons of comparative sex anatomy it must always be much easier for a man to disinfect his (external) organs than a woman hers, which are so largely internal. Still the S.P.V.D. *does* give explicit instructions to women as well as men, as to how to disinfect, and I think we should recognise this. We have no right to deny to any man, even if he *does* resort to prostitution, *protection from v.d. – which does not involve the slavery and additional degradation of women*. You know my feeling

about 'regulation' is as strong as anyone's, but self-disinfection *does not* involve regulation. I should intensely resent any attempt to keep the knowledge of such a possibility from me or any woman friend I was interested in, and we have no right to deny it to men either. Of course I also advocate working *from the roots*, but as we know that is a lengthy process.[47]

In 1918 she tried to persuade the BSSSP to pass a resolution against Regulation 40D under the Defence of the Realm Act that was widely considered to be sneaking the Contagious Diseases Acts back into practice under the guise of war time necessity.[48] In 1922 she was scathing about the report of the National Council of Public Morals Special Committee on Venereal Disease, *The Prevention of Venereal Disease*, which, she wrote, inadvertently revealed 'the entire breakdown of bourgeois morality in the face of venereal disease, the result of ignorance, poverty and prostitution – the three pillars of bourgeois society – and proves up to the hilt the need for sanitary and contraceptive knowledge among the mass of people, as part of the new civilisation.'[49]

As late as 1943 Browne was moved to write to the *Tribune,* concerning the denial of prophylactic instructions to recruits to the women's services, wanting to know why not:

> it is an adult right and an adult duty to know how to prevent disease, and the duty of any civilised contemporary government to supply the knowledge and the means. Venereal diseases cannot be extirpated by knowledge for men only, supplemented by chivying the poorer prostitutes. Both these methods have been tried and failed.[50]

As in her demands for the availability of birth control and the development of improved methods, Browne's approach towards the problem of sexually transmitted diseases was one of providing women (in particular) with information and the means of protecting themselves. They were to be neither stigmatized and penalized nor to be 'protected' by the imposition of ignorance.

The Health of Women

Browne considered that women's health needs were in general grossly neglected, the refusal to provide birth control information being only the most egregious example. On the generally unhealthy conditions under which so many women were doomed to live, she praised Leonora Eyles' *The Woman in the Little House* (1922) in a review in *The New Generation* for depicting the 'disharmony, insufficiency and waste' that constituted the working woman's life: 'housing, insufficient wages and economic dependence, adulterated food, shoddy unhygienic clothing, the methods of small retail tradesmen, and household routine.'[51] She had particularly trenchant things to say about the defects of housing from the perspective of the woman who had to manage a household. '[P]resent domestic construction' (as at 1916, when conditions were perhaps particularly grim due to wartime stringencies) entailed 'the waste of women's time, energy, and very life.' While condemning 'cramped, evil-smelling rooms ... foul sleeping arrangements ... heart-breaking, back-breaking stairs that women climb with water and coal', Browne saw the problem as not simply one of poverty but of the wider neglect of women's domestic needs. 'Not even [in] the most finely-equipped and organised household' had she ever found 'a convenient and well-planned kitchen sink; while as for shelf and cupboard room ...'[52] Concerns such as these were to be directly addressed in the planning of Kensal House in the 1930s, as Elizabeth Darling shows in her chapter.

Browne was unlike those of her contemporaries who idolized a rustic, arcadian vision of England and who, like the writer H. V. Morton, contrasted the domestic cosiness of the cottage with the squalor of industrial environs. Browne did not see bad housing as only an urban phenomenon: in a 1923 article she referred to 'cottages ... whitewashed outside and fragrant with honeysuckle and rose ... within ... full of the degradation and diseases of loathsome overcrowding.'[53] While she had a fondness for the country and natural beauty, she did not subscribe to the pastoral myth of the superiority of the country cottage to the town house. In 1929 she reported on a visit to 'one of the historic Cathedral towns of England', depicting its 'thousand glories of history and poetry, wealth and security, and green English turf and trees.' These were juxtaposed with 'a winding street that writhed down to the Severn, like a slimy reptile: a street of the most inhumanly indecent and insanitary slums I ever beheld', a mere 'stone's throw' from the cosy Trollopean vista.[54] Depictions of such vistas, as Michael Bartholomew shows in his chapter, were much in demand by the inter-war public.

Given the importance society assigned to women's role as mothers, Browne in 1917 deplored 'the disgrace of the maternal death and damage, and the insufficient and unskilled care provided for the poorer women of this country during childbirth.'[55] While generally associated with the prevention of births, she also advocated single motherhood for those with an intense maternal instincts and was concerned over the management of childbirth, keeping up with the latest developments in obstetric analgesia.[56] In 1916, she asked 'When will the great discovery ... [of] twilight slumber ... be as much at the disposal of British women as skilled care and anaesthetics at the service of our wounded soldiers?'[57] A convinced pacifist, she later suggested similarly that 'the synthetic chemistry which can give Governments a choice of 300 different poison gases ... might achieve *one* reliable contraceptive.'[58]

She was extremely critical of existing health provisions, often alluding to the Ministry of Health as the 'Ministry of Disease', and persistently attacking its 'sinister and treacherous incompetence'.[59] It was, she said, 'relentlessly exposed and condemned by its own testimony' as laid out in official reports and statistics.[60] Browne worked for some while in the early twenties at the Ministry's Insurance Department, which she described as 'The House of Bondage'.[61] In an attack on what she described in 1917 as the 'fevered propaganda in favour of what some reactionaries already term "the normal family"', Browne suggested that if the bearing of children was really 'women's supreme duty to the state', this postulated reciprocal duties by the state to guarantee tolerable conditions under which they could bear and rear children. The desiderata which Browne outlined included '[a]n efficient public health service, including a free supply of all appliances, drugs, and services necessary for the care of pregnancy, child-birth and infancy, and equitable and thorough measures for combatting venereal disease.'[62] She did not find that this characterized contemporary public health administration. In 1925, she pointed out that specialist maternity hospitals offered a bare 2000 beds for lying-in and that provision was completely uncoordinated. While praising the work of Infant Welfare Centres in 1925, Browne suggested that being forbidden to give contraceptive advice, they were 'working at some disadvantage'. Infant mortality was actually increasing and maternal mortality declining only very slightly.[63]

Browne was strongly rooted in a Left-wing critique of orthodox medicine that was inspired by alternative health ideas. Orthodox medicine she perceived as riddled with vested interests and in 1926, she protested against 'medical monopoly under pretext of "safeguards", hygienic or "moral"'. Her opinion of the medical profession was not high and she suggested that the doctors' 'reputation for general fair play and disinterested *expertise*' was not of the highest, adding 'quite apart from sexual matters, on which the majority of the profession in Britain are *either* very timid or very uninformed.'[64] Denouncing the Labour politician Dr Ethel Bentham's own 1924 attack on birth control, Browne reminded her 'that the medical profession as a whole derives considerable "private benefit" from unrestricted child-bearing and its consequences.'[65] On various occasions she alluded to the fact that doctors had the smallest families of any class or profession, even while refusing or condemning birth control advice.

She was in no awe of medical science, pointing out in 1924 that 'Official medical opinion has changed its mind very often in the past, and will doubtless do so again!', citing its reversals 'about anaesthetics in childbirth, about asepsis, about psychotherapeutics, about osteopathy'. In addition she pointed to the conflicts between orthodox medical thinking and ideas held by many in the Labour movement (the Labour Party, of course, had recently come to power) on such subjects as 'a diet including flesh meat and the moderate use of alcohol' and 'the fundamental questions of vaccination and vivisection' (Browne had been a member of the Humanitarian League until its demise in the early twenties).[66] While hopeful that the increasing number of women entering medicine might work changes, Browne cautioned that this was only likely if they had 'the courage to refuse ... masculine mythology.'[67]

She referred to herself in 1926 as 'for years extending to the poor the information which their accredited healers mostly refuse.'[68] While in that particular instance she was alluding specifically to birth control, in the following year she made a far broader case against the 'vested interests in women's ignorance and helplessness'. '[I]ll-health, inefficiency and misery' resulted from the ignorance in which women had been left by the medical profession about 'normal general hygiene and the wholesome management of diet during puberty, periodicity, pregnancy and the menopause'.[69] In her lectures on health Browne did her best to alleviate this 'carefully cultivated ignorance of women concerning their own physiology.'[70] She believed in the dissemination of information: writing in 1931 about the recently-discovered Ascheim-Zondek pregnancy test, she commented that this 'could establish the fact of impregnation at an extremely early date' and asked '[b]ut why was this knowledge kept from women who needed it?'[71]

Browne was fully aware of and did not ignore the problems of single working women such as herself. In her article 'Women and the Race', which appeared in *The Socialist Review* in 1917, responding to an anti-feminist article by male socialist S. H. Halford, Browne commented dryly: 'Mr Halford seems to me to over-estimate the magnificence and scope of women's economic prospects!'[72] This was a subject that Browne, a graduate of Somerville and fluent in at least two foreign languages, knew a great deal about: she never seems to have held a good job in her life but had to do a lot of things, many quite uncongenial, in order to make a living.

Although on pacifist principles she had eschewed war work during the First World War, she was sensitive to the anomalous position of women who had assisted the war effort. In 1918, the socialist newspaper *The Call* published her poem 'Scrapped: The Women Munition Workers of Britain, Before and After November 1918', which ended with the ironic:

The world is ours! We've won our War for Right!
Now, women, you can go! You've served our Need!²³

In an article in *The Communist* in 1922 she reiterated this point: 'the women who were gushed at as "splendid" and "saviours of the country" in war time are now realising that it is once more economically a crime to be a woman.' She additionally noted the way in which the 'economic position of women has been injured ... by the deliberate policy of the Government in playing off the temporary women clerks and the ex-servicemen against one another.'⁷⁴ In 1926, she repeated her cautions against tendencies to be 'far too sanguine about the present conditions and immediate prospects of financial independence for women' not only among many men but even among that minority of women already enjoying 'social and economic security'. Women, she suggested, had 'not advanced halfway towards economic justice'.⁷⁵

The Sexual Life

On several occasions, Browne explicitly condemned the social pressures upon the unmarried woman to live, at least in appearance, a desexualized life with 'no publicly recognised and honoured form of sex union which meets both their needs' for independence and for love. Those who engaged in free unions, she commented in 1917, caught '[b]etween the upper and nether millstones of legal marriage and prostitution', were often broken or degraded by 'ceaseless, grinding, social pressure'.⁷⁶ They were forced to struggle against 'the whole social order' for '[their] most precious personal right'.⁷⁷ There was 'huge, persistent, indirect pressure on women of strong passions and fine brains' to find an emotional outlet with other women. Existing social arrangements, Browne suggested, repressed female sexual instincts and militated against women forming either satisfactory and unstigmatized relationships with men or healthy relationships with one another.⁷⁸ Browne's vision of woman as citizen did not divide the sex into two acceptable groups of celibate workers and fertile married women but saw the ideal society as having a place for women with lovers but not babies, women with babies but no husbands, even lesbian mothers.[79] In an ideal society, women would have the opportunity for sexual experimentation as well as for the sexual relationships justified by 'a great love'.[80] She also conceded that a celibate life might entirely suit some individuals.[81]

In her rejection of the marriage/promiscuity dichotomy, Browne was in no way opening the door to unthinking license, but can be positioned as part of an English radical and feminist tradition of critiquing marriage and advocating free love from an elevated ethical standpoint. She wrote to Bertrand Russell in 1917:

> Certainly a great deal of the newer manifestations of sexual liberty are very far from encouraging or attractive, but I think this is partly due to the hateful war atmosphere & conditions, & to other quite adventitious things – e.g. the ignorance & dependence of many women – which have no necessary connection with sexual liberty in itself. One cannot expect people to develop real responsibility, or refinement & discrimination of feeling, in one generation, especially with prostitution so firmly rooted in our social order, as it is & has been.[82]

However, her construction of free love, while remote from frivolity and exploitation, did not confine it simply to permanent monogamous unions unrecognised by church or state. She considered that there were many differing types of sexual nature whose needs should be respected, arguing in 1932 that there were:

> [T]he people whose attitude to sex was casual and incidental, and those to whom sexual experience was intertwined with imagination and affection and one of the greatest things in their life. Both kinds of people existed and both had a reason to exist, and there were also those who were capable of both light love and deep, according to personality and circumstances. No *one* formula would solve sex problems.[83]

While Browne was not sympathetic to the kind of feminism which was more interested in restricting men than freeing women, her attitude towards men was very far from deferential.[84] Indeed, her viewpoint seems definitely that of a sexual subject rather than a sex-object. What a woman required in a man, she believed, was 'splendid physical vitality and virility'. This was 'just as necessary in a sex partner as ideal & intellectual sympathy'.[85] In 1927, she claimed that men of 'creative vigour and intelligence ... sympathy and imagination' who did not feel any necessity to 'fetter and further handicap women' but were able to 'attract and satisfy women as mates, without ... bribery or bullying' were an 'interesting and delightful minority'.[86] She had plenty of criticisms to make of contemporary heterosexual relations: throughout her several articles which appeared during 1916 and 1917, she argued that given a concept of 'conjugal rights' that was outrageous to decency and freedom, the law flagrantly failed to prevent 'exploitation or violation' within marriage.[87] The vast amount of sexual anaesthesia among married women was caused by 'lack of skill, control and sympathy on the husband's part'.[88] Thus many women underwent the 'ordeal of parturition' having enjoyed 'very little definite pleasure in the act of intercourse'.[89]

It is somewhat ironic that some historians have defined Browne as an agent of 'compulsory heterosexuality'.[90] While, in tune with the sexological thinking of her day about 'inversion', she differentiated 'congenital inversion' from an 'artificial tendency to inversion' resulting from 'emotional repression and mismanagement in certain temperaments', she was vigorous in expressing her belief that the 'invert' was entitled to recognition. Browne pleaded for tolerance of deviation: 'Do not persecute or condemn', she demanded in 1928 about the trial of *The Well of Loneliness*, which had come out in July of that year.[91] Indeed, in 1923 she argued that '[w]e are learning to recognise congenital inversion as a vital and very often valuable factor in civilisation, subject of course, to the same restraints as to public order and propriety, freedom of consent, and the protection of the immature, as normal heterosexual desire.'[92] She was even prepared to defend, indeed to recommend the (possibly even more stigmatized) sexual practice of masturbation, suggesting in her 1917 'Sexual Variety and Variability' paper that 'self-excitement and solitary enjoyment ... [are] inevitable in any strongly developed sexual life'. As a disciple (though never an uncritical follower) of Havelock Ellis, she argued that 'normal sexuality includes the beginnings of most abnormal instincts', such as 'inflicting ... or suffering a certain degree of pain' and 'certain forms of fetishism'. She differentiated such 'minor and occasional aberrations' from the damaging effects on women's sexual development of the 'system of silence and repression'.[93]

Like other pressing questions bearing on women's health, the study of menstruation in Browne's view had been neglected: 'the whole periodic function has been as much misunderstood and mismanaged as the maternal', she wrote in 1923.[94] In keeping with the other concepts of women's variety and variability advanced in her

1917 paper, she suggested that there might be diverse types of women who had different experiences in the matter. Browne considered that 'in the social order for which some of us hope and work, provision will have to be made for women's periodic changes' and for the menopause as well as gestation and childbirth. While conceding that 'many experienced medical women ... believe that under fair and healthy conditions, menstruation will gradually become almost negligible', Browne dissented from this view. She agreed that it had been made 'needlessly painful and debilitating' and suggested that 'persistent sexual repression' was one of the 'chief agents in aggravating its symptoms and effects' and that it was often alleviated by sexual relations.[95] In Browne's thought on this issue, there appears to be a subtext that the idea that menstruation should make no difference was colluding in an assumption that women should participate in society as it was organized by and for men. While she never evolved anything as definite as Marie Stopes's theory of the periodical recurrence of female sexual desire, she was certainly sympathetic to the theory of a 'recurrent rhythm in general health, efficiency and mental poise' put forward by Mary Chadwick in 1933.[96]

A Healthy Society

Unlike Marie Stopes, Browne had little sympathy with orthodox eugenics as propounded by the English Eugenics Education Society (EES). She found it class-biassed and misogynistic in its prescriptions, although some writers have rather misleadingly identified her as a eugenist.[97] She queried in 1917 'whether the innate superiority in the governing class, really is so overwhelming as to justify the Eugenics Education Society's peculiar use of the terms "fit" and "unfit"' and she deplored its refusal to extend the knowledge of contraception to the 'exploited classes' (reiterating points made earlier in *The Freewoman*).[98] She makes an interesting contrast to the Communist doctor Eden Paul, who in his contribution to a symposium on birth control in which they both participated in 1922 put a curious, and rather scary, case for a kind of Left-wing eugenics aimed at producing, presumably, the kind of heroic proletarians found on Soviet posters of the period. Paul was particularly virulent about the survival of 'persons with grave eye defects, short-sight, astigmatism, etc, who would, but for spectacles and the absence of a fierce struggle for existence on the biologic plane, be eliminated before they could perpetuate their defective type.'[99]

Browne did not simply replace the desirable racial type as envisaged by the EES with some kind of noble savage or heroic worker. She questioned the value of the whole concept of 'fitness', pointing out that important contributions to society had been made by many who were far from being prime breeding stock. As early as 1912, in the columns of *The Freewoman*, she suggested that problems worthy of contemplation by the EES were 'the occasional union of genius and deformity ... [and] the close connection ... between genius and insanity'.[100] She also queried the basic theories upon which eugenicists founded their programmes: heredity, Browne suggested in 1934, did not seem such a perfectly 'simple, straightforward matter' since Mendel and Bateson had demonstrated its complexities.[101]

Browne joined the Eugenics Society in 1938 (probably in the interests of constructing strategic alliances for the Abortion Law Reform Association) but her membership lapsed in 1942.[102] Her views on eugenics do not seem to have materially altered by the thirties. She constantly refused to countenance 'any *wholesale* sterilising or segregating' and deplored in 1924 the 'raucous hounding of the "unfit" by some supporters of things as they are'.[103] In 1935, during the agitation for legalising sterilization, she also wondered 'why any sane and physically fine adult man or woman should not be able to be sterilised on demand' (i.e. as an efficient form of contraception).[104] In a critique of a 1933 Eugenics Society lecture on 'Race Mixture', she showed herself cognisant of the latest discoveries about blood groups, pointing out the lecturer's neglect of attention to these, 'which are by no means co-terminous with the three primary races', as well as generally dissenting from his conclusions.[105] She was an early admirer of the very different approach to fitness embodied in Innes Pearse and George Scott Williamson's Peckham Experiment of the early thirties, which Abigail Beach discusses in her chapter. Browne however commented that Pearse's and Williamson's 'scale of values seems rather obsessed with Parenthood!'[106]

By the thirties Browne was also aware of and concerned about the rise of Fascism. In 1933 she was condemning the 'sweeping away ... [of] all the achievements of opportunity and equality for German women after the war', as well as the 'burning of the books' and the 'persecution of free inquiry'.[107] Later the same year, she published in the *New Generation* extensive extracts from an 'account of exactly how Fascism works as regards the educated, self-supporting, law-abiding women of Germany'.[108] In the following year, she engaged in a debate with William Joyce (later infamous as 'Lord Haw-Haw') of the British Union of Fascists at the Lyceum Club, proposing the motion that 'the relationship of the sexes is better under

Communism than under Fascism.' Fascism, she argued, although 'honouring and providing for mothers', did so 'on traditional lines by exalting their maternity at the expense of their full humanity'.[109]

Browne consistently depicted the factors that made for ill-health and suffering as structural, innate by-products of the way in which society was organized on all levels, from the planning of kitchens to the highest emotional and spiritual concerns. This did not mean that she saw individuals as completely devoid of agency. Given her critique of medical authority and her democratic and anti-authoritarian position, she believed that individuals could take measures to improve their own health, although in many cases they were left in dire ignorance of the ways they could do so. For example, she suggested in 1931 that 'If all women had access to the best modern knowledge in medicine and hygiene, if all women had means and leisure, and minds freed from fear and medievalism – *how* different things would be.'[110]

Browne held before her a utopian ideal of the 'finer state of life' in which health would be the norm and provision for ill-health freely available rather than grudgingly doled out. However, she did not disdain to fight for immediate and often quite small gains, as we can see from her month by month account in *The New Generation* of the struggle for birth control provision in welfare centres. She does not seem to have believed that working for the revolution took priority over ameliorating the suffering of individuals in the here and now: and indeed she argued that raising women out of a state of dumb suffering was likely to render them capable of working for still greater changes. Her commitment to the individual and her ideal of 'the finer state', characterized by variety and diversity, was voiced throughout her career. In 1924 she explicitly rejected 'a social order which puts necessary work, justice, creative art and science, love and breeding on a cash basis.'[111] What she demanded instead were 'revolutionary changes in all departments ... the development of hitherto isolated human harmonies, or intense and vivid variations of faculty and type.'[112]

Notes

1 Barbara Caine, *English Feminism, 1780-1980*, Oxford, 1997, pp. 102–23; Sandra Stanley Holton, *Feminism and Democracy: Women's Suffrage and Reform Politics 1900-1918*, Cambridge, 1986, pp. 9–28.

2 Ellen Ross, *Love and Toil: Motherhood in Outcast London*, Oxford, 1993, pp. 195–221.

3 Martha Vicinus, *Independent Women: Work and Community for Single*

Women, 1850-1920, London, 1985, pp. 5–6.

4   Lis Whitelaw, *The Life and Rebellious Times of Cicely Hamilton: Actress, Writer, Suffragist*, London, 1990.

5   Biographical details from Public Archives of Nova Scotia, Halifax.

6   Family information kindly supplied by Mr John Dodwell; information from St Felix School; Somerville College archives.

7   F. W. Stella Browne, 'Reflections of a (Female) Briton', *The Malthusian*, January 1916, pp. 10–11.

8   Stella Browne to Olaf Stapledon, 7 February 1949, Olaf Stapledon papers, Sydney Jones Library, Liverpool University Library, STAP HVIIIB.

9   Lucy Bland, *Banishing the Beast: English Feminism and Sexual Morality, 1880-1914*, London, 1995, pp. 206, 211.

10 Bland, *Banishing the Beast*, pp. 214–15; Lesley A. Hall, 'Malthusian Mutations: The Changing Politics and Moral Meanings of Birth Control in Britain', in *Malthus, Medicine and Morality: Malthusianism after 1798*, Brian Dolan (ed.), Amsterdam (forthcoming); Brian Harrison, *Prudent Revolutionaries: Portraits of British Feminists Between the Wars*, Oxford, 1987, 282.

11 Lesley A. Hall, 'The Next Generation: Stella Browne, the New Woman as Freewoman', in *The New Woman: Gendering the fin de siècle*, Angelique Richardson and Chris Willis (eds), (forthcoming).

12 F. W. Stella Browne, 'Some Problems of Sex', *International Journal of Ethics*, 27 (1916): 464–71.

13 Annual Reports of the Women's Social and Political Union, Fawcett Library, London Guildhall University.

14 F. W. Stella Browne, 'Studies in Feminine Inversion', *Journal of Sexology and Psychoanalysis*, 1 (1923): 51–8; Browne, 'Some Problems of Sex'.

15 F. W. Stella Browne, 'Women in Industry' [letter], in *The New Age*, 22 July 1915, 293.

16 F. W. Stella Browne, Review of Havelock Ellis, *The Task of Social Hygiene, English Review*, 13 (1912): 157; and see Lesley A. Hall '"What a Lot there is still to Do': Stella Browne (1880-1955) Carrying the Struggle Ever Onward', in *A Suffrage Reader: Charting Directions British Suffrage History*, Claire Eustance, Joan Ryan, and Laura Ugolini (eds), (forthcoming).

17 Dora Russell, cited in Keith Hindell and Madeleine Simms, *Abortion Law Reformed*, London, 1971, 59.

18 Stella Browne to Havelock Ellis, 9 February 1914, Havelock Ellis papers in the Department of Manuscripts, British Library, Additional Manuscript 70539.

19 Minutes and correspondence in the archives of the British Sexology Society, Harry Ransom Humanities Research Center, University of Texas at Austin (hereafter BSS).

20 Minutes of the Federation of Progressive Societies and Individuals, British Library of Political and Economic Science; notices in *Plan: the Journal of the FPSI*; FPSI ephemera given to the author by Leslie Minchin.

21 Bland, *Banishing the Beast*, pp. 280–6; Lesley A. Hall, 'Suffrage, Sex, and Science', in *The Women's Suffrage Movement: New Feminist Perspectives*, Mary Joannou and June Purvis (eds), Manchester, 1998, pp. 188–200; Margaret Jackson, *The Real Facts of Life: Feminism and the Politics of Sexuality c.1850-1940*, London, 1994, pp. 91–4; Sheila Jeffreys, *The Spinster and her Enemies: Feminism and Sexuality 1880-1930*, North Melbourne, Vic., 1997, pp. 93–101.

22 For a more detailed analysis of Browne's contributions to *The Freewoman*, see Hall, 'The Next Generation'.

23 F. W. Stella Browne, 'Women and Birth Control', in *Population and Birth-Control: A Symposium*, Eden and Cedar Paul (eds), New York, 1917, pp. 247–57.

24 F. W. Stella Browne, 'Poverty and Birth Control', *New Generation*, 4 (1925): 9.

25 F. W. Stella Browne, 'An Open Letter to Dr Ethel Bentham, by a Socialist Woman', *New Generation*, 2 (1924): 84; 'Climb-down or Camouflage: Dr Marion Phillips Answered', *New Generation*, 3 (1924): 115; 'Dr Ethel Bentham Answered', *New Generation*, 3 (1924): 128.

26 F. W. Stella Browne, 'Stocktaking', *New Generation*, 6 (1927): 102.

27 F. W. Stella Browne, 'Our Movement', *New Generation*, 5 (1926): 53.

28 F. W. Stella Browne, 'Birth Control in Parliament', *New Generation*, 4 (1925): 76.

29 Browne, 'Our Movement'.

30 F. W. Stella Browne, 'Current Political Notes', *New Generation*, 7 (1928): 44.

31 F. W. Stella Browne, 'Victory – or Compromise?', *New Generation*, 6 (1927): 39.

32 F. W. Stella Browne, 'Reviews: Endowment of Motherhood', *New Generation*, 4 (1925): 22.

33 F. W. Stella Browne, *Sexual Variety and Variability Among Women and its Bearing on Social Reconstruction*, London, 1917, 3.

34 Browne, 'Women and Birth Control'.

35 F. W. Stella Browne, Review of Marie Stopes, *Married Love: A New*

Contribution to the Solution of Sexual Difficulties, International Journal of Ethics, 29 (1918/19): 112–3.

36   F. W. Stella Browne, 'Current Notes', *New Generation*, 7 (1928): 53.

37   Browne, *Sexual Variety and Variability*, 4.

38   *Ibid.*, 4

39   *Ibid.*, 9.

40   F. W. Stella Browne, 'To the Editor of *The Malthusian*', *The Malthusian*, (July 1916): 64. According to the foreword of *Downward Paths*, the several writers who contributed to the book desired that their names remain unknown.

41   F. W. Stella Browne, 'Review: The Unadjusted Girl', *New Generation*, 3 (1924): 57–8.

42   F. W. Stella Browne, 'The Sex Gospel of Geneva/Civilisation on a Cash Basis', *New Generation*, 6 (1927): 39–40.

43   F. W. Stella Browne, 'A Year of Indiscretion', *New Generation*, 8 (1929): 7.

44   Browne, 'Women and Birth Control'.

45   F. W. Stella Browne, 'A Warning to Women: The Venereal Diseases Peril in Everyday Life', *Beauty and Health*, (July 1915): 23–4.

46   F. W. Stella Browne, 'Women and the Race', *The Socialist Review: a Quarterly Review of Modern Thought*, 14 (1917): 151–7.

47   BSS 'Misc': Stella Browne to Miss Carson, 11 Jul 1920.

48   BSS 'Misc': Minutes Vol [1], 4th AGM [?12] July 1918.

49   F. W. Stella Browne, Review of *The Prevention of Venereal Disease. Being the Report of and the Evidence taken by the Special Committee on Venereal Disease* (1921), *New Generation*, 1 (1922): 13.

50   F. W. Stella Browne, 'Instructions for Women', *Tribune*, 12 March 1943, 14.

51   F. W. Stella Browne, [Review], *'The Woman in the Little House* by Leonora Eyles', *New Generation*, 1 (1922): 12–13.

52   F. W. Stella Browne, 'The Wastage of the Future', *Beauty and Health*, (November 1916): 144–6.

53   F. W. Stella Browne, 'An Open Letter to the Four Suspended MPs by a Socialist Woman', *New Generation*, 2 (1923): 90.

54   F. W. Stella Browne, 'A Cathedral and a Slum', *New Generation*, 8 (1929): 79.

55   F. W. Stella Browne, 'Current Political Notes', *New Generation*, 6 (1927): 29.

56   E.g. in Browne, 'Women and Birth Control'.

57   Browne, 'Reflections of a (Female) Briton'.

58   Browne, 'Climb-down or Camouflage'.

59   Browne, 'An Open Letter to the Four Suspended MPs'.

60   F. W. Stella Browne, 'How the Fight Goes', *New Generation*, 8 (1929): 136.

61   BSS 'Misc': Stella Browne to Janet Carson, 20 September 1920.

62   Browne, 'Women and Birth Control'.

63   F. W. Stella Browne, 'Some Damning Statistics', *New Generation*, 4 (1925): 135–6.

64   F. W. Stella Browne, 'Critics and Champions at Westminster', *New Generation*, 5 (1926): 67.

65   Browne, 'Dr Ethel Bentham Answered'.

66   Browne, 'Climb-down or Camouflage?'.

67   Browne, 'Women and Birth-Control'.

68   Browne, 'Critics and Champions at Westminster'.

69   F. W. Stella Browne, 'Plaistow Meeting', *New Generation*, 6 (1927): 52.

70   Browne, 'Women and Birth Control'.

71   F. W. Stella Browne, 'Miss Browne's Meetings', *New Generation*, 10 (1931): 29.

72   Browne, 'Women and the Race'.

73   F. W. Stella Browne, 'Scrapped: The Women Munition Workers of Britain', *The Call*, 12 December 1918, 7.

74   F. W. Stella Browne, 'The Women's Question', *The Communist*, 11 March 1922.

75   F. W. Stella Browne, 'Mr Joad's Book' [review of C. E. M. Joad, *Thrasymachus, or the Future of Morals*], *New Generation*, 5 (1926): 32.

76   F. W. Stella Browne, 'Review: *The Sexual Crisis: A Critique of our Sex Life*. By Grete Meisel-Hess', *The Malthusian*, (1917): 39.

77   Browne, 'Studies in Feminine Inversion'.

78   *Ibid.*, 5.

79   Discussed further in Lesley A. Hall, '"I have never met the normal woman": Stella Browne and the Politics of Womanhood', *Women's History Review*, 6 (1997): 157–82.

80   Browne, *Sexual Variety and Variability*, pp. 7–8.

81   *Ibid.*, 5.

82   Stella Browne to Bertrand Russell, 12 Sep 1917, Bertrand Russell papers in William Ready Division of Archives and Research Collections, Mills Memorial Library, McMaster University, Hamilton, Ontario, Canada.

83   'British Sexological Society' [report on talk by Miss Browne 'The present Sexual Situation: Achievements and Difficulties'], *New Generation*, 11 (1932): 26.

84   F. W. Stella Browne, 'The Philosophy of the Free Spirit', *New Generation*, 3 (1924): 17.

85   Stella Browne to Havelock Ellis, 25 Dec 1922, BL Add. Mss. 70539.

86   F. W. Stella Browne, 'A Brilliant Boomerang', *New Generation*, 6 (1927): 34.

87   Browne, *Sexual Variety and Variability*, 8; *idem*, 'Some Problems of Sex'.

88   Browne, 'Women and the Race'.

89   Browne, 'Women and Birth-Control'.

90   E.g. Jackson, *The Real Facts of Life*, 125; Jeffreys, *The Spinster and her Enemies*, pp. 115–25.

91   F. W. Stella Browne, 'A Year of Indiscretion: A Triumph of Imbecility' [prosecution of *The Well of Loneliness*], *New Generation*, 8 (1929): 7; see also Browne, 'Studies in Feminine Inversion'.

92   Browne, *Sexual Variety and Variability*, pp. 10–11; see also Hall, '"I have never met the normal woman"', pp. 168–70, for an analysis of Browne's developing views on female homosexuality in the context of her own changing self-definitions.

93   Browne, *Sexual Variety and Variability*, pp. 10–11.

94   F. W. Stella Browne, 'The Age of Bewilderment', *New Generation*, 2 (1923): 80.

95   Browne, *Sexual Variety and Variability*, pp. 9–10.

96   F. W. Stella Browne, 'Review' (Mary Chadwick, *Women's Periodicity*), *New Generation*, 12 (1933): 90.

97   E.g. Jane Lewis, *Women in England 1870-1950*, Brighton, 1984, 105; Greta Jones, 'Women and Eugenics in Britain: the Case of Mary Scharlieb, Elizabeth Sloan Chesser, and Stella Browne', *Annals of Science*, 52 (1995): 481–502.

98   Browne, 'Women and Birth Control'; F. W. Stella Browne, 'A Few Straight Questions to the Eugenics Society', *The Freewoman*, 1 August 1912, 217–8.

99   Eden Paul, 'Birth Control: Communist and Individualist Aspects', *Medical Critic and Guide* (New York), 25 (1922): 212–6.

100   F. W. Stella Browne, 'More Questions', *The Freewoman*, 15 Aug 1912, 258.

101   F. W. Stella Browne, 'Sterilization', *New Generation*, 13 (1934): 126.

102   Eugenics Society archive in the Contemporary Medical Archives Centre at the Wellcome Institute for the History of Medicine: Minutes of Council Meeting of 14 February 1938, CMAC: SA/EUG/L.10, and of 14 April 1942, CMAC: SA/EUG/L.11.

103   F. W. Stella Browne, Review of Miriam Van Waters, *Where Girls Go Right*, in *The New Generation*, 3 (1924): 82.

104   F. W. Stella Browne, Review of J. P. Hinton and Josephina E. Calcutt, *Sterilization: A Christian Approach*, in *Plan for World Order and*

Progress (The journal of the Federation of Progressive Societies and Individuals), vol. 2 no 10, October 1935, 23.

105 F. W. Stella Browne, 'Eugenic Problems and Programmes', *New Generation*, 12 (1933): 75.

106 F. W. Stella Browne, 'Achieving Health', *New Generation*, 11 (1932): 58.

107 F. W. Stella Browne, 'Are We Safer?', *New Generation*, 12 (1933): 64–5.

108 F. W. Stella Browne, 'Woman in Germany', *New Generation*, 12 (1933): 99–100.

109 'Lyceum Club Debate', *New Generation*, 13 (1934): 47.

110 'Miss Browne Replies', *New Generation*, 10 (1931): 99.

111 Browne, 'The Philosophy of the Free Spirit'.

112 Browne, 'Women and Birth Control'.

INDEX

Index

310